Physical Agents
Theory and Practice

Second Edition

Physical Agents Theory and Practice

Second Edition

Barbara J. Behrens, PTA, MS
Coordinator, Physical Therapist Assistant Program
Mercer County Community College
Trenton, NJ

Susan L. Michlovitz, PT, PhD, MS, CHT
Professor, Department of Physical Therapy
Temple University
Philadelphia, PA
Finger Lakes Physical Therapy, PC
Ithaca, NY

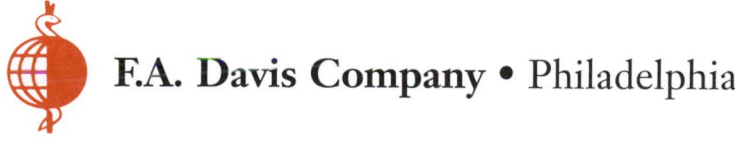

F.A. Davis Company • Philadelphia

F. A. Davis Company
1915 Arch Street
Philadelphia, PA 19103
www.fadavis.com

Printed in the United States of America

Last digit indicates print number: 10 9 8 7 6 5 4 3 2 1

Acquisitions Editor: Margaret Biblis
Design & Illustration Manager: Carolyn O'Brien

As new scientific information becomes available through basic and clinical research, recommended treatments and drug therapies undergo changes. The author(s) and publisher have done everything possible to make this book accurate, up to date, and in accord with accepted standards at the time of publication. The author(s), editors, and publisher are not responsible for errors or omissions or for consequences from application of the book, and make no warranty, expressed or implied, in regard to the contents of the book. Any practice described in this book should be applied by the reader in accordance with professional standards of care used in regard to the unique circumstances that may apply in each situation. The reader is advised always to check product information (package inserts) for changes and new information regarding dose and contraindications before administering any drug. Caution is especially urged when using new or infrequently ordered drugs.

Library of Congress Cataloging-in-Publication Data

Physical agents : theory and practice / [edited by] Barbara J. Behrens, Susan L. Michlovitz.—2nd ed.
  p. ; cm.
Includes bibliographical references and index.
ISBN 0-8036-1134-X (alk. paper)
1. Physical therapy. 2. Physical therapy assistants.
[DNLM: 1. Physical Therapy Techniques. WB 460 P5773 2005] I. Behrens, Barbara J., 1959- II. Michlovitz, Susan L.
RM700.B37 2005
615.8′2—dc22

2005007703

Acknowledgments

We thank the following individuals for their patience, persistence, and assistance with this book:

- All the authors who "tolerated revision well" and participated in making this a wonderful text.
- All the students and clinicians who have participated in our seminars and classes for the past 20 (BJB)/25(SLM) years.
- Laura Balcer, MD, for her knowledge, patience, and compassion in helping BJB to deal with the unknown.
- Ellen Price, PT, MEd, for her insight and unique understanding of electrotherapy that she imparted to BJB.
- Stacie Larkin, PT, MEd, for her valuable assistance in editing many of the chapters for us.
- Larry Petraccaro, Benjamin Hopwood, and Carol Morgan for their wonderful cartoons.
- Our developmental editors, Brigette Wilke and Jennifer Pine, for putting the puzzle pieces together.
- Margaret Biblis, our publisher, and Susan Rhyner, for their support of the new look and conceptual design framework of this project.
- Mel, from BJB, for love, support, and a hug whenever needed.

Barbara J. Behrens
Susan L. Michlovitz

Preface to the Second Edition: For the Student

The Guide to Physical Therapist Practice (2nd edition, APTA 2001) in combination with the increased interest in Evidence-Based Practice have strengthened our quest to provide you, the user of physical agents, with:

- the information you need to know for safe practice,
- the rationale for why it is important to know it,
- guidance on using the information,
- skills to determine if physical agent techniques utilized produced the results that were anticipated, and
- insight into the questions that patients might ask regarding their intervention.

New features include:

- Case study examples, which will facilitate integration of material
- Incorporation of language from *The Guide to Physical Therapist Practice*

We have provided updates on all chapters from our last edition and organized material in a way to enhance learning. Many of the illustrations and photographs are new and enhanced from the last edition. We, the editors, hope to have accomplished our goals and look forward to hearing feedback from you.

Barbara J. Behrens
Susan L. Michlovitz

Contributors

Ute H. Breese, MEd, PT, OCS
Assistant Professor
Physical Therapy Department
East Tennessee State University
Johnson City, Tennessee

Elizabeth Buchanan, PT
Staff Physical Therapist
Spruce Pine Community Hospital
Spruce Pine, North Carolina

Joy Cohn, PT, CLT-LANA
Penn Therapy & Fitness
University of Pennsylvania
Philadelphia, Pennsylvania

Cheryl Gillespie, PT, DPT, MA
Physical Therapist Assistant Program
Suffolk Community College
Selden, New York

Burke Gurney, PT, PhD
Assistant Professor
Physical Therapy Department
University of New Mexico
Albuquerque, New Mexico

Stacie Lynn Larkin, PT, MEd, ACCE
Academic Coordinator of Clinical Education
Department of Physical Therapy
University of Delaware
Newark, Delaware

Ethne Nussbaum, PT, PhD
Department of Physical Therapy
Faculty of Medicine
University of Toronto
Toronto, Ontario
Canada

Peter C. Panus, PT, PhD
Associate Professor
Physical Therapy Department
East Tennessee State University
Johnson City, Tennessee

Russell Stowers, PTA, MS
Director
Physical Therapist Assistant Program
Del Mar College
Corpus Christi, Texas

Kristin von Nieda, DPT, MEd
Associate Professor, Physical Therapy
Temple University
Philadelphia, Pennsylvania

Reviewers

Marja P. Beaufait, PT, MA
Associate Professor, Physical Therapist Assistant Program
Health Education Center
St. Petersburg College
St. Petersburg, Florida

Janet Curran Brooks, EdM, OTR
Lecturer
Boston School of Occupational Therapy
Tufts University
Medford, Massachusetts

Martha Rammel Hinman, PT, EdD
Ruby Decker Professor of Physical Therapy Fellow
Associate Professor, Physical Therapy Program
Sealy Center for the Aging
University of Texas Medical Branch
Galveston, Texas

Stephanie D. Palma, PT, DPT, MEd
Co-ACCE, Physical Therapist Assistant Program
Department of Physical Therapy
Georgia State University
Atlanta, Georgia

Frank B. Underwood, PT, PhD, ECS
Professor, Department of Physical Therapy
University of Evansville
Evansville, Indiana

R. Scott Ward, PT, PhD
Professor and Chair
Division of Physical Therapy
The University of Utah
Salt Lake City, Utah

Peter Zawicki, PT, MS
Chairperson, Physical Therapist Assistant Program
Department of Health Sciences
Gateway Community College
Phoenix, Arizona

Contents

The Concept of Adjunctive Therapies

Objectives

- Define pain.
- Describe the factors that affect an individual's perception of pain.
- Define acute and chronic pain.
- Define analgesia and anesthesia, and differentiate between them.
- Explain the gate control theory of pain; provide examples of the use of physical agents based on this theory.
- Define endogenous opiates, listing events that can trigger the release of these substances.
- Describe therapeutic interventions for a patient in acute pain, including methods of encouraging active patient participation in the recovery process.
- Describe the team approach to the treatment of patients with chronic pain.
- Discuss analgesic and anti-inflammatory medications and their impact on therapeutic interventions.
- Describe key events that occur in the three stages of wound healing.
- Identify precautions for handling wounds during each of the three stages.
- Describe appropriate therapeutic treatment interventions for wounds in each of the three stages.

Key Terms

Acute	Dorsal horn	Ischemia	Pain
Analgesia	Edema	Myotome	Proliferation
Anesthesia	Endogenous	Narcotic	Remodeling
Chronic	Erythema	Nociceptor	Scleratome
Dermatome	Inflammation	Opiate	

Barbara J. Behrens, PTA, MS   *Stacie Larkin, PT, MEd*

Tissue Response to Injury

Outline

"I keep hearing the phrase 'no pain, no gain'; is that really necessary?"

Pain perception is one of the most common reasons or symptoms that cause an individual to seek the assistance of a medical or allied health professional. It can be a sign of physical, physiologic, or psychologic dysfunction. This explains why there are so many different pain assessment instruments developed to measure it.[2] Depending on the individual, pain may be thought of as the body's warning system, the body's way of letting the individual know that something is wrong. Without the sensation of pain, additional tissue damage or injury may occur. Pain may, however, have numerous adverse effects, resulting in symptoms such as muscle guarding or spasm that over time can lead to weakness, decreased range of motion, fatigue, insomnia, increased irritability, anxiety, depression, decreased appetite, sexual dysfunction, and emotional distress.[3-6] Although an individual seeks assistance to relieve his or her pain, it must be remembered that pain management is only one aspect of the complete care of the patient geared toward improving function and reducing disability. Depending on the additional rehabilitation needs of the individual, several therapeutic interventions may be used.

Definitions

Pain is defined as "an unpleasant sensory and emotional experience associated with actual or potential tissue damage, or described in terms of such damage"[7] (Box 1-1). This definition avoids tying pain to just a physical stimulus and instead emphasizes that our willingness to call something painful can be influenced by other factors. These factors include our focus of attention, level of anxiety, degree of suggestibility, level of arousal, degree of fatigue, previous emotional and psychologic experience, and cultural mores.[3,4,8] In other words, although a sensation may start as a physical or chemically mediated stimulus to a nociceptor (pain receptor), our willingness to call the sensation painful or to respond to the painful stimulus is variable depending on past learning and current circumstances and is purely subjective. Only the individual experiencing the "pain" knows the true quality of that sensation and the personal meaning of that sensation. One aspect of a therapeutic intervention for a patient experiencing pain involves controlling the perception and/or sensation of pain. Providing the patient with a way to manage her or his level of discomfort can ultimately lead to improved function.

The body's response to trauma is a complex interaction of sensory, motivational, and cognitive processes that determine a sequence of behavior that characterizes pain[1,6] (Fig. 1-1). On a systemic level, the sympathetic component of the autonomic nervous system responds to the perceived threat by a "fight-or-flight" reaction. This reaction involves numerous

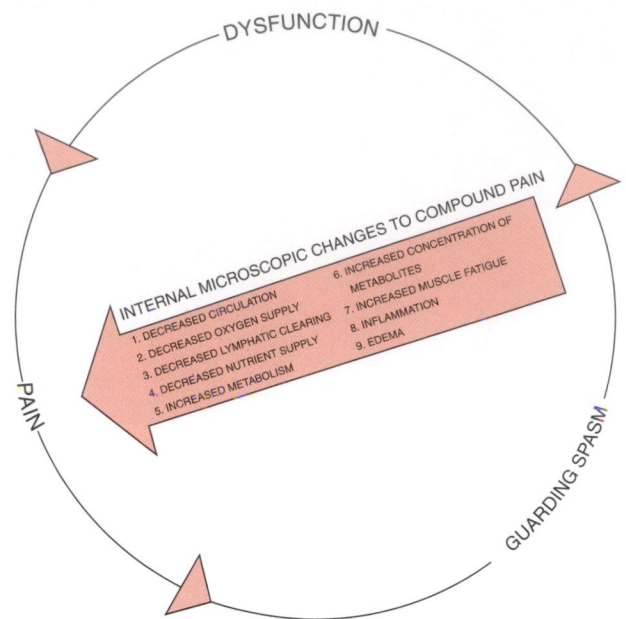

Figure 1-1 Primary pain cycle and associated internal changes. (From Mannheimer, JS, and Lampe, GN, eds. Clinical Transcutaneous Electrical Nerve Stimulation. FA Davis, Philadelphia, 1984, p 10, with permission.)

body systems and typically includes increased heart rate and sweating, expansion of the bronchioles (small airways), dilation of the pupils, shunting of blood from the skin and digestive tract to the muscles and brain, decreased peristalsis, and contraction of the sphincters[9] (Fig. 1-2).

Initially, when experiencing pain resulting from trauma, the person will try to withdraw from the stimulus. Muscle guarding occurs as the body's way to immobilize the injured area and prevent further damage (Fig. 1-3). This reaction of the muscles requires a high level of metabolic activity at the same time as it compresses the blood vessels. The compromised circulation is often inadequate to supply metabolic needs, leading to ischemia, a new source of pain. In addition, the compromised circulation impedes the removal of the metabolic wastes, many of which sensitize nociceptors, resulting in further enhancement of pain.

Edema resulting from injury causes disruption of the capillaries and lymphatics, with an increase in capillary permeability as a result of compression from muscle guarding. This further compounds the problems of nutrient supply and waste removal, thereby causing additional pain perception and subsequent additional muscle guarding. Thus, a vicious circle of pain, spasm, and pain can evolve. Finally, endogenous pain-producing substances such as potassium, serotonin (5-hydroxytryptamine [5-HT]), bradykinin, histamine, prostaglandins, leukotrienes, and substance P are commonly released into the injured area[6,10] (Box 1-2).

These substances can directly activate nociceptors, or they

BOX 1-1   The Terminology of Pain Perception

The use of appropriate terminology is helpful when discussing pain management.

- *Analgesia:* The absence of pain or noxious stimulation; the absence of the sensibility to pain; or the relief of pain without a loss of consciousness.

- *Anesthesia:* A loss of sensation, usually by damage to a nerve or receptor, that is, numbness; or the loss of the ability to feel pain caused by the administration of drugs or medical interventions.

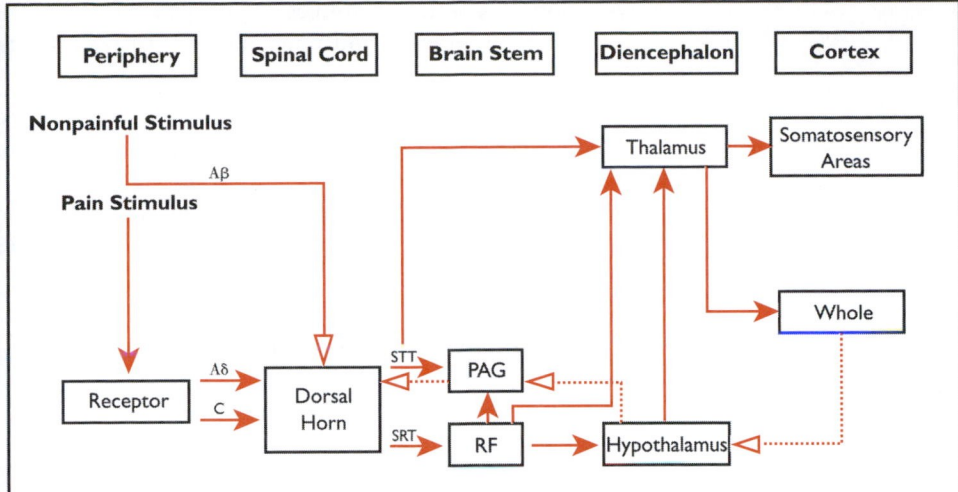

Figure 1-2 Schematic representation of ascending and descending connections responsible for pain sensation. Ascending pathways are represented by solid lines. Pain stimulus triggers a response in the peripheral sensory receptors. Stimulus is sent to spinal cord via the A-delta (Aδ) and C fibers and then to the brainstem (PAG = periaqueductal gray matter and RF = reticular formation) via two tracts (STT = spinothalamic tract and SRT = spinoreticulothalamic pathway). Information is relayed to the thalamus and hypothalamus and then on to the somatosensory areas and other areas of the cortex. Descending, inhibitory pathways are represented by dashed lines. Descending modulation of pain perception is thought to block pain signal transmission in the dorsal horn of the spinal cord. Nonpainful sensory stimulus (transmitted via A-beta [Aβ]) is also thought to block pain signal transmission in the dorsal horn.[10,21]

may act alone or in combination to sensitize nociceptors to other agents. For example, histamine excites polymodal nociceptors, bradykinin increases the synthesis and release of prostaglandins from nearby cells, and prostaglandin E produces hyperalgesia and sensitizes nociceptors.[6] The body responds to trauma by an acute inflammatory response. The symptoms associated with the inflammation are a warning to the individual, indicating tissue damage. The symptoms experienced are the cardinal signs of inflammation, pain, heat, erythema, edema, and loss of function.

Acute and Chronic Pain

Pain can be classified as acute or chronic.[6,11–13] Acute pain is most often the result of infection, injury, or internal disease. It is predictable in characteristics, easily localized by the patient, relatively easy to diagnose and treat, and often readily relieved. Chronic pain, however, may or may not relate to an actual physical injury and may persist well beyond the presence of obvious physical findings to support it. The longer the pain persists, the more likely it is to be referred away from the site of the actual cause or lesion.[11] The pain associated with an injury can also result in decreased function of the injured body part. Range of motion may be limited as

a result of increased pain with motion due to the added stress at the site of injury. Also, muscle contraction produces pain because of the "tension" created at the injury site by the contraction. Pain may cause protective muscle guarding, which further increases pain perception. The end result is the pain-spasm cycle.[10] The prolonged protective guarding of a muscle can lead to ischemia of the tissue because of compression of the blood vessels. The ischemia can also further sensitize already irritated nociceptors and increase pain perception. The combination of the prolonged painful event and resultant muscle guarding may lead to an inability to use the body part without pain.

Chronic pain is pain that lasts longer than 3 months[1] and

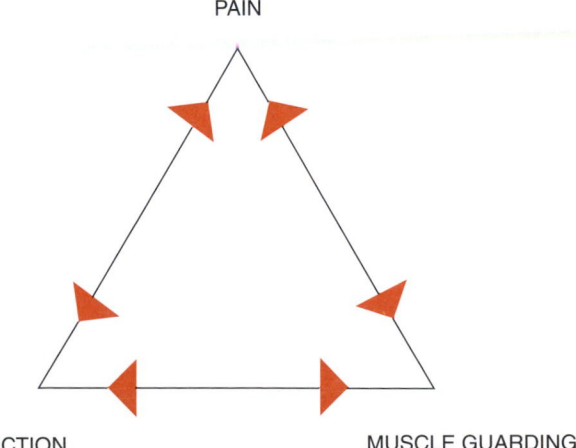

Figure 1-3 The Pain Triangle depicts an interrelationship between each of the points of the triangle. Pain perception has the ability to increase muscle guarding, which could then cause a decrease in circulation and impair the healing process. Conversely, treatment interventions that address pain in addition to its cause and the dysfunction itself will help to break the cycle, increasing circulation by decreasing protective muscle guarding.

Before You Begin

Remember that on a local level, the body reacts to injury in three primary ways through

1. Muscle guarding
2. Edema formation
3. Release of endogenous pain chemical mediators

BOX 1-2   *Pain-Producing Substances Triggered by Injury*

Injury triggers the release of the following endogenous pain-producing substances into the injured area[6,10]:

Potassium

Serotonin (5-HT)

Bradykinin

Histamine

Prostaglandins

Leukotrienes

Substance P

---

leads to a long-term loss of function, as well as imposing many psychosocial stresses on the patient and his or her friends and family. The mechanism by which acute pain is similar to or different from chronic pain is not fully understood. The extent to which pain is perceived and responded to may be a function of the influences of biologic, psychosocial, behavioral, neurohormonal, and neurochemical factors.[1-3,11-15] There are reasons postulated for this that are not yet completely understood. Various mechanisms have been proposed to account for chronic pain. The most commonly described mechanisms are as follows[6,10,13]:

 What Do I Need to Know About...

Cardinal Signs of Inflammation

ERYTHEMA

Vascular changes occur with an inflammatory response that allows fluid and cells to exude from the blood vessels that promote phagocytosis, fibroblastic activity, and the beginning of the formation of new capillary beds.

INCREASED TISSUE TEMPERATURE

Increased tissue temperature and erythema are the result of the vasodilation of the blood vessels, allowing more blood to pass through the area and increasing metabolic rate.

EDEMA

The fluid exudate in the extravascular space accumulates due to the increased permeability and vasodilation of blood vessels.

PAIN

The resultant pain perception is due to the stimulation of the pain receptors and free nerve endings of A-delta and C fibers by the chemicals present at the site and the mechanical pressure of the edema.

LOSS OF FUNCTION

This is the ultimate result of sensitization of pain receptors, tissue damage, fluid retention impeding range of motion, and an active unchecked inflammatory response.

---

1. *Mechanical:* Clinical examples of mechanical irritation include entrapment syndromes such as carpal tunnel syndrome.

2. *Chemical:* Chemical irritation in the injured area occurs as the body releases various substances in reaction to trauma, inflammation, or ischemia. These substances increase the sensitivity of the nociceptor,[6] enhance each other's action, and facilitate the release of prostaglandin E. A positive-feedback loop of pain causing inflammation causing more pain results.

3. *Regeneration:* As nerves are regenerating following surgery or trauma, there can be a period of marked increase in discharges from the peripheral nerve fibers that transmit pain signals (A-delta and C fibers[6,13]).

4. *Reflexes:* Motor reflexes that normally act to protect tissue from acute pain can persist and produce changes associated with chronic pain such as muscle guarding. This can result in ischemia and nerve compression. Overactivity of sympathetic reflexes can result in vasoconstriction, ischemia, and trophic changes.

5. *Inhibitory failure:* Inhibitory failure involves a breakdown in the usual response of the central nervous system (CNS).[6] In response to significant pain, the CNS normally releases chemicals called endogenous opiates. These chemicals exert control at the first relay of incoming injury signals in the dorsal horn of the spinal cord and decrease or block the transmission of further pain signals. Some examples of this inhibitory failure are thalamic pain, pain associated with brain or spinal cord injury, and pain associated with demyelinating diseases such as multiple sclerosis.

The transition from acute to chronic pain has not been well defined. If pain meets the following three criteria, however, it is usually termed chronic pain[6]:

1. The cause is uncertain or not correctable.

2. Medical treatments have been ineffective.

3. Pain has persisted for longer than 3 months.

Chronic pain is often treated by a team approach with a heavy emphasis on psychologic support, behavior modification techniques, and guidance.[11,16-21] The team can include a coordinating physician and/or nurse practitioner, a psychologist, a physical therapist, an occupational therapist, a social worker, and a vocational rehabilitation counselor. Recreational therapists, dietitians, biofeedback technicians, and other health professionals also play roles on some teams. The team attempts to empower the patient and his or her family through education. Physical therapy treatment intervention emphasizes active management of the pain[17] through the proper use of activity alternating with rest, body mechanics, posture education, stretching, strengthening, cardiovascular conditioning,[16] relaxation techniques, work condtioning or hardening, and home use of physical agents such as heat, ice, and transcutaneous electrical nerve stimulation (TENS).[17] Manual techniques and physical agents are kept to a minimum but may include joint or soft tissue mobilization techniques, ultrasound, and electrical stimulation. Other members of the team deal with drug dependency, stress management, assertiveness training, behavioral modification, family therapy, and vocational counseling as needed.

Psychologic Implications

On a psychologic level, the individual reacts to the ongoing misery and stress of chronic pain, the failure of adequate pain relief, changes in role and social status, and financial hardship. Many people experience depression in the face of these problems. Patients with chronic pain may also engage in pain behavior and pain games as maladaptive behavioral responses to their situation[5,6] (Fig. 1-4).

Medical Management after Painful Insult to Soft Tissues

Medical management often involves the use of prescription or over-the-counter analgesic medications to help alleviate acute symptoms associated with pain. It is hoped that their use will decrease the potential for progression into a chronic condition and the associated difficulties previously described. Medications used to relieve pain are referred to as analgesics, which may be of two classifications: non-narcotics and narcotics.

Examples of non-narcotic drugs are aspirin and nonsteroidal anti-inflammatory drugs (NSAIDs). Narcotic analgesics include codeine and morphine. Each class of drug affects the body in different ways to alter the painful experience. Non-narcotic pain medications selectively affect the hypothalamus of the brain. In addition, the synthesis of prostaglandins is inhibited and bradykinin is prevented from stimulating pain receptors at the site of injury. NSAIDs interrupt the inflammatory response by making cell membranes less permeable and inhibiting prostaglandin synthesis. Narcotic analgesics are used to alleviate severe pain. The mechanism of action affects the CNS to decrease anxiety and the response to pain. The drugs do not affect the peripheral nerves and receptors, so the pain stimulus is still present. In effect, the patient does not respond to the stimulus because of the depression of the CNS.[6]

The adverse effects of this group of medications include gastrointestinal irritation, toxicity, mental confusion, drowsiness, and hypersensitivity. Narcotic analgesics, in addition to the adverse effects previously mentioned, can produce tolerance and physical addiction to the drug. In some cases, the use of electrical stimulation for pain control and continuous low-level heat therapy has decreased the need for the use of analgesic medications.[18,21]

Electrical stimulation is believed to produce analgesic

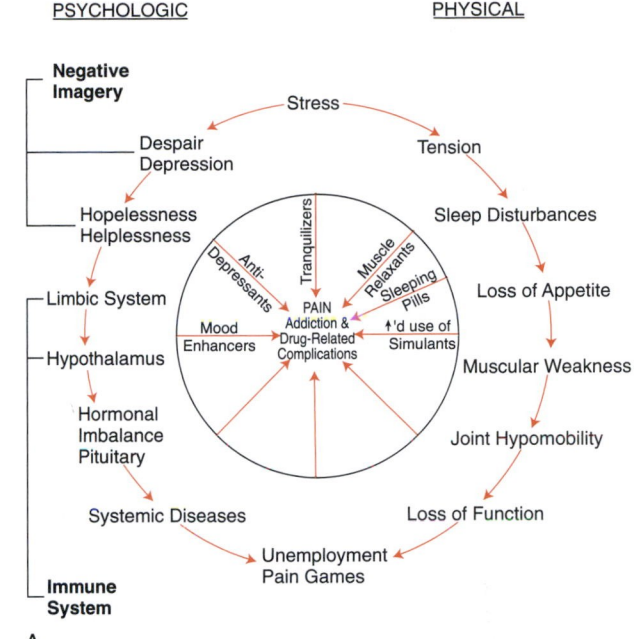

A.

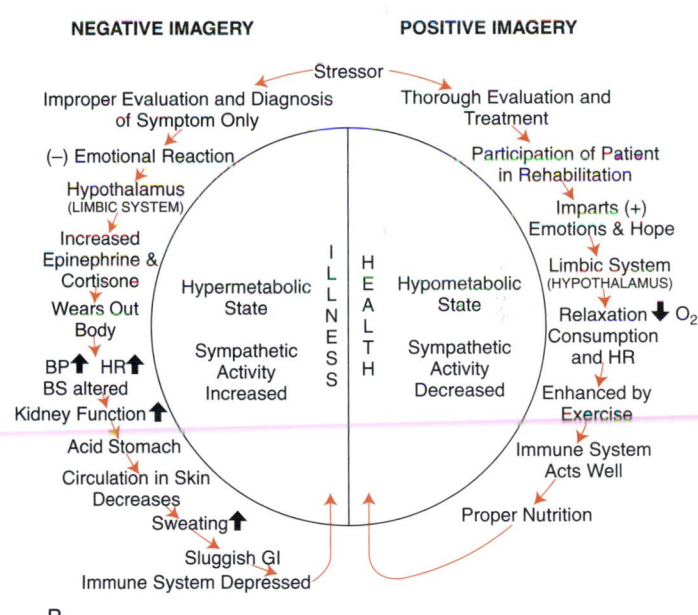

B.

Figure 1-4   Chronic pain cycle. (A) Psychologic and physical impact. (B) Psychologic feelings or attitudes toward illness. (Adapted from Mannheimer, JS, and Lampe, GN, eds. Clinical Transcutaneous Electrical Nerve Stimulation. FA Davis, Philadelphia, 1984, pp 12–13, with permission.)

effects through stimulation of the peripheral and central nervous systems. Electrical stimulation devices are available for use in the clinic and as portable models (see Chapters 10 and 12) that the patient can use at appropriate times during the day as needed. The portable units are generally the size of a "beeper" and run on rechargeable batteries. The portability of the electrical stimulators allows the patient greater

Patient Perspective

Remember that your patient is the only individual who can actually quantify what he or she is feeling. The answers you provide to the questions below can have a positive or an adverse affect on the results of the therapeutic intervention for a given patient. Fear is often linked with pain, despite the fact that a patient might not express it.

PATIENTS' FREQUENTLY ASKED QUESTIONS

1. How can such a small area hurt so much?

2. Why is it that some people don't seem to "suffer" as much with pain?

3. Why does someone who is having a "heart attack" feel pain down his or her left arm?

4. Why does "swelling" happen?

5. Why does healing take so long to happen with some people and not with others?

autonomy in his or her own care and the option for use of extended periods of stimulation. When the unit and electrodes are used appropriately, side effects are minimal. There is a chance for a chemical burn at the stimulation site, hypersensitivity reactions to the stimulation, or allergic reactions to the adhesives used to hold an electrode in place.[7,8] These are minimal in comparison to the adverse reactions that may result from ingested medications.

Referred Pain

Pain arising from deep body structures but felt at another, distant site is called referred pain.[19,21,23,24] It is considered an error in the localization of pain.[23,24] Mechanisms that cause the referral of pain are based on the convergence of cutaneous (skin) and visceral (internal organ) afferent nerve fibers within the spinal cord. Areas of skin that are innervated by a particular nerve root are referred to as dermatomes. Areas of bone that are innervated by a specific nerve root are known as sclerotomes, and myotomes are the areas of muscle innervated by a nerve root.

These areas may overlie each other, complicating the diagnostic process. Referred pain may be an indicator of the spinal segment in which there is a problem.[23] Pain in the L5 dermatome (buttock, leg, and foot) could arise from irritation around the L5 nerve root, the L5 disc, any facet involvement of L4 to L5, any muscle supplied by the L5 nerve root, or any visceral structure having L5 innervation.[23] Another common example of referred pain is the pain associated with angina (ischemia of the heart) and with myocardial infarction (heart attack). An individual experiencing these conditions may feel pain radiating down the arm in the T1 and T2 dermatomes.[21,25] Pain is felt here because the pain fibers innervating the heart arise from the T1 to T5 nerve roots (Fig. 1-5).

Not all referred pain follows a segmental (spinal nerve) pattern. Pain referred from an active trigger point follows a predictable and characteristic pattern for the muscle that is harboring the trigger point. These trigger points are defined by their referred pain pattern.[25] It is important to be aware of common referral patterns to identify the anatomic source of pain correctly and treat it appropriately.[20] Also, because pain that is perceived by the patient appears to arise from the area of referral and not the deeper, more distant structures, it is important to be able to explain to the patient why you may not be treating him "where it hurts" but rather that you are treating the source of the pain. Failure to educate the patient regarding the pain pattern and source may feed into feelings of helplessness and of not being heard. The patient has informed you that his "leg hurts," but you seem to ignore him and instead treat his back. The perception of the patient may be that you are not listening or that you do not care about his or her recovery. Patient education can make a substantial difference in improving your rapport with your patient and enhance overall treatment effectiveness.

Pain Assessment

Pain is a subjective experience, and as such it is difficult to measure. It is essential, however, to have some means of monitoring an individual's perception of pain at any given time to monitor response to treatment and activity. The McGill Pain Questionnaire (MPQ),[20,24,26] visual analog scales (VASs),[3] and numeric pain-rating scales (NPRSs)[3,27] are some pain assessment tools commonly used in the assessment of pain perception (see Chapter 2).

McGill Pain Questionnaire

The MPQ is made up of several parts and attempts to measure the patient's perception of pain. Body diagrams for pain location and word descriptors for pain quality are included. The patient's description of pain intensity and the pattern of pain related to activity compose the remainder of the questionnaire. The advantages of using the MPQ include collecting quantitative and qualitative information regarding pain and providing information on the effects of different treatments and activities on pain perception.

Visual Analog Scales

Although not as sensitive as the MPQ, the VAS is a quick means by which patients can rate pain.[3,6] The patient is given a piece of paper marked with a line that is 10 cm long. At one end is written "the worst pain I ever felt," and at the other, "no pain at all." The patient is asked to mark the line at the point corresponding to the intensity of pain felt at that moment. Records can be kept by measuring the position of

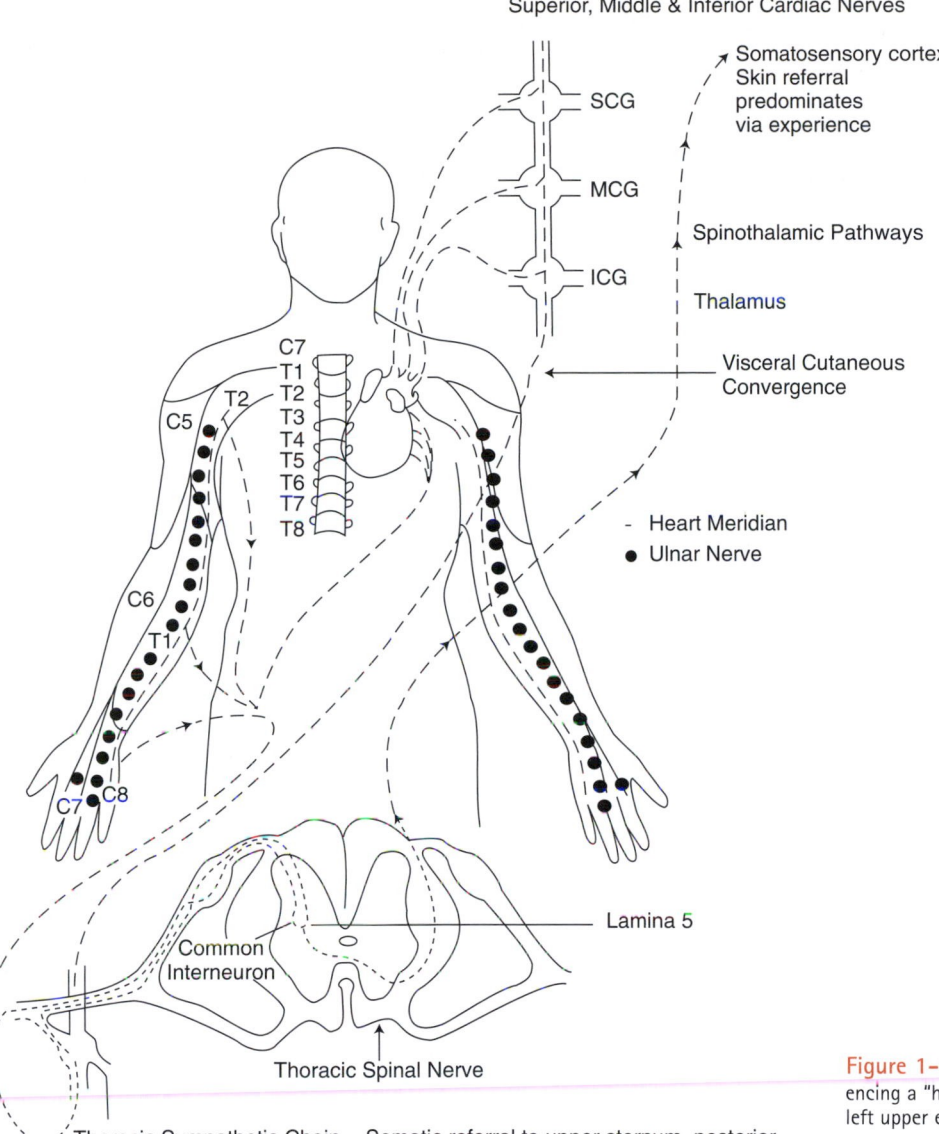

Superior, Middle & Inferior Cardiac Nerves

Somatosensory cortex
Skin referral
predominates
via experience

SCG

MCG

Spinothalamic Pathways

ICG

Thalamus

Visceral Cutaneous
Convergence

- Heart Meridian
• Ulnar Nerve

Lamina 5

Common
Interneuron

Thoracic Spinal Nerve

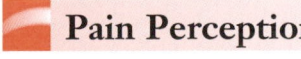

Thoracic Sympathetic Chain

Somatic referral to upper sternum, posterior
& anterior chest, arm, neck, jaw, occiput &
epigastrim.

Figure 1-5 Diagram of dermatomes. When someone is experiencing a "heart attack," pain can be perceived throughout the left upper extremity, which corresponds to the overlap of dermatome, myotome, and scleratome. (Adapted from Mannheimer, JS, and Lampe, GN, eds. Clinical Transcutaneous Electrical Nerve Stimulation. FA Davis, Philadelphia, 1984, p 109.)

the marks on the scale from treatment to treatment. An NPRS is a variation of the VAS. The patient is asked to rate his or her pain "on a scale of 1 to 10, 10 being the worst pain imaginable, 1 being no pain." This information is then recorded in the patient's chart. Further description of pain assessment is detailed in Chapter 2.

Pain Perception

The mechanisms of pain perception are not completely understood,[6] although some pieces of the puzzle are better identified and understood than others. "Pain signals" must be picked up by sensory receptors in the periphery, and the signals must be transmitted to the brain for us to perceive pain. This is not a simple stimulus-response situation.[6,10] Many factors modify the signal before and after it reaches the brain.[6,28–32] The following is a brief review of the neural mechanisms of pain perception.

Pain Receptors

Specialized receptors called nociceptors signal actual or potential tissue damage.[6,9,21] The receptors in the skin are understood better than the receptors found in the viscera and cardiac and skeletal muscle.[6] The nociceptors are actually three distinct types of free nerve endings that respond to

TABLE 1-1 **Types of Nociceptors**

TYPE	RESPONDS TO	FIBER CONNECTION	SENSATION	SPEED OF CONDUCTION
High-threshold mechanoreceptor	Strong mechanical stimulation	A-delta	Sharp "Pricking" Well localized	Fast
Mechanothermal nociceptor	Strong mechanical stimulation Noxious heat	A-delta	Sharp "Pricking" Well localized	Fast
Polymodal nociceptor	Strong mechanical stimulation Noxious heat Irritant chemicals	C	Dull Aching Burning Poorly localized	Slow

different stimulus modalities (Table 1-1). The nociceptors do not normally respond to sensory stimuli in nondamaging ranges. For example, high-threshold mechanoreceptors (HTMs) do not usually respond to light touch. The sensitivity of HTMs increases following mild injury, however, causing the surrounding tissue to become more sensitive to pressure. Polymodal nociceptors become increasingly sensitive following repeated heat or chemical activation,[30–32] possibly accounting for the hyperalgia experienced in injured skin. Pain sensation is elicited by a noxious stimulus that is the result of excitation of the various sensory receptors and free nerve endings of the skin and internal structures. The nerve fiber types that are the mediators of pain impulses in the CNS are the A-delta and C fibers. A-delta fibers transmit discriminative touch stimuli from the skin. A-delta fibers are sensitive to crude touch, pain, and temperature. C fibers are the afferent fibers coming from pain receptors.[9]

Pain Fiber Types and Central Pathways

Once a pain receptor is stimulated, the nerve fiber transmits a signal to the dorsal horn of the spinal cord. A few ascending and descending fibers branch off to form Lissauer's tract and communicate with neighboring spinal segments. The main fiber continues in the dorsal horn to make connections with neurons of lamina I, II, III, IV, and V. Lamina III is also known as the substantia gelatinosa. Synaptic connections are then made with neurons, giving rise to the lateral spinothalamic tract. These neurons cross over to the opposite side of the spinal cord at the ventral white commissure (Fig. 1-6). The fibers of the lateral spinothalamic tract ascend the spinal cord and enter the brainstem, where some fibers send branches to the reticular formation. Other fibers continue to the thalamus, where they form synapses with neurons that ascend to the primary and secondary somatosensory cortex. The fibers that have been projected to the reticular formation then synapse with other fibers that relay pain information to the thalamus, hypothalamus, and limbic sys-

tem. The end result of all these connections is the perception of pain.[1,9]

Peripheral Fibers

Each type of nociceptor is attached to one of two distinct types of primary afferent (sensory) neurons: small myelinated A-delta fibers and small unmyelinated C fibers. The A-delta fibers conduct impulses at a rate faster than the C fibers. Stimulation of A-delta fibers evokes a sharp and pricking pain sensation that is well localized and of short duration (sometimes referred to as "first pain"[23]). Stimulation of C fibers produces a longer-lasting burning sensation, which is dull and poorly localized (sometimes referred to as "second pain"[23]).

Dorsal Root Ganglia

The cell bodies of the A-delta and C fibers, together with those of the larger sensory fibers (A-β), are found in the dorsal root ganglia at the various levels of the spinal cord. Primary afferent (sensory) signals are transmitted from these ganglia by axonal processes to specific areas of the spinal cord.

Doral Horn of the Spinal Cord

A-delta and C fibers carrying pain signals travel through the lateral division of the dorsal root. They may then ascend several spinal segments before entering the spinal gray matter. "The dorsal horn of the spinal cord acts like a computer that processes the incoming sensory signals, rearranging and modulating them before sending them on to the next higher level."[21] Many factors influence which signals are emphasized and which are ignored.

Within the dorsal horn, A-delta and C fibers communicate with several different types of neurons in different layers of the gray matter.[24] These include nociceptive-specific neurons that receive input only from A-delta and C fibers (pain fibers) and wide-dynamic-range neurons that receive input from

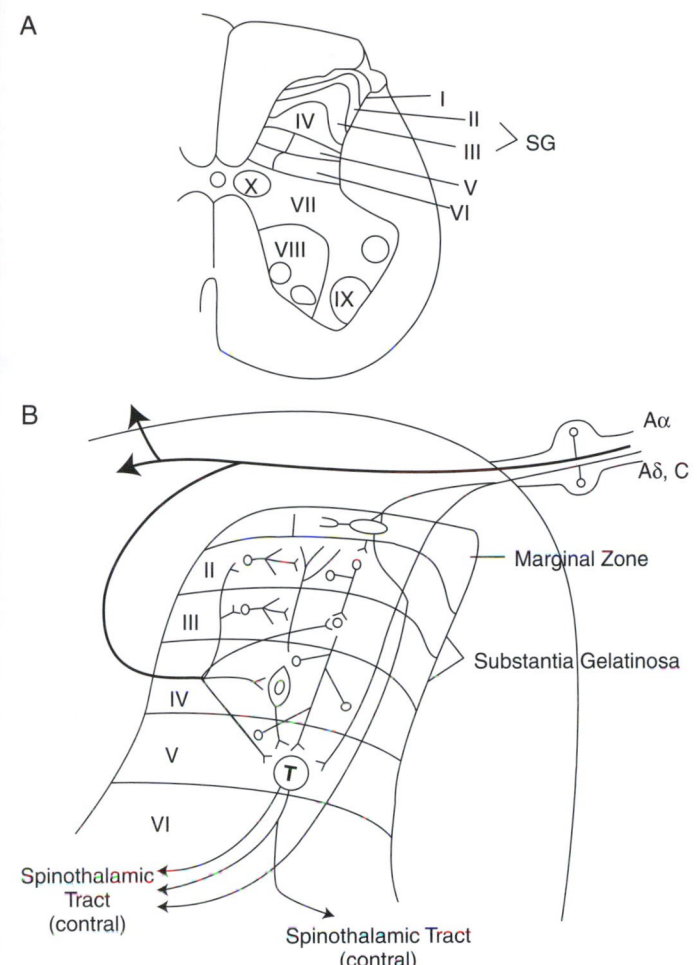

A

B

Aα

Aδ, C

Marginal Zone

Substantia Gelatinosa

T

Spinothalamic
Tract
(contral)

Spinothalamic Tract
(contral)

Figure 1-6   Spinal cord dorsal horn illustration with crossover of information. The main fiber continues in the dorsal horn to make connections with neurons of lamina I, II, III, IV, and V. Lamina III is also known as the substantia gelatinosa. Synaptic connections are then made with neurons, giving rise to the lateral spinothalamic tract. These neurons cross over to the opposite side of the spinal cord at the ventral white commissure. The fibers of the lateral spinothalamic tract ascend the spinal cord and enter the brainstem, where some fibers send branches to the reticular formation. Other fibers continue to the thalamus, where they form synapses with neurons that ascend to the primary and secondary somatosensory cortices. The fibers that have been projected to the reticular formation then synapse with other fibers that relay pain information to the thalamus, hypothalamus, and limbic system. The end result of all these connections is the perception of pain.[1,9] (Adapted from Manheimer, JS and Lampe, GN <eds> Clinical Transcutaneous Electrical Nerve Stimulation. FA Davis, Philadelphia, 1984, p 45. Originally adapted from Heavner, JE: Jamming spinal sensory input: effects of anesthetic and analgesic drugs in the spinal cord dorsal horn. Pain 1:239, 1975.)

A-delta mechanoreceptive (nonpainful) fibers as well as from A-delta and C fibers. Nociceptive-specific neurons assist in discrimination of the specific type of pain, that is, thermal, mechanical, or chemical, but do not localize the pain sensation well. The wide-dynamic-range cells contribute to the localization of burning or pricking pain, as well as the discrimination between touch and noxious pinching. These cells receive input from both the viscera and the skin. It is thought that this convergence of noxious stimuli may be the basis for

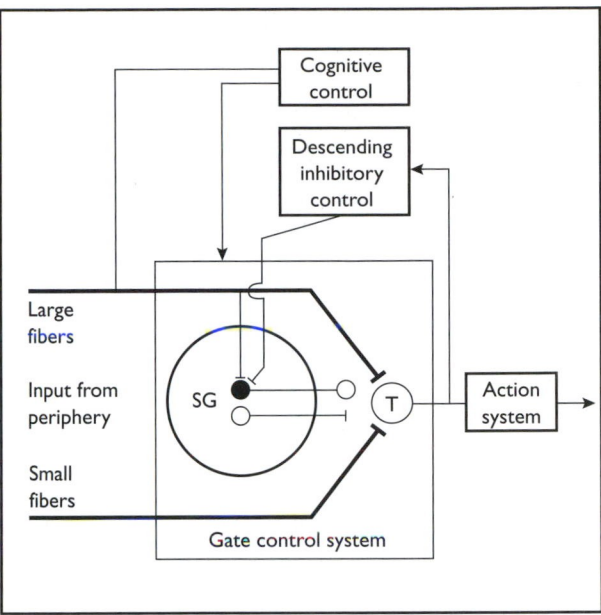

Figure 1-7   The gate control theory. The new model includes excitatory (open circle) and inhibitory (shaded circle) links from the substantia gelatinosa (SG) to the transmission (T) cells, as well as descending inhibitory control from brainstem systems. The round knob at the end of the inhibitory link implies that its actions may be presynaptic, postsynaptic, or both. All connections are excitatory, except the inhibitory link for the SG to T cell. (From Bonica,[6] p 10, with permission.)

referred pain, because the brain may be unable to discriminate between a visceral and a cutaneous source of stimuli. Wide-dynamic-range cells are also called T (transmission) cells and form the basis for the gate control theory[20,24] (Fig. 1-7).

Pain Pathways

Ascending

For an individual to be aware of pain, the noxious input to the dorsal horn of the spinal cord must travel to the brain. Several ascending tracts are responsible for the transmission of pain signals.[9] The axons of most of the transmission cells cross over and ascend via the spinothalamic tract. This tract transmits the pain signal to the thalamus. The thalamus acts as a general relay station for sensory information and has precise projections to the portion of the brain called the somatosensory cortex.[9] Once the signal reaches the cortex, it is perceived as a sharp, discriminative, and relatively localized sensation.[9] The second pathway is called the spinoreticulothalamic pathway. As the name implies, signals travel from the spine to the reticular formation of the brainstem and to the thalamus. Signals are also thought to connect to nuclei in the periaqueductal gray area of the midbrain and to areas of the limbic system. The information that this pathway conveys is perceived as diffuse, poorly localized somatic and visceral pain[9,33] (Fig. 1-8).

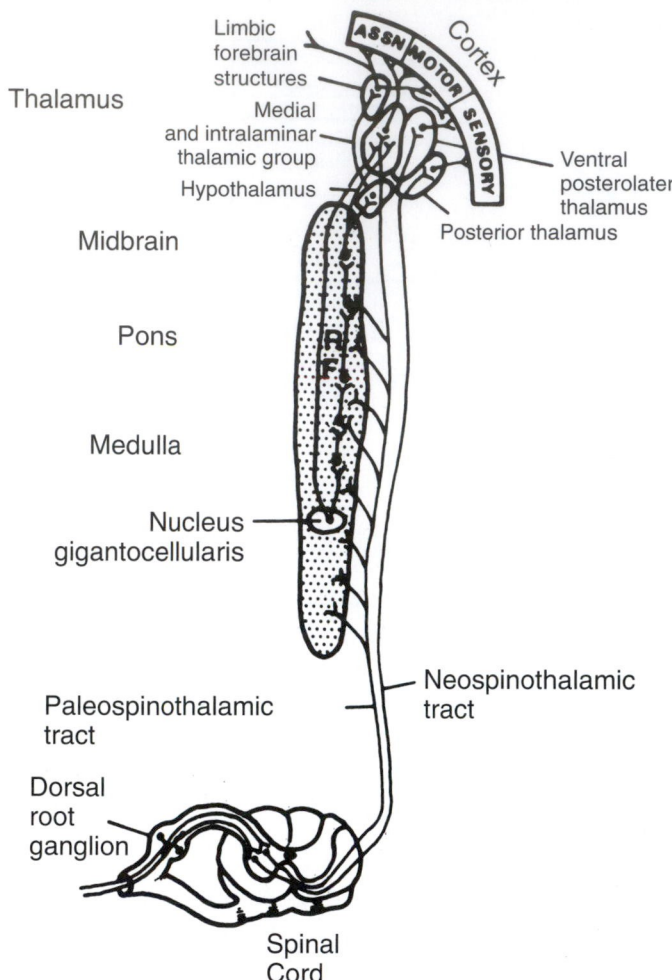

Figure 1-8   Generalized conceptualization of projections from pain pathways traversing the neuraxis.

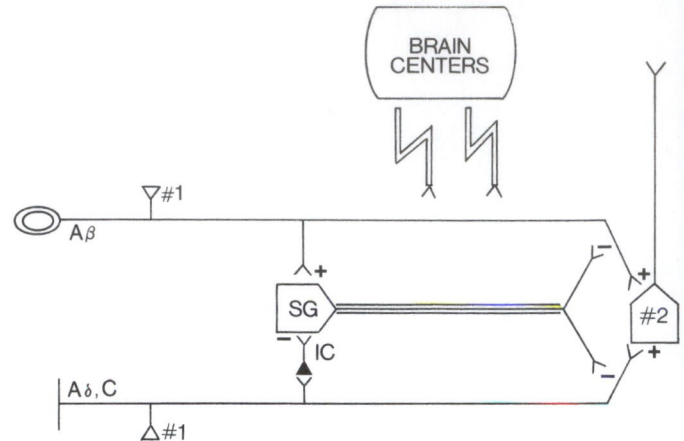

Figure 1-9   Gate control theory. (From Michlovitz, SL: Thermal Agents in Rehabilitation, ed 3. FA Davis, Philadelphia, 1996, p 45.)

pain.[24] The reader should be aware, however, that knowledge of the nature of pain and the mechanisms of its perception continues to expand.

Gate Control Theory

The gate control theory was proposed in 1965 by Melzack and Wall[20] and was modified in 1975[26] and 1982[24] (Fig. 1-9). They stated that sensory mechanisms alone failed to account for the fact that nerve lesions do not always cause pain. Instead, they proposed a more complex interaction of peripheral and central mechanisms. Injury activates small-diameter myelinated afferent nerve fibers (A-delta fibers) and small-diameter unmyelinated afferent fibers (C fibers). These nerve impulses excite central transmission cells (T cells) that were proposed to be in the substantia gelatinosa of the dorsal horn of the spinal cord. These T cells receive a convergence of excitatory and inhibitory influences, some from nociceptors and some from other sensory nerve endings. Whether further transmission occurs and the pain signal is sent on to higher centers to be perceived by the individual depends on the summation of inhibitory and excitatory influences. In addition, Melzack and Wall proposed that descending control from the brainstem and cortex also strongly influenced the excitability of the transmission cells. They stated that "psychological factors such as past experience, attention, and emotion influence pain response and perception by acting on the gate control system."[27]

Endogenous Opiates

In the years since 1965, much has been learned about pain control mechanisms. The accuracy of the original statement by Melzack and Wall that facilitation and inhibition occur and influence the perception of pain is clear; where and how this facilitation and inhibition occur are not clear. A new

Descending

The descending control system for modulation of pain is not completely understood. There is evidence that naturally occurring substances called endogenous opiates exist that inhibit the perception of pain.[6,10] Examples include methionine enkephalin (met-enkephalin), beta-endorphin (β-endorphin), serotonin, dynorphin,[34,35] and dopamine. They work via various mechanisms and are effective for different lengths of time. Release of endogenous opiates is stimulated by systemic pain, intense exercise, laughter, relaxation, meditation, acupuncture, and electrical stimulation.[6]

Pain Theories

A number of theories have been proposed to explain the nature of pain and how it is perceived. The gate control theory is considered by some the most complete model of

class of neurotransmitters called endogenous opiates[6,10] has been discovered. These naturally occurring "pain killers," including enkephalins, endorphins, serotonin, and dopamine, operate in different parts of the nervous system and are effective for varying lengths of time. They may partially account for the "descending control mechanisms" referred to by Melzack and Wall. Enkephalins, which are short-acting endogenous opiates that operate at the spinal cord level, are now thought to "block the gate" by interfering with A-delta and C fiber signal transmission to T cells. They have a very short half-life, meaning that they are effective while actually present in the tissue and for only a short time afterward. Nonpainful sensory stimulus is effective in triggering the release of enkephalins.

Endorphins are another class of endogenous opiates. They act in several different areas of the nervous system (including the dorsal horn) to inhibit pain signal transmission or to decrease the amount of chemical irritants present in the system.[6,10] The half-life of these neurotransmitters is 4 hours. The release of endorphins is stimulated by a variety of factors, including intense pain, intense exercise, acupuncture, laughter, meditation, and relaxation.

Serotonin (5-HT) and dopamine are also capable of influencing pain perception; however, the mechanisms of their actions are not well understood. Serotonin is released from platelets and activates the primary afferent pain fibers,[6,35,36] which would seem to increase the number of pain signals. However, serotonin is also involved in the descending (brain to spinal cord) system that inhibits signals from peripheral nociceptors.[37] Serotonin is a necessary link in the analgesic system.[35–37] Dopamine, a neurotransmitter well known for its role in influencing movement through basal ganglion functioning, may also be used by the body to synthesize morphine and codeine.[30] More continues to be learned regarding these substances and the roles they play in the human body.

Clinical Versus Experimental Pain

Experimental pain is pain that is induced to study physiologic, psychologic, emotional, and behavioral responses to stimuli. Subjects are often healthy volunteers who are aware of the controlled nature of the study or patients with pain who are submitting to induced pain to have their responses or pain tolerance measured. Although experiments with pain have greatly expanded our knowledge of the responses to such stimuli, the controlled nature of the stimulus and the situation may very well bias subjects' responses. Care should be taken in extrapolating experimental results to clinical situations. As Wall stated, "In the real world outside the laboratory, the variation in the relationship between pain and injury occupies all portions between injury with no pain and pain with no injury."[38]

Pain Relief

Pain as a Symptom of Dysfunction

Rehabilitation typically focuses on pain that is caused by physical dysfunction or is the result of disease. Pain is usually a symptom of dysfunction. The underlying dysfunction or problem, as well as the symptom of pain, should be treated. A complete approach to working with a patient experiencing pain should include the following[39,40]:

1. Gathering background information, including mechanism of injury (if applicable), prior medical problems, work background, recreational activity, health habits, and sleep patterns

2. Assesment of pain location, temporal aspects, quantity, and quality. Pain assessment forms, including pain-rating scales, should be part of routine documentation.

3. Physical examination, including range-of-motion measurements, volume and girth assessments (if applicable), strength assessments, postural evaluation, joint alignment and mobility, soft tissue examination, and functional ability

The intervention plan that results from this evaluation should prioritize, then address, all pertinent problems. Effective initial therapeutic treatment intervention with pain-relieving modalities or medications prescribed by a physician is important to minimize the pain-dysfunction-guarding cycle (see Fig. 1-3) and can be critical to the success of the plan; however, limiting the treatment of pain to medication or physical modalities such as ice massage, hot packs, ultrasound, and/or soft tissue massage is seldom effective in addressing all of the underlying causes of pain and restoring lost function.

Frequently, poor posture and body mechanics, decreased flexibility, and an overall decline in fitness are contributing factors to the dysfunction causing pain.[39] Common examples include the patient with a severe forward head and rounded shoulders who complains of neck pain or shoulder pain due to tendinopathy and the truck driver with shortened hamstring muscles who complains of low back pain. If these patients are only treated symptomatically with pain-relieving modalities and the issues related to posture, overuse, and muscle length are not addressed, there is a high likelihood that they will either achieve poor control of their pain or become "revolving-door patients" who return on a frequent basis with the same or related pain complaints.

It is also important that the psychologic and emotional aspects of the patient's pain problem not be ignored. Positive reinforcement of pain behavior may increase the likelihood of an acute pain problem be coming a chronic pain problem.[14,16] Involvement in decision making and treatment activities by the patient is important to foster a sense of personal responsibility over dependency. If properly administered, even the physical modalities may include education and active involvement on the part of the patient. For example, instruction in proper body mechanics, positions of rest, the appropriate use of heat, and relaxation techniques including deep breathing and visualization can all be part of an effective home program.

Therapeutic Intervention—Clinical Decision Making

The form that treatment takes, the timing with which it is administered, and the attitude of the health care professional toward the patient and his or her problem are all critical to the successful treatment of pain. The importance of correcting dysfunction as a means of treating pain was previously discussed. The various tools that can be used as therapeutic treatment interventions to provide analgesia are briefly reviewed next. They are discussed in greater depth in subsequent chapters of this text.

Thermal Agents

Thermal agents include the following:

1. Superficial heating agents such as hot packs, paraffin, Fluidotherapy, infrared lamps, and warm whirlpool baths (>98.6°F)[41,42]
2. Deep heating agents such as ultrasound and shortwave diathermy
3. Cold agents such as cold packs, ice massage, ice towels, and cold baths

The decision of which thermal modality to use should include consideration of several factors, most notably, goal of treatment, stage of healing of the injury, depth of the target tissue, patient tolerance and preference, and ease of application (especially for home use).

Electrotherapeutic Devices

Transcutaneous electrical nerve stimulation (TENS) is an application of electrotherapy specifically designed for pain managment.[43–45] TENS units are small, portable, battery-powered pulsed stimulators. The stimulus parameters used with these devices are based on the theories of pain perception. Two of the more commonly used protocols are sensory-level (conventional or high-rate) TENS, which is set at 75 to 100 pulses per second (pps), a short pulse duration, and sensory paresthesia level of intensity[38] to "block the gate," and low-rate TENS, which is set at a low rate (1 to 4 pps), a moderate duration, and a motor threshold level of intensity to stimulate the release of endorphins.[38] Electrical stimulation as a treatment intervention and form of pain management is discussed in more detail in Chapter 12.

Biofeedback is another electrotherapeutic device modality that is frequently used in the management of pain. Biofeedback is used to monitor various functions in the body, including muscle activity, skin temperature, skin conductance, heart rate, respiratory rate, blood pressure, and brain waves. The information picked up by the biofeedback unit in the form of electrical potentials is then translated into an audio and/or a visual signal that the patient can relate to activity of the body. The idea is to bring physiologic functioning that normally occurs below our level of awareness to our conscious attention so that we can learn to control various body systems. A common application in physical therapy is the monitoring of muscle function[46] to enhance muscle activity in a weak muscle or to promote relaxation in a tense muscle.

Tissue Repair

A predictable sequence of reactions of the body occurs from injury through the completion of healing. There are both physical and psychologic factors that may influence the phases of this sequence. Estimates of the length of each phase vary,[47,48] but it is generally agreed that they overlap.[48,49] Certainly factors such as the size of the insult or wound, the presence of cardiovascular and pulmonary system diseases, infection and immunosuppressive disorders, and the administration of immunosuppressant drugs influence the course of recovery.

The goals of this next section are to (1) describe the normal response to tissue trauma, (2) discuss factors that affect wound healing, and (3) introduce ways in which physical agents and electrotherapy can be used to influence tissue healing.

Tissue Response to Trauma: Inflammation and Repair

The body responds to injury of vascularized tissue with a series of events, collectively called inflammation and repair.[47] Vascular, cellular, hormonal, and immune system responses occur to minimize tissue damage and restore function. Skin, muscle, peripheral nerves, and bone can regenerate to a certain extent following cell death; other human tissue, such as the brain and spinal cord, cannot. Scar tissue replaces damaged tissue that cannot regenerate. Although scar tissue may restore a certain structural integrity to the tissue, it is not as strong as the original tissue (maximal tensile strength of scar tissue is between 70% and 80% of normal tissue[50,51]), is poorly vascularized, may disrupt organ functioning, may restrict movement (especially if it occurs near a joint), and may be disfiguring.

Inflammation (Days 1 to 10)

The initial phase of healing is described as the inflammatory, or "self-defense," response. This normal process, which is a prerequisite to healing, does have uncomfortable and sometimes distressing symptoms, including the "cardinal signs of inflammation": redness, heat, swelling, and pain. In addition, there is typically a loss of function.[49] These signs are the result of complex interactions of the vascular, hemostatic, cellular, and immune systems. (Refer to the *Cardinal Signs of Inflammation* box on page 6.)

Immediately following injury, changes in severed vessels occur as the body attempts to wall off the wound from the external environment.[49] Platelets aggregate, blood coagulation is initiated, severed lymph channels are sealed off, and arterioles constrict. These brief but important compensatory mechanisms serve to protect the individual from excessive blood loss and increased exposure to bacterial contamination.

Within a few minutes of injury, vasodilation of the injured vessels occurs, resulting in increased blood flow, redness, and heat. Noninjured vessels dilate in response to chemicals such as histamine and prostaglandins released from injured tissues.[48] An increase in the hydrostatic pressure also occurs within the vessels. At the same time, the capillaries and venules become more permeable (because of chemicals called bradykinins and histamine), allowing the release of cells, macromolecules, and fluid from the vascular system into the interstitial spaces. Lymph vessels that normally clear osmotically active particles from this area are unable to keep up with the demand. Edema occurs as fluid moves in to the interstitium to restore the balance of osmotic pressures.

The make-up of the edema fluid changes as the stages of inflammation progress and with the magnitude of injury. Initially the fluid is a clear, watery substance called transudate. As more cells and plasma proteins enter the interstitial space, the edema fluid becomes viscous and cloudy and is called exudate. If the exudate contains large numbers of leukocytes (white blood cells), it is called pus.[49]

For healing to commence, the wound must be decontaminated (through phagocytosis) and a new blood supply must be established (revascularization).[50] Phagocytosis is carried out first by polymorphonuclear leukocytes. In a few days, another type of phagocyte called a macrophage appears. These cells remain in the wound until all signs of inflammation are gone. Macrophages attack and engulf bacteria and dispose of necrotic tissue in the wound. They have been called the "director cells" of repair because, by emitting certain chemical signals, macrophages recruit fibroblasts to form scar tissue. The number of fibroblasts relates to the amount of scar tissue. If there are not enough macrophages or they cannot function well enough because of a lack of oxygen, there will be no signal to stimulate the fibroblasts, and a chronic wound results.

Another important component of healing is the release of growth factors. Growth factors stimulate the production of many of the necessary components of the tissue extracellular matrix. These growth factors are referred to as cytokines. Growth factor beta-1 stimulates collagen production.[52] Fibroblasts are also intricately involved in wound healing and scarring. Fibroblast growth factors (FGFs) appear to be a key component during the beginning of cellular proliferation, differentiation, migration, and matrix deposition phases of wound healing.[53,54] Hepatocyte growth factor (HGF) is involved in antifibrotic activities, assisting in the prevention of excessive fibrous deposition of healing tissues.[55] There are also osteogenic growth factors involved in the enhancement of bone repair. Gene therapy for recombinant osteogenic growth factor is now available and has the potential for use in nonunion fractures and the enhancement of bone repair[55] (Box 1-3).

As this phase comes to a close, chemicals are released from blood vessels to dissolve clots. The lymphatic channels open to assist in reducing wound edema.[50]

Proliferative Phase (Days 3 to 20)

Revascularization and rebuilding of the tissue occur in the proliferative phase. Revascularization is thought to be triggered by the macrophages through the release of growth factors ("director cells" of the inflammation phase). Intact blood vessels at the edges of the wound develop small buds and sprouts that grow into the wound area. These outgrowths eventually come in contact with and join other arteriolar or venular buds and form a functioning capillary loop. These loops are what create the bright pink color seen throughout healing wounds. They are extremely fragile when first formed and can be easily disrupted. Immobilization or protected movement is important to prevent bleeding. Vigorous heating at this time may also cause increased bleeding and is contraindicated.

Rebuilding of the structure of the wound occurs through resurfacing with epithelial tissue and restrengthening with connective tissue. This phase is extremely active and is highly dependent on the oxygenation of the tissue. Hypoxic wounds build poor-quality scars. Fibroblasts, which form scar

BOX 1-3	Growth Factors (Cytokines) Involved in Tissue Repair
Growth factor beta	*for collagen production*
Fibroblast growth factors	*for cellular proliferation*
	differentiation
	migration
	matrix deposition phases of wound healing
Hepatocyte growth factor	*for antifibrotic activity*
	prevents excessive fibrous depositions
Osteogenic growth factors	*for bone repair*

TABLE 1-2	Three Stages of the Proliferative Phase of Healing	
STAGES OF PROLIFERATIVE PHASE	**CHANGES WITHIN THE WOUND**
Epithelization (granulation)	Wound is filled in with granulating tissue, from the edges in and from structures like hair shafts and sweat glands out
	Epithelial cells seek out a moist, oxygen-rich environment
	Epithelial cells can only cover 2 cm of open wound
Wound contraction	Myofibroblasts pull the entire wound together
	Occurs from 4 to 14–21 days
Collagen production	Wound tensile strength is dependent on crosslinking
	Weak electrostatic forces hold edges together

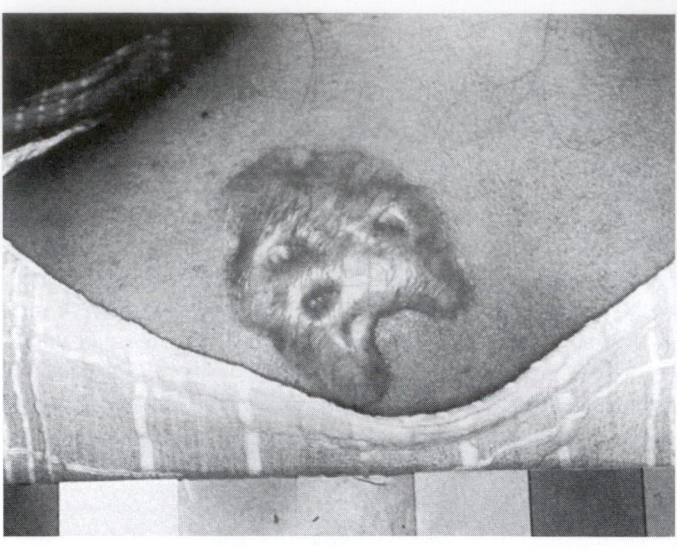

Figure 1-10 A keloid of the left posterior scapula area that is the result of thermal injury to the back. This thermal injury occurred as the result of carbon dioxide laser treatment of a decorative tattoo. (Courtesy of David B. Afelberg, MD, Palo Alto, CA, as shown in Reed and Zarro,[47] p 11.)

tissue, respond to changes in the electrical potential at the wound (chemotactic influence) and migrate into the inflamed area along fibrin strands.

Three processes occur simultaneously to close the wound and are outlined in Table 1-2. The process of wound contraction deserves special mention. The purpose of this process is to decrease the open area that the skin must ultimately cover. It occurs through action of the myofibroblasts located at the edge of the wound. This is a normal part of the healing process, starting around day 4 postinjury and continuing to days 14 through 21. Depending on the location of the wound, the results of this contraction process may or may not restrict movement. For example, the contraction of a large scar in the hand may cause functional problems, whereas the contraction of a large scar on the buttocks may not. Wound contraction is one of many different forces that may lead to a contracture and subsequent loss of passive motion.

Remodeling or Maturation Phase (Day 9 Onward)

The long-term goal of wound healing is the return of function. During the final phase of healing, remodeling of the scar tissue occurs. Ideally, there should be a balance between the formation of new collagen and the breakdown of old collagen. As long as the scar looks "rosier" than normal, remodeling is under way[56]; this process may continue for years. The desired outcome is a scar that is pale, flat, and pliable. Abnormal scars form when more collagen is produced than is reabsorbed. Overproduction of collagen can result in a hypertropic scar or keloid scar (Fig. 1-10). These scars appear red, raised, and rigid.

During remodeling, randomly oriented collagen fibers are replaced with fibers that are oriented both linearly and laterally. Through processes that are not fully understood, the scar takes on some of the characteristics of the structure it is replacing: repaired ligamentous tissue will ultimately have a different structure than the repaired joint capsule only millimeters away. Two theories have been proposed to explain how collagen realigns appropriately. The induction theory hypothesizes that scar tissue tries to mimic the characteristics of the tissue it is healing. The tension theory hypothesizes that the collagen fibers that lay down during remodeling respond to internal and external stresses that are placed on the wound and align accordingly. The application of dynamic splints, serial casting, continuous passive motion (CPM) machines, neuromuscular electrical stimulation (NMES), scar massage, and positional stretching techniques to wounds or scars to increase flexibility and range of motion is based on this theory. NMES is detailed in Chapter 10.

Delays in Wound Healing

Delayed closure of a wound simply means that a wound is taking longer than expected to heal.[56] There are two types of delayed closure. The first is intentionally created by the medical staff when a choice is made to not suture a wound closed (healing by first intention) but rather to leave it open to granulate and reepithelialize on its own (healing by second intention). Reasons for promoting healing by second intention include dirt in the wound, infection, and excessive drainage. The second type of delayed closure is not deliberate and involves many factors affecting the conservative treatment of a wound. It is important to consider whether the delay is caused by (1) a factor related to the patient's general physical

<table>
<tr><td colspan="2">

BOX 1-4   Factors that Increase the Likelihood of a Wound Becoming Chronic

1. Medications such as certain nonsteroidal anti-inflammatory drugs, steroids, and immunosuppressive drugs used for transplant patients
2. Comorbidities such as acquired immunodeficiency syndrome (AIDS), diabetes, cancer, and peripheral vascular disease[56]
3. Cellular toxicity of commonly used antimicrobial agents such as povidone-iodine (e.g., Betadine; Benton-Dickinson Acute Care, Franklin Lakes, NJ), hydrogen peroxide, and acetic acid
4. Radiation therapy
5. Chemotherapy
6. Malnutrition

</td></tr>
</table>

or mental condition or (2) an iatrogenic factor, such as the way the wound is physically managed and treatments, including drugs and therapies (see Box 1-5).[52,56] Factors that can be changed should be addressed (see Tables 1-2, 1-3, and 1-4).

An important area beyond the scope of this chapter is

TABLE 1-3   Effect of Local Factors on the Promotion or Impairment of Wound Healing

LOCAL FACTORS	PROMOTION OF WOUND HEALING	IMPAIRMENT OF WOUND HEALING
Surgical technique	Close approximation of wound edges	Excessive tension
Blood supply	Patent	Devitalized tissue
		Atherosclerosis
		Venous stasis
		Tissue ischemia
Infection	None	Bacteria
		Mycobacteria
		Fungi or yeast
Medications	Some topical antibiotics (e.g., mupirocin-Bactroban)	Topical steroids
		Many systemic and topical antibiotics
		Antineoplastic drugs
		Hemostatic agents (aluminum chloride or Monsel's solution)
Trauma	None	Chronic trauma
		Foreign body
		Factitial trauma
Microenvironment	Occlusive dressings	Dry dressings
		Photo-aged skin
		Radiation injury
Ulcer type		Decubitus ulcers
		Tumor (Marjolin's ulcer)
		Neuropathic ulcers (malperforans ulcers)

From Daly,[50] P 41, with permission.

TABLE 1-4   Effect of Systemic Factors on the Promotion or Impairment of Wound Healing

SYSTEMIC FACTORS	PROMOTION OF WOUND HEALING	IMPAIRMENT OF WOUND HEALING
Nutrition	No deficiencies	Deficiency of protein, calories, vitamins (especially A and C), trace metals (especially zinc and copper)
Age	Young	Advanced chronic illness (hepatic, renal, hematopoietic, cardiovascular, autoimmune, carcinoma)
Illness	None	Endocrine disease (e.g., diabetes mellitus, Cushing's disease)
		Systemic vascular disorders (periarteritis nodosa, vasculitis, granulomatosis, atherosclerosis)
		Connective tissue disease (e.g., Ehlers-Danlos syndrome)
Systemic medications		Corticosteroids, aspirin, heparin, coumadin, penicillamine, nicotine, phenylbutazone, and other nonsteroidal anti-inflammatory drugs; antineoplastic agents

Source: From Daly,[50] P 41, with permission.

wound coverage with dressings. The traditional concept of promoting wound healing by "airing" the wound has given way to an understanding of the importance of maintaining a moist environment at the wound bed. Semiocclusive or occlusive dressings are now used to promote reepithelization, avoid the formation of a crust (scab or eschar), decrease bacterial exposure, and decrease the secondary trauma of frequent dressing changes.[56–58]

Chronic wounds are wounds that are not healing despite conservative or surgical treatment.[56] This does not mean that healing is impossible but that intervention will be needed to improve the chances of successful wound closure. Some of the factors that are likely to increase the chance of chronicity of a wound are summarized in Box 1-4.

Age is also a factor in wound healing. The neonate may have a modified response because of the immaturity of organ system functioning. Children have a greater capacity for tissue repair than adults but lack the reserves necessary to counteract any significant trauma. This is shown by "an easily upset electrolyte balance, sudden elevation or lowering of body temperature, and rapid spread of infection."[59] Older adults undergo the same healing process as young adults but do so more slowly. They are, however, "more susceptible to wound healing problems due to the interactions of body sys-

PHASES OF HEALING	EFFECTS OF AGING
TABLE 1-5 The Effects of Aging on the Healing Response [53,56]	
Inflammatory, "self-defense" phase	• ↓ 'd and disrupted vascular supplies → ↓ 'd clearance of metabolites, bacteria, and foreign materials
	• ↓ 'd supply of nutrients
	• ↓ 'd inflammatory response
	• → ↑ 'd likelihood of "chronic wounds"
	• ↓ 'd rate of wound capillary growth
Proliferative phase	• ↓ 'd metabolic response
	• ↓ 'd migration and proliferation of cells
	• Delayed maturation of cells
	• Delayed wound contraction
Remodeling phase	• Delayed collagen remodeling
	• ↑ 'd tertiary cross-linking of collagen → less flexible and weaker scars

tems, environmental stresses, and disease with an aging process that takes place over many years."[60] Aging leads to decreased efficiency in many body systems, including the cardiovascular, pulmonary, immune, and integumentary systems.[60] This decrease in efficiency affects healing. It is important to remember, however, that there is more variability in the older population than in any other age group: what may be true for a fragile, debilitated 60-year-old with diabetes mellitus may not be true for a healthy, robust 80-year-old (Table 1-5). (Box 1-5)

BOX 1-5   Factors that Influence Wound Healing

1. Balance is critical to the success of the healing process.
2. If there is no inflammatory response, there is no healing.
3. If there is too little inflammatory response, healing is slow.
4. If there is too much inflammatory response, healing is prolonged and excessive scar tissue forms.

Other Factors:

5. Virulence of the bacteria
6. Presence of foreign objects
7. Presence of necrotic tissue
8. Poor oxygen supply
9. Dehydration
10. Certain vitamin deficiencies (vitamin C, vitamin E,[70] vitamin D[71])
11. Lack of protein[70]
12. Irradiated tissues[72]
13. Immunosuppression

Physical Therapy Interventions for Soft Tissue Healing

Physical agents play a vital role in the management of soft tissue injuries (for both closed and open wounds). For closed wounds, including sprains and strains, physical therapy management initially involves rest, ice, compression, and elevation (RICE) of the affected part. As the inflammatory stage resolves, other therapeutic interventions can be applied, including ultrasound, hot packs, whirlpool, shortwave diathermy, and electrical stimulation, to further promote healing, increase soft tissue extensibility, and decrease any pain that may be present. Range-of-motion exercises, strengthening exercises, and functional activities are added as the soft tissue heals and is better able to tolerate these forces.

If the trauma includes an open wound, therapy may include the following:

1. Hydrotherapy (whirlpool or now, more commonly, pulsatile lavage with suction) to cleanse and debride the wound
2. Electrical stimulation to promote wound healing[56,61–65]
3. Vacuum-assisted closure (VAC) to assist with the closure of acute, subacute, and chronic wounds[66]
4. Pulsed ultrasound to promote wound healing during the proliferative and remodeling phases[66–68]
5. Hyperbaric oxygen chambers[66,69] to promote healing of chronic wounds
6. Ultraviolet-C radiation (UVC) for the treatment of infected wounds[56]
7. Early controlled mobilization of the injured part, including management of bracing with adjustable locks and exercise to prevent contractures and minimize muscle atrophy
8. Positioning programs to protect healing tissue and avoid the development of pressure sores or contractures
9. Design of seating systems (if applicable) to prevent the development of pressure sores and provide optimal mobility
10. Advising staff, patients, or family members in the selection of pressure-relieving devices (specialty beds, mattresses, and seat cushions)
11. Patient and family education in appropriate home activities

Summary

This chapter has dealt with the topics of pain and wound healing. It is important to be aware that knowledge of pain perception, pain management mechanisms, and wound healing continues to expand rapidly. To provide the most effective therapeutic treatment interventions for patients, health care providers must be ready to modify choices as new information and interventions become available.

Pain is a frequent concern for patients involved in rehabilitation. Skillful management of the physical, physiologic, and psychologic aspects of the patient with pain is a responsibility of all members of the rehabilitation team. An understanding of pain mechanisms will lead to appropriate choices of treatment interventions and approaches.

Wound healing progresses through a series of predictable stages, each of which may require different handling. Wound closure may be intentionally delayed if there is debris in the wound, infection, or excessive drainage. Errors in wound management, as well as factors relating to the patient's underlying physical and mental condition, may lead to the development of chronic wounds. The rehabilitation team may be involved in numerous aspects of wound care ranging from debridement to the prevention of secondary complications to optimization of mobility during the patient's recovery.

Discussion Questions

1. If a patient asked you to explain the nature of pain, how would you explain why some people seem to feel more discomfort than others? What terminology would you use to ensure that your explanation is easily understood by the patient?
2. How would the psychologic implications of pain perception influence your approach to a patient with chronic pain? Would this approach change in any way if this were an acute pain syndrome rather than a chronic pain syndrome?
3. If the patient asked you why he or she was feeling pain in an amputated limb or pain that travels down an arm or a leg, how would you explain it? Be careful to use terminology that a patient would understand.
4. How would you explain the inflammation and tissue repair process to a patient? Be careful to use terminology that the patient would understand. Your explanation should address the significance and necessity of the process.
5. Prepare an explanation for a patient that would discuss the importance of proper nutrition and wound care to promote tissue healing. Your explanation should include the rationale for keeping the wound moist as opposed to the patient's expressed desire to "let the wound dry."

References

1. Loeser, JD, and Melzack R: Pain: An overview. Lancet 353:1607–1609, 1999.
2. Turk, DC, and Melzack, R: Handbook of Pain Assessment. Guilford Press, New York, 1992.
3. Tyrer, SR (ed): Psychology, Psychiatry and Chronic Pain. Butterworth Heinemann, Oxford, 1992.
4. Sternbach, R: Psychology of Pain, ed 2. Raven Press, New York, 1986.
5. France, RD, and Krishnan, KRR: Chronic Pain. American Psychiatric Press, Washington, DC, 1988.
6. Bonica, JJ: The Management of Pain, Vols I and II, ed 2. Lea and Febiger, Malvern, PA, 1990.
7. Merskey, HM: Pain terms. Pain 3(suppl):S215–S221, 1986.
8. Kwako, J, and Shealy, CN: Psychological consideration in the management of pain. In Mannheimer, JS, and Lampe, GN (eds): Clinical Transcutaneous Electrical Nerve Stimulation. FA Davis, Philadelphia, 1984, p 29.
9. Gilman, S, and Newman, SW: Manter & Gatz's Essentials of Clinical Neuroanatomy and Neurophysiology, ed 10. FA Davis, Philadelphia, 2003.
10. Kandel, ER, Schwartz, JH, and Jessell, TM: Principles of Neural Science, ed 3. Elsevier, New York, 1991.
11. Sternbach, RA: Acute versus chronic pain. In Wall, PD, and Melzack, R (eds): Textbook of Pain. Churchill Livingstone, New York, 1994, p 173.
12. Bowsher, D: Acute and chronic pain and assessment. In Wells, PE, Frampton, V, and Bowsher, D (eds): Pain Management in Physiotherapy. Butterworth Heinemann, Oxford, 1996.
13. Tandon, OP, Malhotra, V, Tandon, S, and D'Silva, I: Neurophysiology of pain: Insight to orofacial pain. Ind J Physiol Pharmacol 47:247–269, 2003.
14. Brookoff, D: Chronic pain: 1. A new disease? Hosp Pract (Off Ed) 35:Jul 15, 2000.
15. Aronoff, GM: Evaluation and Treatment of Chronic Pain. Williams & Wilkins, Baltimore, 1992.
16. Sculco, AD, Paup, DC, Fernhall, B, and Sculco, MJ: Effects of aerobic exercise on low back pain patients in treatment. Spine J 1:95–101, 2001.
17. Barr, RB: Physical modalities in chronic pain management. Nurs Clin North Am 38:477–494, 2003.
18. Nadler, SF, Steiner, DJ, Erasala, GN, Hengehold, DA, Abein, SB, and Weingand, KW: Continuous low-level heatwrap therapy for treating acute nonspecific low back pain. Arch Phys Med Rehabil 84:329–334, 2003.
19. Graven-Nielsen, T, and Arendt-Nielsen, L: Induction and assessment of muscle pain, referred pain, and muscular hyperalgesia. Curr Pain Headache Rep 7:443–451, 2003.
20. Melzack, R, and Wall, PD: Pain mechanisms: A new theory. Science 150:971, 1965.

CASE STUDY

Phil is a 40-year-old Federal Express driver who has been referred to physical therapy subsequent to intermittent pain, weakness, and cramping in his dominant left hand thumb. Extension and abduction of the thumb reproduce his pain. There are no fractures, and he describes the onset of the pain as gradual. The hand is edematous with exquisite tenderness over the anatomical "snuff box."

- What could potentially cause his pain to be intermittent?
- At 40, would you expect this injury to heal as quickly as if Phil was 20? Why or why not?
- Because this is Phil's dominant hand, how does the *Pain Triangle* fit into his recovery?

21. Bowsher, D: Central pain mechanisms. In Wells, PE, Frampton, V, and Bowsher, D (eds): Pain Management in Physiotherapy. Butterworth Heinemann, Oxford, 1996.
22. Nadler, SF, Steiner, DJ, Erasala, GN, Hengehold, DA, Abein, SB, and Weingand, KW: Overnight use of continuous low-level heatwrap therapy for relief of low back pain. Arch Phys Med Rehabil 84:335–342, 2003.
23. Bowsher, D: A note on the distinction between first and second pain. In Mathews, B, and Hill, RG (eds): Anatomical and Physiological Aspects of Trigeminal Pain. Excerpta Medica, Amsterdam, 1982.
24. Melzack, R: Pain: Past, present and future. Can J Exp Psych 47:615–629, 1993.
25. Travell, JG, and Simmons, DG: Myofascial Pain and Dysfunction: The Trigger Point Manual. Williams & Wilkins, Baltimore, 1983.
26. Melzack, R: The McGill Pain Questionnaire: Major properties and scoring methods. Pain 1:277, 1975.
27. Wall, PD: On the relation of injury to pain. Pain 6:253, 1979.
28. Melzack, R, and Wall, PD: Pain mechanisms: A new theory. Science 150:971, 1965.
29. Cepeda, MS, Africano, JM, Polo, R, Alcala, R, and Carr, DB: Agreement between percentage reductions calculated from numeric rating scores of pain intensity and those reported by patients with acute or cancer pain. Pain 106:439–442, 2003.
30. Loomis, CW, et al: Monomaine and opioid interactions in spinal analgesia and tolerance. Pharmacol Biochem Behav 26:445, 1987.
31. Roberts, MH: Involvement of serotonin in nociceptive pathways. Drug Des Deliv 4:77, 1989.
32. Matsubara, K, et al: Increased urinary morphine, codeine and tetrahydropapaveroline in parkinsonian patient undergoing L-3,4-dihydroxyphenylalanine therapy: A possible biosynthetic pathway of morphine from L-3,4-dihydroxyphenylalanine in humans. J Pharmacol Exp Ther 260:974, 1992.
33. Takeuchi, Y, and Toda, K: Subtypes of nociceptive units in the rat temporomandibular joint. Brain Res Bull 61:603–608, 2003.
34. Jansen, AS, Farkas, E, MacSams, J, and Loewy, AD: Local connections between the columns of the periaqueductal gray matter: A case for intrinsic neuromodulation. Brain Res 784: 329–336, 1998.
35. Gardell, LR, Ibrahim, M, Wang, R, Ossipov, MH, Malan, TP, Porreca, F, et al: Mouse strains that lack spinal dynorphin upregulation after peripheral nerve injury do not develop neuropathic pain. Neuroscience 123:43–52, 2004.
36. Witta, J, Palkovits, M, Rosenberger, J, and Cox, BM: Distribution of nociceptin/orphanin FQ in adult human brain. Brain Res 997:24–29, 2004.
37. Miranda, HF, Lemus, I, and Pinardi, G: Effect of the inhibition of serotonin biosynthesis on the antinociception induced by nonsteroidal anti-inflammatory drugs. Brain Res Bull 61:417–425, 2003.
38. Melzack, R, and Wall, PD: The Challenge of Pain. Basic Books, New York, 1983.
39. Magee, DJ: Orthopedic Physical Assessment, ed 4. WB Saunders, Philadelphia, 2002.
40. Saunders, HD: Orthopedic Physical Therapy: Evaluation, Treatment, and Prevention of Musculoskeletal Disorders. Educational Opportunities, Edina, MN, 1985.
41. Ceylan, Y, Hizmetli, S, and Lilig, Y: The effects of infrared laser and medical treatments on pain and serotonin degradation products in patients with myofascial pain syndrome. A controlled trial. Rheumatol Int 24:260–263, 2004. Epub 2003 Nov 20.
42. Walsh, MT: Hydrotherapy: The use of water as a therapeutic agent. In Michlovitz, SL (ed): Thermal Agents in Rehabilitation, ed 3. FA Davis, Philadelphia, 1996.
43. Chesterton, LS, Foster, NE, Wright, CC, Baxter, GD, and Barlas, P: Effects of TENS frequency, intensity and stimulation site parameter manipulation on pressure pain thresholds in healthy human subjects. Pain 106:73–80, 2003.
44. Sluka, KA, and Qalsh, D: Transcutaneous electrical nerve stimulation: Basic science mechanisms and clinical effectiveness. J Pain 4:109–121, 2003.
45. Rakel, B, and Frantz, R: Effectiveness of transcutaneous electrical nerve stimulation on postoperative pain with movement. J Pain 4:455–464, 2003.
46. Colborne, GR, Olney, SJ, and Griffin, MP: Feedback of ankle joint angle and soleus electromyography in the rehabilitation of hemiplegic gait. Arch Phys Med Rehabil 74:1100–1106, 1993.
47. Reed, B, and Zarro, V: Inflammation and repair and the use of thermal agents. In Michlovitz, SL (ed): Thermal Agents in Rehabilitation, ed 3. FA Davis, Philadelphia, 1996.
48. Hardy, MA: The biology of scar formation. Phys Ther 69:1014, 1989.
49. Kloth, LC, and McCulloch, JM: The inflammatory response to wounding. In Kloth, LC, and McCulloch, JM (eds): Wound Healing: Alternatives in Management, ed 3. FA Davis, Philadelphia, 2002.
50. Daly, TJ: The repair phase of wound healing: Re-epithelialization and contraction. In Kloth, LC, and McCulloch, JM (eds): Wound Healing: Alternatives in Management, ed 3. FA Davis, Philadelphia, 2002.
51. Cooper, DM: Optimizing wound healing. Nurs Clin North Am 25:165, 1990.
52. Alaish, SM, Yager, DR, Diegelmann, RF, and Cohen, IK: Hyaluronic acid metabolism in keloid fibroblasts. J Pediatr Surg 30:949–952, 1995.
53. Cool, SM, Snyman, CP, Nurcombe, V, and Forwood, M: Temporal expression of fibroblast growth factor receptors during primary ligament repair. Knee Surg Sports Traumatol Arthrosc 12:490–496, 2004. Epub 2003 Dec 23.
54. Hirano, S, Bless, DM, Massey, RJ, Hartig, GK, and Ford, CN: Morphological and functional changes of human vocal fold fibroblasts with hepatocyte growth factor. Ann Otol Rhinol Laryngol 112:1026–1033, 2003.
55. Baltzer, AW, and Lieberman, JR: Regional gene therapy to enhance bone repair. Gene Ther 11:344–350, 2004.
56. Feedar, JA, and Kloth, LC: Conservative management of chronic wounds. In Kloth, LC, and McCulloch, JM (eds): Wound Healing: Alternatives in Management, ed 3. FA Davis, Philadelphia, 2002.
57. Hollinworth, H: Wound care: Pathway to success. Nursing Times 88:66, 1992.
58. Bayley, EW: Wound healing in the patient with burns. Nurs Clin North Am 25:205, 1990.
59. Garvin, G: Wound healing in pediatrics. Nurs Clin North Am 25:181, 1990.

60. Jones, PL, and Millman, A: Wound healing and the aged patient. Nurs Clin North Am 25:263–273, 1990.

61. Kloth, LC: How to use electrical stimulation for wound healing. Nursing 32:17, 2002.

62. Kloth, LC: Electrical stimulation in tissue repair. In Kloth, LC, and McCulloch, JM (eds): Wound Healing: Alternatives in Management, ed 3. FA Davis, Philadelphia, 2002.

63. Feedar, JA, Kloth, LC, and Gentzkow, GD: Chronic dermal ulcer healing enhanced with monophasic pulsed electrical stimulation. Phys Ther 71:639, 1991.

64. Akai, M, and Hayashi, K: Effect of electrical stimulation on musculoskeletal systems: A meta-analysis of controlled clinical trials. Bioelectromagnetics 23:132–143, 2002.

65. Houghton, PE, Kincaid, CB, Lovell, M, Campbell, KE, Keast, DH, Woodbury, MG, et al: Effect of electrical stimulation on chronic leg ulcer size and appearance. Phys Ther 83:17–28, 2003.

66. Hess, CL, Howard, MA, and Attinger, CE: A review of mechanical adjuncts in wound healing: Hydrotherapy, ultrasound, negative pressure therapy, hyperbaric oxygen, and electrostimulation. Ann Plast Surg 51:210–218, 2003.

67. Ziskin, MC, McDiarmid, T, and Michlovitz, SL: Therapeutic ultrasound. In Michlovitz, SL (ed): Thermal Agents in Rehabilitation, ed 3. FA Davis, Philadelphia, 1996.

68. Dyson, M: The role of ultrasound in wound healing. In Kloth, LC, and McCulloch, JM (eds): Wound Healing: Alternatives in Management, ed 3. FA Davis, Philadelphia, 2002.

69. McWhorter, JW: Hyperbaric oxygen in wound healing. In Kloth, LC, and McCulloch, JM (eds): Wound Healing: Alternatives in Management, ed 3. FA Davis, Philadelphia, 2002.

70. MacKay, D, and Miller, AL: Nutritional support for wound healing. Altern Med Rev 8:359–377, 2003.

71. Passeri, G, Pini, G, Troiano, L, Vescovini, R, Sansoni, P, Passeri, M, et al: Low Vitamin D status, high bone turnover, and bone fractures in centenarians. J Clin Endocrinol Metab 88:5109–5115, 2003.

72. Payne, WG, Walusimbi, MS, Blue, ML, Mosielly, G, Wright, TE, and Robson, MC: Radiated groin wounds: Pitfalls in reconstruction. Am Surg 69:994–997, 2003.

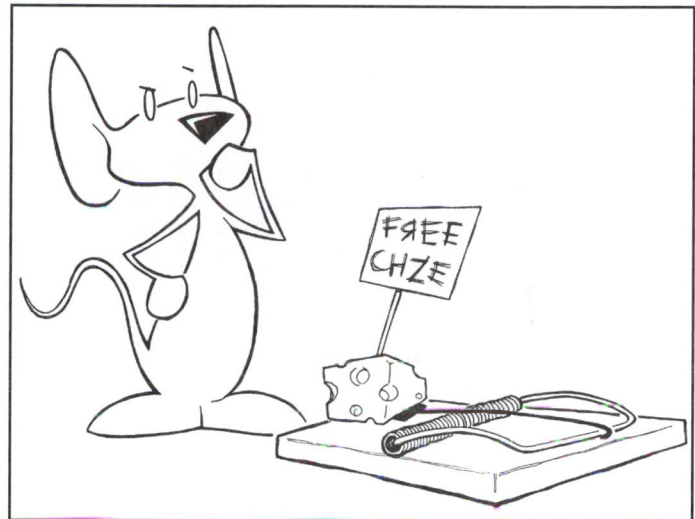

Objectives

- Describe the potential patient responses to therapeutic treatment interventions.
- Outline examination techniques for pain, edema, muscle spasm, range of motion, and muscle strength.
- Select appropriate tests and measures to determine effectiveness of a treatment.

Key Terms

Analog scale	Evaluation	Mottling	Observations
Assessment	Examination	Muscle guarding	Palpation
Capillary refill	Girth	Muscle spasm	Skin blanching
Edema	Melanin	Muscle tone	Volumeter
Erythema			

Barbara J. Behrens, PTA, MS   *Stacie Larkin, PT, MS*

Patient Responses to Therapeutic Interventions

Outline

"Is this really supposed to make my knee so red?"

The importance of assessing a patient's response to treatment cannot be overstated. It is critical in determining the success of any treatment intervention with a patient. This chapter will focus on the clinician's role in assessing the patient's response to interventions with physical agents. The purposes of these observations are to ensure safety in administration of treatment, monitor patient progress, and adjust dosage when necessary.

Examination, Evaluation, and Intervention

For consistency's sake, the definitions given for examination, evaluation, and intervention are those that can be found in the *Guide to Physical Therapist Practice*, second edition (2001).

Examination: "The process of obtaining a history, performing relevant systems reviews, and selecting and administering specific tests and measures"

Evaluation: "A dynamic process in which the physical therapist makes clinical judgments based on data gathered during the examination"

Intervention: "Purposeful and skilled interaction of the physical therapist with the patient/client...using various physical therapy methods and techniques to produce changes in the condition that are consistent with the diagnosis and prognosis"

After a thorough initial examination and evaluation, a plan of care is created by the physical therapist that includes anticipated goals and expected outcomes. Physical agents and mechanical modalities are most commonly used for the goals of

- Decreasing pain
- Reducing soft tissue/joint swelling and inflammation
- Increasing blood flow and enhancing delivery of nutrients to tissue
- Promoting muscle relaxation
- Increasing the extensibility of connective tissue
- Increasing muscle strength

Skin (Integument) Assessment

Assessment of the skin's (integument's) characteristics, including color continuity and temperature, is necessary when determining the condition of the soft tissue being treated. Skin color is based on the amount of melanin and hemoglobin that is present. Fair-skinned individuals have less melanin, and changes in blood flow will be more obvious compared with an individual with darker skin. Temperature of the skin surface indicates the current state of the tissue. Elevated skin temperatures indicate either a burn, inflammation in the area, or possibly infection. Decreased skin temperatures may indicate vascular compromise. One also should inspect for any wounds, blisters, or rashes, as they will also affect the decision of which interventions are most appropriate and safe to use.

Skin Color

Pigmentation of human skin is determined by the presence of a biochemical compound known as *melanin*. Persons with darker skin tones have a greater amount of melanin. Fairer-skinned individuals will appear to respond differently to the increases in subcutaneous circulation than will individuals with "olive" or "black" skin tones. The skin of "fair-skinned" patients will appear "pink" or "red" after prolonged exposure

to the sun or heat. This coloration is readily visible due to the lack of melanin. Darker-skinned individuals also respond to prolonged exposure to the sun or heat; however, the changes in skin color and in local circulation will be less apparent. Patients who have areas of skin that have been continually exposed to severe weather conditions, and have marked "weathering" of their skin, will also respond less noticeably to changes in local circulation.

Skin coloration may vary due to the day-to-day elements, including temperatures, to which the skin is exposed. Skin texture will also vary depending on the forces it encounters. Scars in the treatment area make the skin respond in a particular way to physical, mechanical, or electrotherapeutic treatment interventions. For example, where there is scar tissue, there is altered circulation and the response to heat will be different. Clinicians must become cautious observers of the skin and surrounding tissues they are treating, noting subtle changes when they occur.

Uniformity of skin coloration provides information regarding the local circulation and the potential sensitivity of the skin to thermal agents. Skin that is pale or bluish in appearance indicates a decrease in blood flow to that area (for example, frostbite). Skin that is pink or red indicates an increase in blood flow to that area (for example, a thermal burn or an acute injury). It is important to be sure that the modality chosen for a given patient takes into consideration the current status of the tissue being treated. Heating agents are commonly applied to promote circulation, which will enhance the nutrient base for tissue healing. However, use of a heating agent would not be indicated if the skin is already red and inflamed, as this would only increase the blood flow to the area.

The presence of scars must also be observed and taken into consideration when choosing a modality. Immature scar tissue, which is pink, is well vascularized. When immature scars are exposed to heat, they will turn bright red in response. Mature scar tissue, which is often pale in appearance, is not as well vascularized as is noninjured or repaired tissue and will likely retain a white appearance regardless of being heated or cooled. Sensation may also be impaired around the scar. For these reasons, the presence of a scar and skin coloration in the treatment area are important to note and to monitor closely during the application of any thermal agent.

Circulatory Irregularities

Because circulatory changes can be noted to some degree by appearance, it is important for the clinician to observe and identify various skin types and their responses to local changes in circulation. One simple test for circulatory impairment is known as the capillary refill test or "blanching." Blanching of the skin is the term used to describe the response to applied pressure on the surface of the skin. Those with normal circulation will temporarily lose color when pressure is applied, and as the capillary beds refill with blood, the color returns. This return of the normal pink skin color should occur in less than 3 seconds.[1] Areas where arterial circulation is impaired may not respond by blanching when pressure is applied; they may remain unchanged, or the return to pink color make take longer than 3 seconds, indicating that the underlying tissue has impaired circulatory function. Mature scar tissue is another example where blanching may not be observed. The mature scar will remain pale when pressure is applied to it. This may indicate that the patient will have an increased sensitivity to heat or cold. The application of pressure to the skin is a simple activity that provides quick information regarding the ability of the capillary beds and arterioles to respond to this form of stimuli.

Mottling of the Skin

Spotting patches of erythema that occur after the application of thermal agents is referred to as mottling of the skin. It may be indicative of overheating or overcooling of the skin. It may also be indicative of repeated or prolonged use of superficial thermal agents. Mottling should be considered a warning sign of potential inability of the tissue to respond to the thermal agent. If mottling occurs, the application time and/or intensity of the thermal agent should be decreased during the next application (Fig. 2-1).

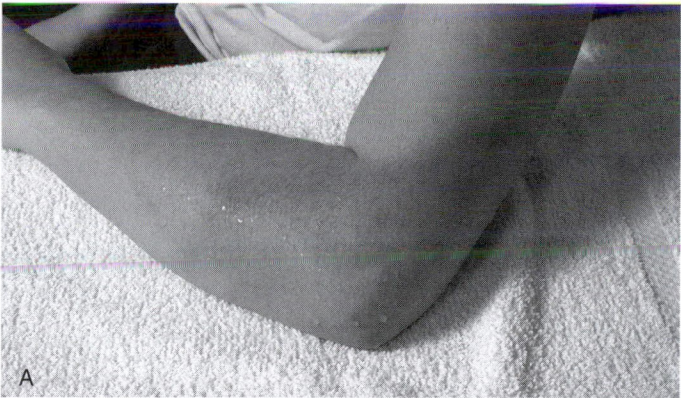
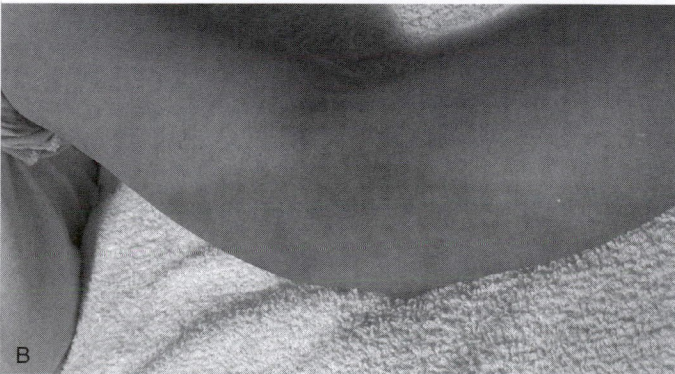

Figure 2-1   *A, B,* The extremity exhibits signs of uneven erythema with white patches, indicating excessive exposure to a thermal agent. The condition is referred to as "mottling" of the skin.

Patient Perspective

Remember that your patient is curious about all of the tests and measurements that clinicians take and record. Your patient wants to know what some of the test results mean and why you are taking the time to record the information. Also, the word "test" may increase anxiety and therefore increase muscle guarding, which may have a negative impact on the results of your testing. Keeping the patient informed as to what you are doing and why you are doing it will most often decrease any anxiety that your patient might be feeling.

PATIENTS' FREQUENTLY ASKED QUESTIONS

1. Why are you taking so many different types of measurements?
2. What do all of the numbers mean?
3. Why is the treatment area "red" after treatment; does that mean something 'bad' has happened?
4. Why can't I bend my elbow as much when it's my shoulder or hand that is injured?
5. What is the difference between that water tank and a tape measure for swelling?
6. Why does "the injured area" feel hot after I exercise?
7. Why doesn't the pain relief that I get in therapy last longer after the first visit?
8. What difference does poor posture make on neck or back problems?
9. Why is it so hard to get dressed in the morning, but after I have been up for a while, I seem to be able to move more easily?

Skin Surface Temperature

As with skin color observation, the temperature of the skin surface can provide information regarding the circulatory status of the underlying tissue. Warmth may indicate inflammation, whereas coolness may indicate poor circulation. Surface temperature of the skin should change in response to environmental influences. The application of heat will cause local vasodilation, an increase in the surface temperature of the skin, accompanied by erythema and possibly perspiration. The application of cold will cause a decrease in the surface temperature of the skin accompanied by a reflex vasodilation erythema (after about 8 minutes of application time). These responses can be detected via observation of the color changes of the skin and via palpation of the surface temperature of the skin.

Before You Begin

VISUAL OBSERVATIONS

If there are any alterations in the appearance or temperature of the skin, these areas are prone to a *different* response to thermal agents. Watch these areas more closely!

Skin temperature, color, and overall integrity provide the clinician with valuable information regarding the patient's response or his/her potential response to the application of a thermal agent. This information will help determine if a given intervention is appropriate and safe to perform. Visual inspection before and after treatment should be a routine aspect of patient care.

 ## Pain Assessment

Pain represents the most difficult complaint to quantify and objectively document. Pain assessment encompasses a variety of techniques used to quantify and measure the impact it has on the patient's ability to perform functional activities. There may be a strong psychologic component to the expression of pain. The patient is the only individual who can describe the intensity of his or her experience. Due to these complexities, many researchers and clinicians have attempted to compile an objective set of baseline measures to reflect the experience of pain. Pain scales have been used in an attempt to quickly measure the level or quantity of discomfort a patient is experiencing.

Pain Scales: Visual Analog and Numeric Pain Rating

Visual analog scales (VASs) involve the use of a 10-cm line drawn on a piece of paper, with a beginning and an end anchor identified by word descriptors like "no pain" and "pain as bad as it can be," respectively. Patients are asked to place a mark on the line indicating their level of discomfort (Fig. 2-2). The clinician then measures the distance in centimeters from the start of the line and records the measurement. After treatment, the patient is given a new, unmarked 10-cm line and asked to reassess the level of discomfort and to mark the new line (Fig. 2-3). The clinician then measures the distance to the new mark and again records the length of the line in centimeters. For each assessment, the patient is given a clean, new line to indicate his or her level of discomfort so that past responses do not influence how the patient rates his or her current pain level. If the results of the line measurements are recorded regularly, then it will be possible for the clinician to actually chart the patient's progress. This may assist the clinician in determining if the selected treatment interventions have been appropriate and effective for relieving the patient's pain according to the patient's reported responses.

A similar assessment may be done with numbers from 0 to 10 marked along a 10-cm line, and thus is a numeric pain-rating scale (NPRS). A change of 3 points on the NPRS or a change of 28 mm on the VAS is needed for it to be considered a detectable change.[2] The drawback with marking the num-

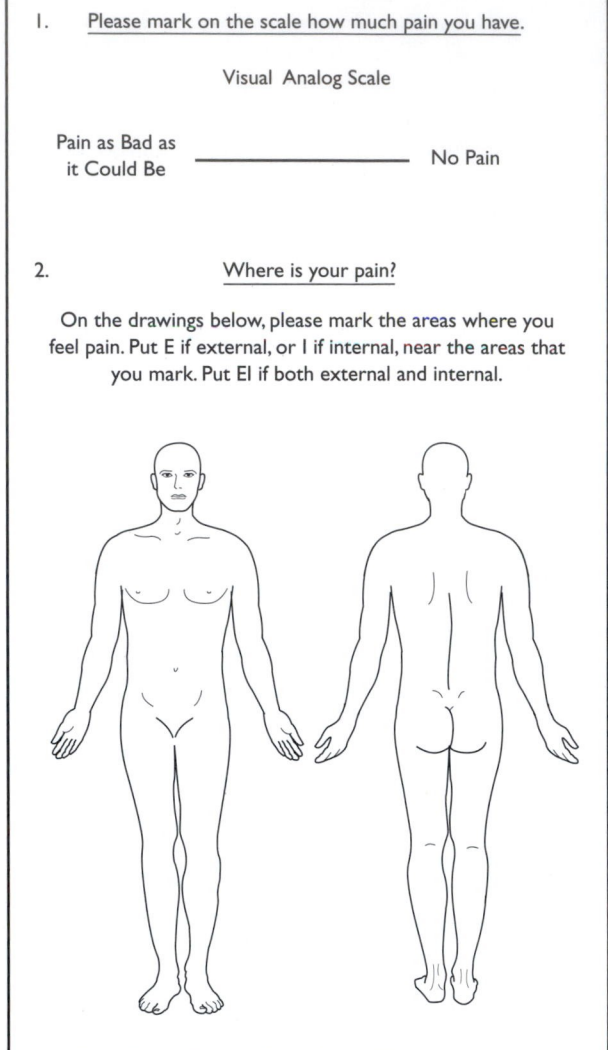

Figure 2-2 (*1*) Visual analog scale. Patients are to indicate the level of pain they are experiencing by marking on the 10-cm line. The distance from the start point of the line is measured and recorded for future assessment comparisons. (*2*) Anatomic pain drawings. (Parts 1 and 2, excerpted from of the McGill Pain Questionnaire, Courtesy of R. Melzack.)

bers is that the patient has a reference point to refer to, which may influence how he or she marks the line. Clinically, however, it is the NPRS that is most commonly used, as it is very quick to use.

Factors that Influence Pain Ratings

Use of either the VAS or the NPRS involves assessment of the level of discomfort before and after treatment to determine if the treatment had any effect on the patient's pain. The type of questions asked of the patient are important, and clinicians must be careful to encourage the patient to respond not to the presence of pain but rather to the presence of whatever the sensation or symptom is the greatest. Optimally, a

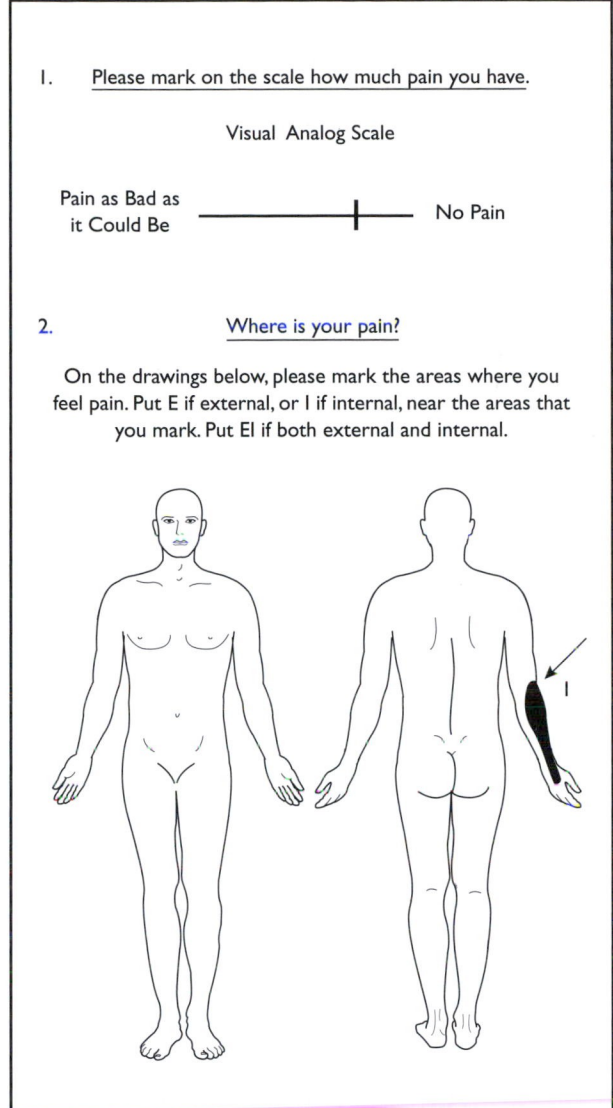

1. Please mark on the scale how much pain you have.

Visual Analog Scale

Pain as Bad as   ———————|———   No Pain
it Could Be

2.   Where is your pain?

On the drawings below, please mark the areas where you feel pain. Put E if external, or I if internal, near the areas that you mark. Put EI if both external and internal.

Figure 2-3   Drawing of a 10-cm line that a patient has used, indicating the level of discomfort. The beginning of the line has the descriptor "no pain" and the end of the line has the descriptor "pain as bad as it can be." (Parts 1 and 2, excerpted from the McGill Pain Questionnaire, Courtesy of R. Melzack.)

pain, as he reports it, returns to a level of "3." If using the unmarked line, he or she may arbitrarily decide that his assessment of pain must be one third of the distance from the starting point. This decision may be made by the patient before he will be satisfied that he can return to work. This is another reason why pain ratings are just one factor in pain assessment. Pain scales are simple, quick, subjective measures for a pain complaint. They are not flawless, however, and should not be used as the sole source for pain assessment.

Pain Inventories

Inventories for pain assessment represent another tool for quantifying and documenting the subjective complaints of pain. The McGill-Melzack Pain Questionnaire was formulated in an attempt to create an instrument that would be universally applicable for many cultures, diagnoses, and multiple levels of cognitive understanding. Patients who reported that they were experiencing pain and had been diagnosed with a painful condition were surveyed to describe their pain with whatever words they could use to adequately capture their individual experience. The patient reactions or expressions were categorized as affective, emotional, and behavioral responses to the painful experience. Participants in the survey were then asked to rank order the phrases or words that were offered, from least annoying to the worst experience. Many translations took place so that the information could be used with virtually any culture. A standardized version of the test was formulated, and a methodology for grading or interpreting it was also developed. Individual categories of descriptors are graded according to their ranking within the category. Thus, if there are four words in a category, the first word listed is ranked as the least bothersome, and the fourth word, as the most annoying and potentially serious.

Some of the descriptors include words such as "sharp" or "dull," which will assist the clinician in assessing the ease of localization of the discomfort. As discussed in Chapter 1, pain receptors can be A-delta fibers, transmitting fast "pain or injury," or they can be C-fibers, which are responsible for the transmission of the "pain of suffering" or a difficult-to-identify or -localize aching sensation. The McGill-Melzack Pain Questionnaire records information about and evaluative components of the patient's pain experience and is quite comprehensive[5,6] (Fig. 2-4).

Anatomic Pain Drawings

Line drawings of the anatomy allow the patient to locate just where he or she is experiencing discomfort. If a patient is instructed to fill in the areas that correspond to the pain, the completed drawing guides the clinician to the primary area(s) of discomfort. This type of information can be extremely important if radiating pain is present, because it may indicate the original source. It also acts as a road map for clinicians

clinician would ask the patient to rate his or her discomfort and, after treatment, let the clinician know just what he or she is feeling. The questions should not reinforce the perception of pain by using the word "pain" in the question.[3,4] Rather than asking a patient, "Are you still in pain?" or "Do you still hurt?" ask "What are you feeling now?" to find out about the primary complaint the patient is experiencing.

Patients who are not motivated to recover may skew their responses and invalidate their subjective responses to treatment. The patient may also attempt to control the "recovery time" by assigning an arbitrary number to his or her "acceptable" level of pain to be able to return to work. He or she may decide that he is only willing to discontinue therapy when his

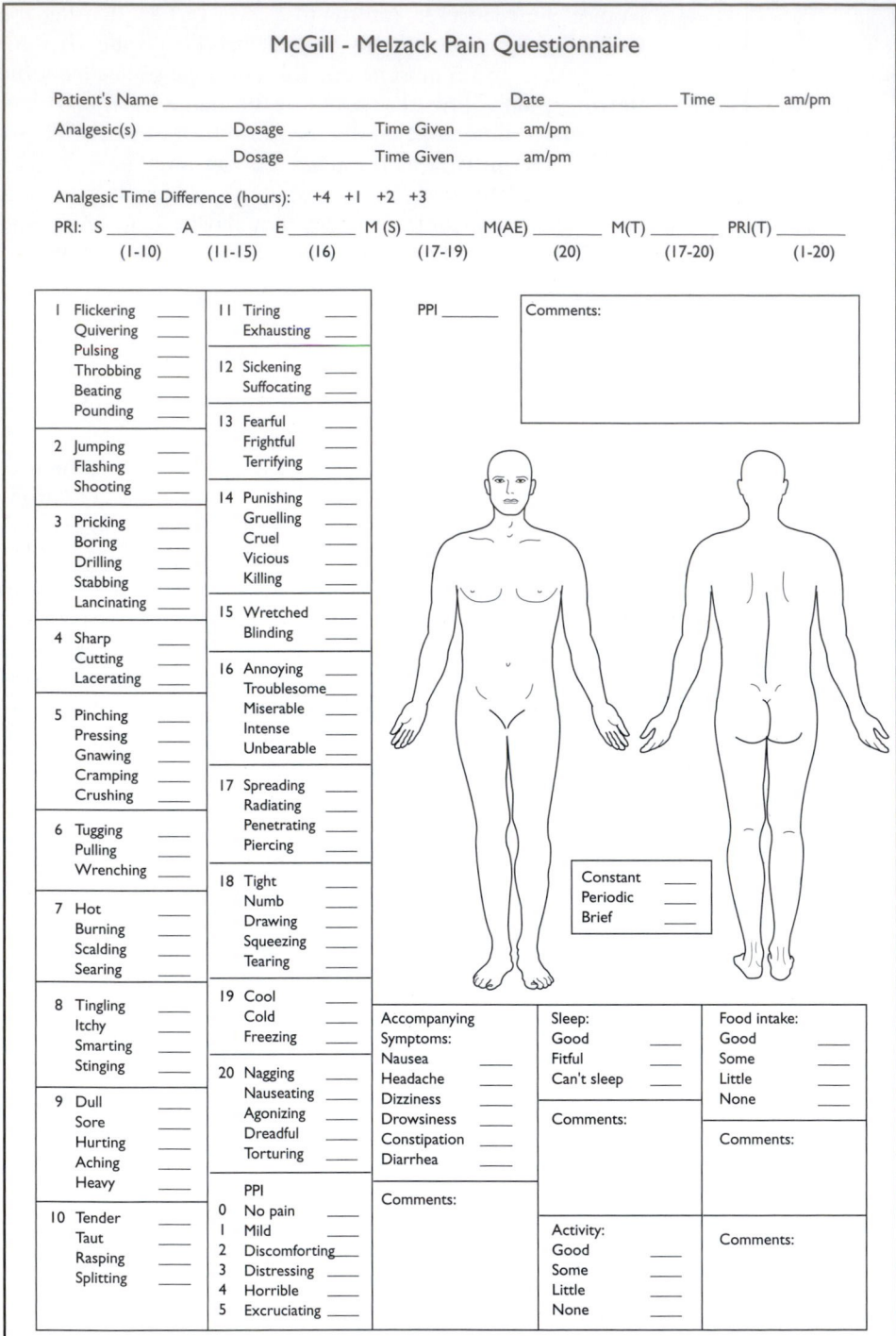

Figure 2-4 The McGill-Melzack Pain Questionnaire. (Courtesy of R. Melzack.)

working with patients who are experiencing multiple areas of involvement, because the patient is instructed to "color in" the worst area first. Caution should be observed when interpreting these drawings if the clinician is unable to solicit responses directly from the patient. Some patients may have difficulty recognizing a particular part of the body on the line drawing. This would be another reason that the drawing should be completed in the presence of a clinician who is able to answer questions as they arise. Technology has introduced computer animation to pain drawing and pain drawing analysis, which may lead to further refinement of the data obtained.[7-12]

Word inventories, not anatomic drawings, should be completed by patients while they are comfortably positioned and relaxed, possibly while they are waiting to be seen by the clinician. The anatomic pain drawings, however, should be completed in the presence of a clinician so that any sequencing can be noted. Although the information obtained in these inventories is useful, it is by no means complete and should be accompanied by other performance-related assessments.

Pressure Algometers

Objective tools have been developed to help determine tissue sensitivity in the form of strain gauges; however, their use clinically is not widespread. Most of the determinations that are made are based on the experience of the clinician. Strain gauges are calibrated to detect the amount of applied pressure administered to a patient. They then can objectively quantify just how much force was exerted on the surface of the skin before the patient complained of discomfort. These devices are referred to as dolorimeters or pressure algometers.[13–17] Refer to Box 2-1.

Other Means to Assess Pain

Facial expression can be another way of assessing a patient's subjective complaint of pain. Facial musculature, particularly in the forehead and around the eyes, will contract in response to pain perception. A patient may not verbally express discomfort because of his or her cultural background but will "look like" he or she is in pain. After treatment, the patient appears more comfortable, despite other objective responses indicating that there has been no change in the level of discomfort that he or she is experiencing. This is truly an interpretation but may provide the clinician with additional information regarding the patient's pain (Fig. 2-5).

The ability to perform a functional activity or perform a certain range of motion can also provide information regarding a patient's current level of pain. Rather than focusing on the patient's pain through pain scales as a means to determine progress, it becomes even more important to focus treatment goals on returning the patient to his or her prior functional level. Range-of-motion (ROM) measurements taken before

BOX 2-1	**Pain Assessment**

1. Pain is only quantifiable by the individual WHEN they are experiencing it.
2. Diagrams work well for some patients to describe their pain; they do not work for all patients.
3. Some patients may not objectively assess their discomfort.
4. Some patients may be motivated not to report that they feel better. This is why you need to assess more than just their subjective response to a treatment intervention.

and after a treatment intervention can provide clear objective data regarding the patient's ability or willingness to move. When ROM is limited, the cause of that limitation needs to be identified. Pain secondary to muscle guarding, joint restriction, nerve impingement, and edema are some possibilities. After treatment for these impairments, it is necessary to reassess the patient's ROM to see if a change has occurred in the quantity and the quality of the motion. Pain should also be assessed to see if the increase in ROM results with a decrease in pain, as one would expect. If there was no change in pain, yet gains were made in ROM, this is still considered a positive outcome as functional gains have been made.

Another means to determine if progress is being made is to assess the frequency, dosage, and types of pain medication a patient is taking. When a patient reports a decrease in use of pain medications or switches from a prescription to an over-the-counter pain medication, this is valuable information that indicates a positive change in the patient's pain level.

When Patients Are Not Improving as Expected

Most patients who seek assistance in the management of pain have legitimate complaints. However, there are occasions when the potential for secondary gain, or the potential of a legal battle, may influence a patient's response to treatment. When a patient is not progressing as anticipated, it is important to reevaluate and determine if any change has occurred or if any new problems have arisen. Working with patients who are influenced by outside sources to prolong the course of treatment may be particularly frustrating. Resources such as *The Guide to Physical Therapist Practice*, second edition (2001), can provide the therapist with the general range of therapy visits needed to achieve the anticipated goals and expected outcomes for a given diagnostic classification. When therapy progress is happening slowly or not at all, the physical therapist must reexamine the patient to evaluate progress, modify the treatment plan, or possibly consider discontinuation of therapy if it is no longer providing any benefit to the patient.

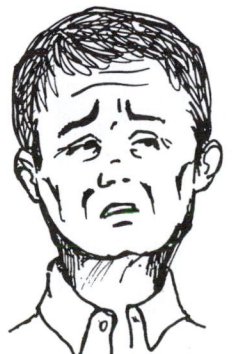 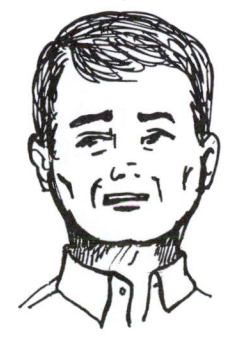

Figure 2-5   Facial expression can indicate whether an individual is experiencing pain.

Edema Assessment

Edema, or swelling, is an abnormal increase in the amount of interstitial fluid. It may be diffuse throughout the area or localized to the injury site. When swelling is contained within a joint capsule, it is referred to as "joint effusion." Edema in small quantities is a normal response to trauma, and it is necessary for the repair process of tissue healing. Prolonged and/or massive edema can interrupt repair by impeding the diffusion of nutrients to cells or perhaps by leading to tissue fibrosis. To accurately assess the quantity of edema present in an area, there are several options available, depending on the location of the edema. The options include*

- Circumferential or girth measurements
- Volumetric water displacement
- Joint mobility
- Functional performance

Circumferential or Girth Measurements

Using a tape measure can be one of the quickest, easiest, and most accurate ways to assess the presence of edema. For consistency of measurement, the following factors must be adhered to.

1. Use a tape measure that does not stretch.
2. Measure with the same tape measure each time.
3. The same therapist should record the measurements each time.
4. Measurements are most accurate and comparable when taken at the same time of day.
5. Use bony landmarks as reference points for measurement.
6. Use the same measurement technique each time you measure.
7. Remember to use the same unit of measurement each time a measurement is taken (centimeters or inches).

If these factors are adhered to, then there will be a reasonable degree of accuracy and reliability of the measurements

 Before You Begin

EDEMA ASSESSMENT

There is more than one way to assess edema.
Make sure that you use the same measurement tools each time.

---

*Refer to Chapter 7 for an in-depth explanation of the physiology of edema.

 Why Do I Need to Know About...

SKIN SURFACE TEMPERATURE

Consider the following before treatment:

1. If the skin of the area being treated is warm and red in appearance (compared with its surrounding area), then inflammation or infection may be present. This would be a contraindication for the use of heating agents.

2. If the skin of the area being treated is cooler and paler (compared with its surrounding area), then circulation may be compromised. Vascular insufficiency is a contraindication for all heating and cooling agents.

3. If there is scar in the area, then be sure sensation has been tested. This is important when using modalities where you are dependent on the patient's response to guide the intensity and duration of treatment.

(Fig. 2-6). Further details regarding circumferential measurement are provided in Chapter 7.

Volumetric Water Displacement

When edema is confined to distal extremities, volumetric measurements are considered practical and accurate. A volumeter is a device that measures water displacement to record the volume that a distal extremity occupies when submerged

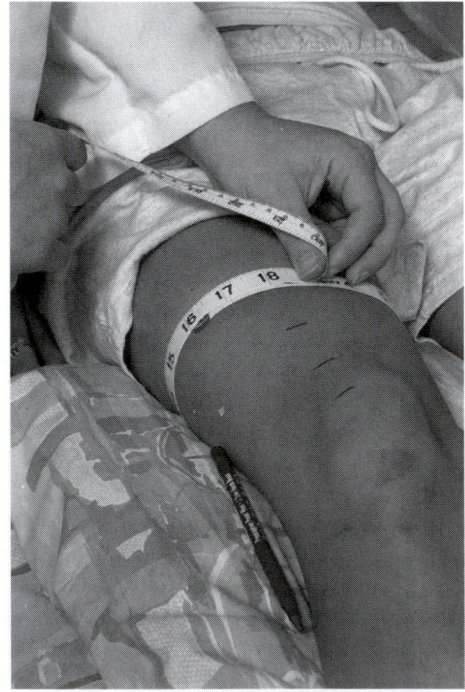

Figure 2-6 The clinician is performing circumferential girth measurements using a tape measure. She is using bony landmarks as reference points and areas distal and proximal to them that have been marked.

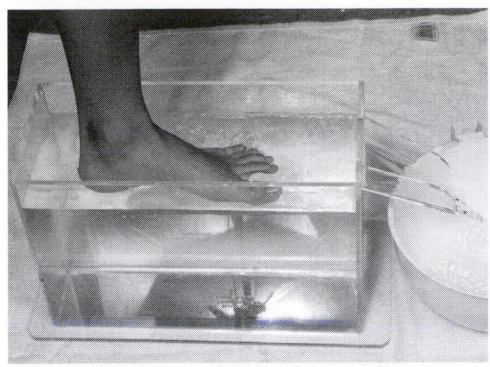

Figure 2-7   Volumetric assessment of edema can be performed using a volumeter and water displacement. The patient places the edematous extremity into the water, and the displaced water is measured to determine the volume of the edema.

in water. If an edematous extremity is placed in a known volume of water and the displaced water is measured, then the volume of that part of the extremity can be determined (Fig. 2-7). Subsequent measurements will reveal the status of the edema and whether the volume of displaced water increases, decreases, or remains unchanged. Some critical factors for accuracy of this form of measurement include the following:

1. The time of day for subsequent measurements should be the same as the initial time of measurement.
2. The same temperature of water should be used for each measurement.
3. The unit of measurement must remain constant (ounces or milliliters of water).

Hand and foot volumeters are commercially available in Plexiglas (Volumetrics Limited, Idylwild, CA). Commercial devices have known values for accuracy.

There can be several disadvantages to volumetric measurements if they are used as the sole source of assessment of edema. This form of assessment looks at total volume of the part immersed but does not account for individual areas of excessive edema relative to the diffuse edema. It does not enable the clinician to document precisely where the edema is located, simply that **there is edema**. It is not as practical to use for the assessment of an entire extremity, as would be circumferential measurements. Despite the disadvantages, it can be a useful and time-efficient form of edema assessment for the foot and ankle, wrist, or hand.

Functional Performance Limited by Edema

A patient's ability to perform activities of daily living (ADLs) may be impaired by the presence of edema. Limitations in movement caused by an increase in edema may inhibit the patient's ability to don a garment. Putting on socks or stockings may be very difficult if there is a significant quantity of edema in the lower extremity. These specific activities can also be a means to access progress toward functional goals.

What Should Be Monitored for Edema Management?

Assessment of edema will take into account all of the elements that apply to the individual patient. If the possibility of volumetric and circumferential measurements is feasible, then both should be monitored. To be considered valid, the form of assessment should be kept consistent for a given patient. If a patient had an acute ankle sprain and the initial evaluation used volumetric measurements for edema, then any reassessment of the edema should also use volumetric measurements. Likewise, if the initial evaluation used circumferential measurements, then subsequent assessments of edema should use circumferential measurements.

 Soft Tissue Assessment

Muscle guarding can inhibit or delay a patient's recovery. The assessment of soft tissue requires palpation of muscle tone and observation of posture. Each of these assessments helps define the total picture of the patient's condition.

Muscle Guarding

Muscle guarding is an indication of the degree of motor unit firing present in a muscle that exists to protect the area from further trauma. Prolonged muscle guarding can result in a shortening of the underlying tissue and a feeling of "hardening" so that the muscle now feels harder than the surrounding tissue. The actual number of sarcomeres in the muscle may decrease due to the prolonged immobility and shortened position of the muscle.[18]

Patients may report that they "feel a muscle spasm"; there is still a degree of controversy regarding the nature of the physical existence of the phenomenon the patient describes. Some thermal agents are used to help reduce or eliminate perceived increases in muscle guarding or "spasms." It is important to palpate the area before and after applying a therapeutic intervention to determine whether the treatment technique produced any changes in the muscle tone. Palpation of the treatment area before and after a treatment intervention is also a way to validate the outcome of the chosen approach. If the clinician examines the area via palpation before the initiation of treatment and fails to reexamine the area after the application, it is difficult to determine if change occurred as a result of the selected intervention (Fig. 2-8).

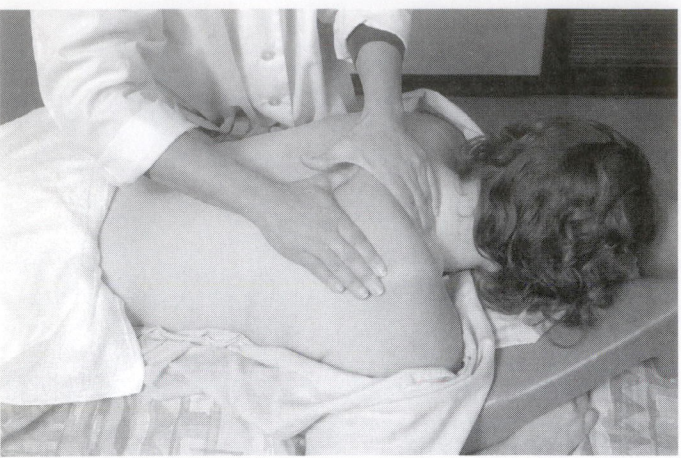

Figure 2–8   This clinician is palpating the area to be treated before the application of any physical agent. The same approach will be repeated after the administration of a therapeutic intervention to assist the clinician in determining whether a soft tissue change occurred.

Muscle Tone

Muscle tone refers to the resistance of the muscle to passive stretch or elongation, or how "tight" it feels. When a muscle guards, it assumes a shortened state to help protect the area from further injury. Its tone may therefore be increased protectively, causing it to feel harder than uninvolved tissue when palpated. Ease in reaching the determination that a muscle is guarding comes with experience in palpating a multitude of soft tissue injuries on a wide variety of patients. Muscle tightness and its causes are difficult to assess objectively without an external source of measurement such as a surface electromyographic (EMG) reading of the electrical activity taking place within the muscle.

Tissue tone assessment relies heavily on the experience of the clinician monitoring it. In many acute conditions, the patient will experience some degree of tenderness in the injured soft tissue. Tissue tone changes may or may not be one of the first palpable signs of injury. If muscle guarding is present, then it will typically occur in both the agonist and the antagonistic muscle groups crossing or surrounding the injured area. Palpation comparison of the involved with the uninvolved side will provide further insight as to the level of discomfort or tightness that the patient is experiencing.

Postural Assessment

Postural changes are likely to be observed in patients who are experiencing pain and muscle guarding. This is especially noticeable when the injured area involves postural muscles. For example, many patients who have injured their cervical spine or who have had a "whiplash" or cervical strain exhibit different sitting/standing postures than individuals who have

not experienced this type of trauma. In this situation, the cervical muscles guard in both anterior and posterior regions supporting the head and limit the mobility of the head. This may visually look as if they have a stiff neck, avoiding any active cervical movements. If this problem is not assessed and treated, a "forward head" posture may result, where the head is displaced anteriorly on the cervical spine because of the increased muscle tone or guarding in the upper posterior cervical musculature resulting in an increased cervical lordosis[19] (Fig. 2-9).

Range-of-Motion Assessment

As with other forms of assessment, the measurement of joint ROM can provide an objective measure of the available movement within a given joint. It is important to look at both the quantity of motion available and the quality of that motion. In the case of muscle guarding, an agonist muscle may limit the antagonistic direction of joint ROM. The presence of edema can also impede joint movement, resulting with a decrease in ROM. This simple assessment tool should be a part of every peripheral joint assessment and its reassessment to determine whether progress had been made with a particular treatment technique. Measurements of available joint ROM with a goniometer can provide additional objective baseline information with which to make a comparison after therapeutic treatment interventions.

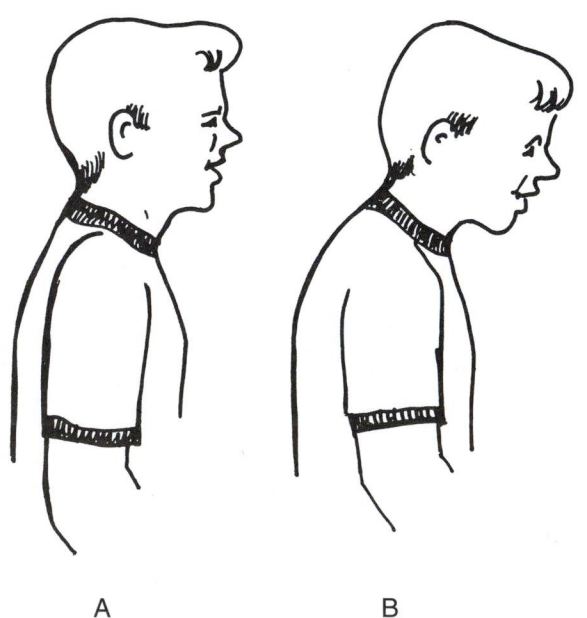

A   B

Figure 2–9   Illustration depicts (A) normal cervical posture and (B) "forward head posture."

Muscle Strength Assessments

Muscle strength assessment can be accomplished either manually or with the use of sophisticated equipment to record force or torque production. A manual muscle test (MMT) assesses the strength of specific muscles or gross muscle actions. MMTs are performed when the area to be tested is stabilized and both active and passive ROMs have been measured. Manual resistance is then applied as the patient attempts the motion. The patient is provided with verbal instructions to resist the movement or force being applied to the area. The patient's response to the resistance is graded from trace to normal depending on the patient's position, completed ROM, and ability to perform against resistance.

More reproducible testing of muscle performance may involve the use of a commercially manufactured dynamometer that measures the force applied at a given speed of motion. This is referred to as isokinetic force testing. "Iso" refers to the speed, which can be set to a fixed number, and "kinetic" refers to the fact that motion takes place. This type of equipment provides for proximal stabilization when resistance is applied to the distal extent of the tested extremity. One advantage of this type of device is that the patient will experience resistance only if he or she meets the preset speed of the resistance arm. In other words, if the patient is unable to contract quickly enough to "catch up" with the resistance arm, the patient will not experience any resistance. This means that if a patient experiences pain with a resisted contraction, he or she will not injure themselves further with an isokinetic device. If the patient does not "push," there is nothing to push against. This is quite different than the use of "free-weights" to assess muscle strength, where the patient may be able to "lift" the weight but not let it down without injury. Isokinetic dynamometers provide a torque or force reading to indicate the maximal level of torque exerted by the muscle. Subsequent tests should reveal increases in torque output if a patient is progressing and all testing factors are kept constant, such as test position, speed, and stabilization.

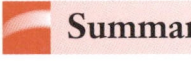

Summary

This chapter has presented many areas where specific tests and measures can provide valuable information regarding the condition of a patient. It is important to gather information from multiple sources, to help provide the clearest picture of the condition and progress that a patient is making. Without objective measures, the subjective complaints of the patient cannot be substantiated. The future of the profession of phys-

ical therapy rests on our ability to accurately quantify and qualify what we do for our patients. Capturing that information is critical.

CASE STUDY

Richard is a 55-year-old retired truck driver who has been referred to physical therapy for treatment to relieve pain and stiffness in his right knee. Radiographs revealed arthritic changes in both knees. He had a medial meniscectomy in the right knee 2 years ago. His recent complaints of pain and stiffness are related to his present leisure and work activities. Richard is an avid golfer, country and Western dancer, and chauffeur.

- What types of assessments would be important for this patient?
- What symptoms would you be interested in pursuing, and how would you do that?
- Describe how you would approach Richard to determine the degree of discomfort that he is experiencing and when.

Discussion Questions

1. Describe at least two pain assessments that evaluate the quality of a patient's pain experience.
2. Describe at least two pain assessments that attempt to quantify a patient's pain experience.
3. What are the components of edema assessment?
4. Which assessment tool(s) would provide data for the determination of multiple symptoms, for example, edema and muscle spasm? How is this possible?

Research Tips

The Guide to Physical Therapist Practice published by the American Physical Therapy Association is the most comprehensive and well-organized source of information; it deals with signs and symptoms and what to do with the information.

References

1. Kloth, LC, and McCulloch, JM. Wound Healing—Alternatives in Management, ed 3. FA Davis, Philadelphia, 2002, p 180.
2. Finch, E, Brooks, D, Stratford, P, and Mayo, N: Physical Rehabilitation Outcome Measures, ed 2. Lippincott, Williams, and Wilkins, Philadelphia, 2002, pp 180 and 244.
3. Warfield, CA (ed): Manual of Pain Management. JB Lippincott, Philadelphia, 1991, pp 20–23.
4. Loeser, JD, and Melzack, R: Pain: An overview. Lancet 353:1607–1609, 1999.

5. Melzack, R: McGill Pain Questionnaire (1975). In Turk, DC, and Melzack, R (eds): Handbook of Pain Assessment. Guilford Press, New York, 1992, pp 154–161, 165–166.

6. Melzack, R: Short form McGill Pain Questionnaire (1987). In Turk, DC, and Melzack, R (eds): Handbook of Pain Assessment. Guilford Press, New York, 1992, pp 161–163.

7. Lowe, NK, Walker, SN, and MacCallum, RC: Confirming the theoretical structure of the McGill Pain Questionnaire in acute clinical pain. Pain 46:52, 1991.

8. Holroyd, KA, et al: A multi-center evaluation of the McGill Pain Questionnaire: Results from more than 1700 chronic pain patients. Pain 48:301, 1992.

9. Mann, HN, et al: Initial-impression diagnosis using low-back pain patient pain drawings. Spine 18:41, 1993.

10. Swantson, M, et al: Pain assessment with interactive computer animation. Pain 53:347, 1993.

11. North, RB, et al: Automated "pain drawing: Analysis by computer-controlled, patient interactive neurological stimulation system. Pain 50:51, 1992.

12. Toomey, TC, et al: Relationship of pain drawing scores to ratings of pain description and function. Clin J Pain 7:269, 1993.

13. Fischer, AA: Clinical use of tissue compliance meter for documentation of soft tissue pathology. Clin J Pain 3:23, 1987.

14. Fischer, AA: Pressure threshold measurement for diagnosis of myofacial pain and evaluation of treatment results. Clin J Pain 2:207, 1987.

15. Atkins, CJ, et al: An electronic method for measuring joint tenderness in rheumatoid arthritis. Arthritis Rheum 35:407, 1992.

16. Bryan, AS, Klenerman, L, and Bowsher, D: The diagnosis of reflex sympathetic dystrophy using an algometer. Bone Joint Surg (Br) 73:644, 1991.

17. Cott, A, et al: Interrater reliability of the tender point criterion for fibromyalgia, Rheumatology 19:1955, 1992.

18. Soderberg, GL: Skeletal muscle function. In Currier, DP, and Nelson, RM (eds): Dynamics of Human Biologic Tissues. FA Davis, Philadelphia, 1992, pp 92–93.

19. Calliet, R: Neck and Arm Pain, ed 3. FA Davis, Philadelphia, 1991, pp 74–75.

Additional References

American Physical Therapy Association: A Normative Model of Physical Therapist Assistant Education: Version 99. American Physical Therapy Association, Alexandria, VA, 1999.

American Physical Therapy Association: Guide to Physical Therapist Practice, ed 2. American Physical Therapy Association, Alexandria, VA, 2001.

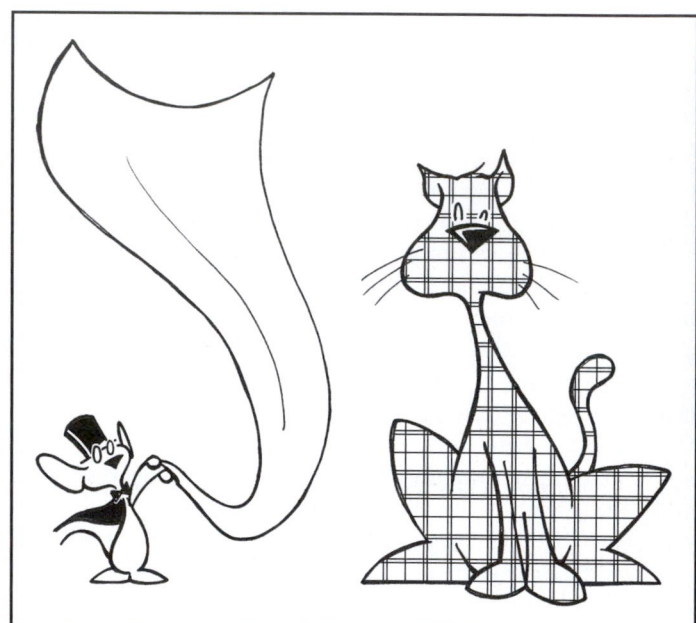

Thermal and Mechanical Agents

Objectives

- Describe the different types of heat and cold agents.
- Discuss the application techniques for heat and cold agents.
- Differentiate between the possible choices of heat and cold agents.
- Discuss the clinical decision making involved in using heat or cold agents to optimize therapeutic benefit.
- Describe safety considerations for the use of heat and cold agents.

Key Terms

Acute inflammation	Evaporation	Muscle guarding or spasm	Radiation
Afferent neurons	Homeostasis	Muscle spindle	Raynaud's disease
Axon reflex	Hot pack	Nerve conduction velocity	Shortwave diathermy
Capacitance	Hydrocollator pack	Pain threshold	Specific heat
Cold vasodilation	Hyperthermia	Paraffin bath	Subcutaneous tissue
Conduction	Hypothalamus	Perfusion	Temperature regulation
Connective tissue	Inductance	Peripheral vascular disease	Thermal conductivity
Convection	Inflammatory	Physiologic effects of heat	Thermoreceptors
Conversion	Joint capsule	Radiant energy	Vasoconstriction
Counterirritation	Magnetic field		Vasodilation
Cryotherapy	Mechanoreceptors		
Efferent neurons	Metabolic rate		

Susan Michlovitz, PT, PhD, CHT   Kristin von Nieda, DPT, MEd

Therapeutic Heat and Cold

Outline

> *"To relieve pain, is it better to use heat or cold?"*

Heat and cold agents are age-old remedies for pain control. Each has a role during the phases of tissue healing and recovery and with disorders such as arthritis that lead to muscle ache and joint stiffness. This chapter provides the background for developing problem-solving skills for appropriate and safe clinical application of heat and cold agents. Knowledge of the body's physiologic responses to heat and cold in combination with patient goals provides the basis for decisions regarding the use, method of application, and intervention duration of heat agents.

Temperature Regulation

Temperature regulation occurs to maintain homeostasis through the interaction of local and central neural mechanisms. Sensory receptors in the skin, muscles, and joints respond to changes in temperature. Sufficient intensity of and exposure to the stimulus are needed for activation of the temperature-regulating center in the hypothalamus. The hypothalamus acts as the "body's thermostat" to maintain a normal range of human body temperature from 36° to 38°C (96.5° to 99.5°F). When sensory information reaches the hypothalamus, the information is integrated and interpreted along with information on the temperature of the blood circulating through the hypothalamus. This results in the activation of temperature-regulating mechanisms, including the following[1]:

1. Changes in circulation (e.g., vasodilation or vasoconstriction of blood vessels)

2. Shivering, to maintain heat

3. Sweating, to lose heat

Several mechanisms come into play for the body to lose heat (Table 3-1). Knowledge of basic neuroanatomy and neural transmission is necessary to understand temperature regulation in the body. Neural transmission is a function of first-, second-, and third-order afferent and efferent neurons or nerve fibers. Afferent neurons conduct sensory information from the periphery to the spinal cord and brain. Efferent neurons conduct motor information from the brain to the periphery. First-order neurons transmit information from thermal receptors or free nerve endings and terminate in the dorsal horn of the spinal cord. Second-order neurons transmit information along ascending or descending tracts of the white matter of the spinal cord and terminate in the thalamus. Third-order neurons transmit ascending sensory and descending motor information between the thalamus and the cerebral cortex. For example, the affect of stepping on a nail has the effect of withdrawing from a nail. The sensory afferent input to the cerebral cortex stimulates an efferent response resulting in a motor effect (Figs. 3-1 and 3-2). Chapter 1 of this text provides detailed information about the neurophysiology of pain.

Physical Mechanisms of Heat Exchange

The means by which therapeutic heat or cold is delivered to the target tissue is attributed to the following physical mechanisms: conduction, convection, radiation, conversion, or evaporation. The extent of temperature change results from several of the following factors:

1. Temperature difference between the heat agent and the intervention tissue

2. Time of exposure to the heat agent

3. Thermal conductivity of the intervention tissue

4. Intensity of the heat agent

Adipose tissue, skeletal muscle, bone, and blood have different levels of conductivity to heat or cold. Adipose tissue acts as insulation to underlying tissues, thus limiting the degree of temperature change in deeper tissues. Blood and muscle, which contain relatively high water contents, readily absorb and conduct heat.

Conduction

Heat loss or gain through direct contact between materials with different temperatures is called conduction. Heat absorbed by the body when using a hot pack is an example of heat exchange by conduction. When cold packs are applied to the skin, heat is lost from the skin via conduction.

Convection

Convection is defined as the transference of heat to a body by the movement of air, matter, or liquid around or past the body. An example of convective heat is a hot-air furnace. A furnace circulates warmed air around a room, and the temperature of the contents changes. A clinical example is the use of Fluidotherapy, whereby warm air is circulated through a bed of fine-grained cellulose particles. The movement of the warm cellulose particles around a body part results in a temperature change of the skin and underlying subcutaneous tissue.

TABLE 3-1 **Pathways of Heat Loss**	
PATHWAY	**MECHANISM**
Skin (major pathway)	• Radiation and conduction—heat is lost from the body to cooler air or objects. • Convection—air currents move warm air away from the skin. • Sweating—excess body heat evaporates sweat on the skin surface.
Respiratory tract (secondary pathway)	• Evaporation—body heat evaporates water from the respiratory mucosa, and water vapor is exhaled.
Urinary tract (minor pathway)	• Urination—urine is at body temperature when eliminated.
Digestive tract (minor pathway)	• Defecation—feces are at body temperature when eliminated.

From Scanlon, VC, and Sanders, T: Essentials of Anatomy and Physiology, ed 4. FA Davis, 1991, Philadelphia, p 379.

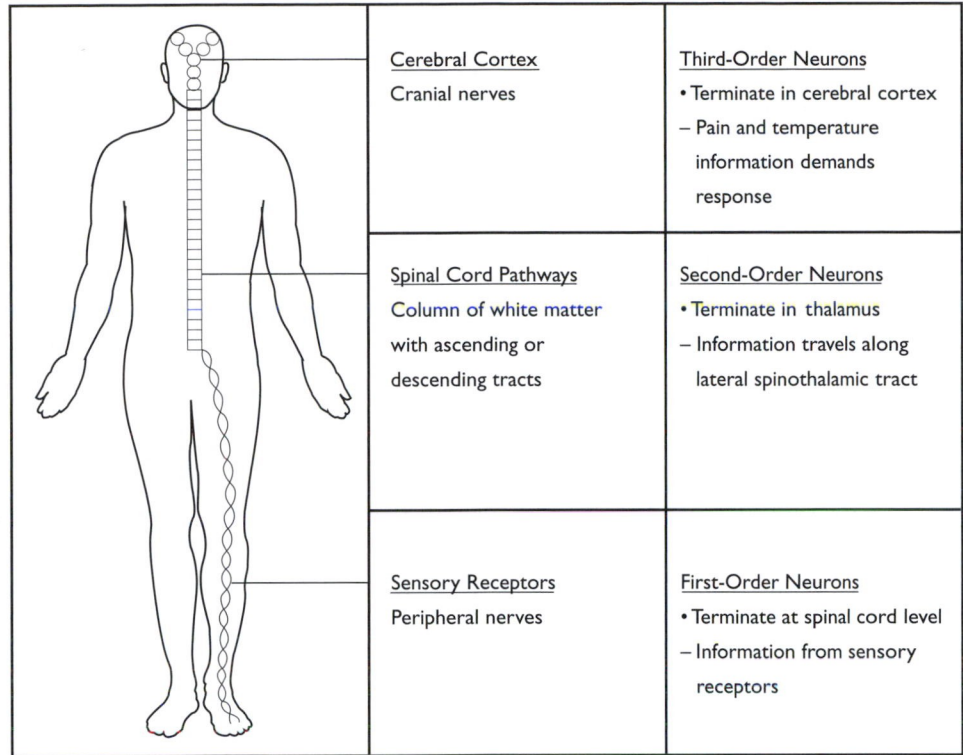

Cerebral Cortex
Cranial nerves
	Third-Order Neurons
	• Terminate in cerebral cortex
	– Pain and temperature
	  information demands
	  response

Spinal Cord Pathways Column of white matter with ascending or descending tracts	Second-Order Neurons • Terminate in thalamus – Information travels along lateral spinothalamic tract
Sensory Receptors Peripheral nerves	First-Order Neurons • Terminate at spinal cord level – Information from sensory receptors

Figure 3–1   First-, second-, and third-order neuron transmission pathways for sensation perception.

Radiation

Radiation or radiant energy transfers heat through air from a warmer source to a cooler source. Examples of radiant heat include the glowing coals of an open fire or the heating element on an electric stove. A therapeutic example is an infrared heat lamp. (The infrared lamp, though, is not in common use in clinical practice.) The infrared element in the lamp does not come in contact with the tissue. When radiant heat is generated from the lamp, only those body areas in the immediate vicinity of the lamp receive direct heating effects.

Conversion

Conversion refers to the temperature change that results from energy transformed from one form to another, such as the conversion from mechanical or electrical energy to heat energy. A clinical example is continuous-wave therapeutic ultrasound, in which sound waves (mechanical energy) are transformed to heat (thermal energy) as they are absorbed by the tissue.

Evaporation

Evaporation is defined as the transformation from a liquid state to a gas state. This transformation requires an energy exchange. Heat is given off when liquids transform to gases. Sweating results from heat production within the body.

Cooling occurs as the perspiration evaporates from the surface of the skin. Vapocoolant sprays cause the cooling of the skin via evaporation.

 Therapeutic Heat

Several heat agents are available for heat application to tissues. Generally, two categories are described: superficial and deep heating agents. Superficial heating agents, such as hot packs, air-activated heat wraps, warm whirlpool, Fluidotherapy, and paraffin, primarily increase the temperature of the skin and subcutaneous tissues with less effect on deeper structures. Deep heating agents, such as continuous ultrasound and continuous shortwave diathermy, can increase the temperature of tissues at depths of 3 to 5 cm. Shortwave diathermy is discussed later in this chapter. Ultrasound is addressed in Chapter 4.

Physiologic Effects of Heat

Physiologic changes in response to heat application vary according to the intensity of the agent, the duration of application, and the area being treated. Therapeutic levels of heating are categorized as mild and vigorous. Heating is considered mild when tissue temperatures are less than 40°C,

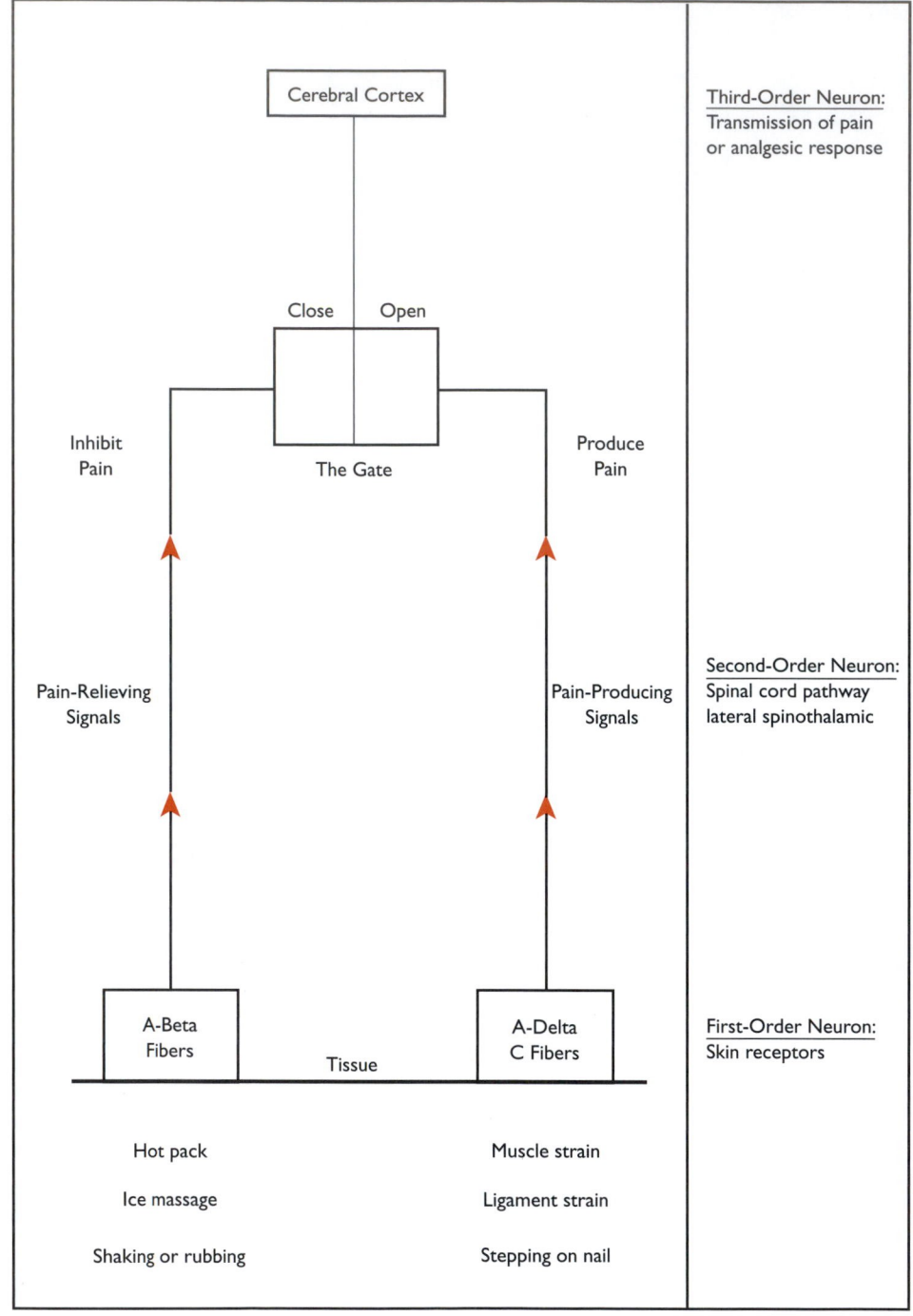

Third-Order Neuron:
Transmission of pain
or analgesic response

Cerebral Cortex

Close   Open

Inhibit
Pain

The Gate

Produce
Pain

Pain-Relieving
Signals

Pain-Producing
Signals

A-Beta
Fibers

Tissue

A-Delta
C Fibers

Hot pack

Ice massage

Shaking or rubbing

Muscle strain

Ligament strain

Stepping on nail

Figure 3-2   Schematic representation of
the gate control theory of pain.

and vigorous heating occurs when tissue temperature reaches 40° to 45°C.[2] At these temperatures, hyperemia or redness is noted, which indicates an increase in blood flow. Temperature increases greater than 45°C have the potential to result in thermal pain and irreversible tissue damage.[3,4]

Elevating the tissue temperature results in an increase in blood flow to the area, attributable in part to the vasodilatory response in surface blood vessels.[5] The increase in blood

flow removes heat from the area, whereas blood that is relatively cooler flows into the area, thus preventing excessive heat accumulation. Conversely, therapeutic heating levels may not be reached because the increased blood flow may not allow for adequate heat buildup in the area. Heat accumulation is affected by the intensity and duration of the stimulus, as well as the rate of heat absorption by the tissue. If therapeutic heating levels are reached with local application, reflex heating in other areas of the body may also occur. Local heat application has both direct and indirect heating effects. For example, when heat was applied to the low back area, an increase in subcutaneous blood flow and vasodilation to the distal extremities was reported.[1,5,6] An older technique involved trying to increase circulation to the extremities of someone with peripheral vascular disease via the "indirect" effect. This is not commonly used in contemporary practice.

The application of superficial heating agents generally does not allow for increases in muscle temperatures, unless those structures are themselves superficial or the conductive heat agent is left on for 30 minutes or longer. Increased temperature in the muscles and tendons of the hand and foot may occur with the use of superficial heating agents, because insulation from adipose tissue is not prevalent in these areas.

Changes in metabolic rate in association with changes in tissue temperature have been reported. An increase in tissue temperature correlates with an increase in metabolic rate.[1] This increase in metabolic rate may be used advantageously to facilitate tissue healing. Conversely, in the face of acute inflammation, heat can exacerbate the inflammatory process due to the increase in metabolic rate. In that case, cold, which slows metabolic rate, can thus reduce potential tissue damage.

Heat may have a beneficial role in wound healing based on the increase in blood flow. The increase in blood improves perfusion of the wound and periwound tissue. Improved perfusion results in an increase in oxygen tension of the wound, and the increase in oxygen allows for greater clearing of bacteria from the wound site.[7] Increasing tissue temperature to therapeutic levels (40° to 45°C)[2] can facilitate the release of oxygen from the blood's hemoglobin, thus improving tissue nutrition

Intervention Goals

Based on the physiologic effects of therapeutic heat, intervention goals are easy to identify. Therapeutic heating agents are used as adjunctive intervention techniques for achieving functional goals. Heat contributes to the alleviation of pain and to pain management, which may allow increased functional activity or improved range of motion. The increase in motion may in turn lead to improvement in activities of daily living. When heat is used for reduction of muscle guarding or spasm, it may lead to pain reduction and further improvement in mobility. By affecting the viscoelastic properties of tendon and muscle with the use of heat, tissue extensibility is enhanced, potentially allowing for return of lost motion.

Each of the therapeutic goals—pain reduction and management, reduction of muscle guarding and spasm, and increased tissue extensibility—are addressed in relationship to the specific heat agent. It is important to recognize the connection between these therapeutic goals and the overall functional goals.

Pain Reduction

The use of superficial heat for the alleviation or management of pain is well recognized, but the mechanism by which heat produces analgesia is not fully understood. Several mechanisms have been proposed to explain pain relief in response to therapeutic heat.

Melzack and Wall[8] proposed the gate control theory of pain, in which a spinal "gating" mechanism was responsible for pain mediation. Small A-delta fibers and C fibers are primary afferents that transmit pain impulses from free nerve endings or nociceptors to the spinal cord. When therapeutic heat is used, the thermal stimuli provide input to the spinal gating mechanism, which in effect overrides the painful stimuli. When there is greater non-noxious input (heat) than noxious input (pain), the "gate" is in a relatively closed position, thus inhibiting transmission of pain to second-order neurons or ascending tracts. The theory proposed by Melzack and Wall has not been proved but serves as a good conceptual framework to discuss the application of physical agents (see Fig. 3-2).

Gammon and Starr[9] postulated that thermal stimuli (heat or cold) produced counterirritation. Pain was not as readily perceived because the thermal input "countered" painful stimuli. This may explain why a common response to initial injury is rubbing or pressure, both of which could be considered counterirritants.

Heat has also been shown to elevate the pain threshold[9,10] and increase nerve conduction velocity.[11] An elevated pain threshold may delay the onset and perception of pain. Clinical relevance associated with the change in nerve conduction velocity has not been demonstrated.

Reduction of Muscle Guarding or Spasm

Muscle guarding or spasm may occur in response to (1) trauma, as a protective mechanism to guard against the potential pain and further injury or pain associated with joint movement, or (2) a painful stimulus that activates or perpetuates the pain-spasm-pain cycle.[12] Heat has been used to relieve muscle guarding and spasm[13,14] and to increase tissue flexiblity.[15] When muscle temperature is sufficiently elevated, as can be seen with the use of deep heating agents, the firing rate of the muscle spindle afferents (type II) is decreased, whereas that of the Golgi tendon organs (type Ib) is increased.[16] The resultant decrease in alpha motor neuron activity leads to a decrease in tonic muscle activity. In other words, there is a decrease in muscle guarding resulting from decreased stimuli to the muscle.

The reduction in muscle guarding and spasm as the direct result of elevated muscle temperature does not explain the reduction seen with the use of superficial heating agents. This muscle relaxation may be explained by an indirect reduction in muscle spindle firing as a direct result of elevating skin temperature. The increase in skin temperature causes a decrease in gamma efferent activity, thus altering stretch on the muscle spindle and producing a decrease in the firing rate and an overall decrease in alpha motor neuron activity.[7]

Heat application has a direct affect on pain and muscle spasm such that the pain-spasm-pain cycle[13] can be interrupted by influencing pain as well as the muscle spasm. A reduction in pain can lead to a reduction in spasm, thus further reducing pain.

Tissue Extensibility

Shortening of connective tissue may result from injury or immobilization. The viscoelastic properties of muscle, tendon, and ligament are affected.[18] The use of heat has been shown to decrease viscosity and increase the elastic properties of connective tissue, specifically muscle, tendon, and joint capsule.[2] However, a sufficient load must also be applied to produce residual elongation of the tissue over a long time.[17] The temperature range needed for residual length changes is 40° to 45°C.[2] Furthermore, the potential for irritation and tissue damage is lessened when heat is applied during the stretching procedure.

Residual elongation of connective tissue is dependent on a sufficient increase in tissue temperature, the timing of the application, and the type of stretch applied. The stretch is best applied during heat application, if possible, or immediately after removal of the heat source. A low-load prolonged stretch was reported as preferable to a high-load brief stretch because it resulted in less tissue damage and greater increases in range of motion.[18–21]

Patients with arthritis who have pain and limited motion associated with joint stiffness may benefit from the use of therapeutic heat. The direct effect of heat is an increase in the elastic properties of the joint capsule,[22] and the reduction of associated pain may also contribute to the resultant increased range of motion.

Heat and Exercise

A greater increase in blood flow is reported with heat and exercise than with either heat or exercise alone.[23] An initial decrease in isometric muscle strength was seen during the first 30 minutes after deep heat application, and subsequent increase in strength was measured during the next 2.5 hours.[24] Endurance was shown to decrease after heat applications.[25,26] These findings are of particular interest because muscle performance may be altered in response to heat. The clinical implications of the relationship between the use of heat and exercise are important considerations for planning and implementing exercise programs and for evaluating patient performance. To assess progress or limitations in strength and endurance accurately, measurements should be taken consistently either before or after exercise. If an initial measurement is taken before exercise and a subsequent measurement is taken after exercise, comparison of the results may

 Before You Begin

Make sure you know the goal of the treatment. If the patient has a muscle spasm, you may wish to position to reduce "stretch" on muscle. If heat is being used to increase range of motion, you may position with joint at or near the end range of available motion.

lead to erroneous conclusions about the patient's performance and the efficacy of the intervention.

Methods of Heat Application

Superficial Heating Agents

Heat from superficial heating agents generally penetrates to depths of less than 2 cm from the surface of the skin. Subcutaneous tissue that is well vascularized reaches its maximum temperature increase within 8 to 10 minutes of application.[27–29] Skin and subcutaneous tissue temperatures increase 5° to 6°C after 6 minutes and are maintained up to 30 minutes after application. An intervention duration of 15 to 30 minutes is necessary for an increase in muscle temperature of 1°C at depths up to 3 cm.[27,28,30] Temperature of a joint capsule in the foot increased 9°C in response to 20 minutes of heat exposure at 47.8°C.[31] It is therefore possible to heat joint structures using superficial heating agents when these structures are closer to the skin surface Therefore, in this instance; heat should be applied for 15 to 30 minutes for maximal benefit.

Hydrocollator Packs

The commercial hydrocollator pack, or hot pack, is one of the most common ways to deliver superficial moist heat. Generally, hot packs contain a hydrophilic substance, such as silica gel or betonite, encased in channeled canvas covers. They are stored in thermostatically controlled units that are filled with water at a temperature range of 71° to 79°C.[2] Frequent use, low water levels, and faulty thermostats can affect the temperature of the hot packs, so it is important to check the water level (replenishing water levels frequently) and temperature to ensure optimal heat delivery so therapeutic heat levels are achieved. The hot packs should be checked for ruptures in the canvas or mold formation, which can weaken the canvas and allow leakage. When a hot pack leaks, it should be discarded and replaced with a new one.

The temperature of the hot pack itself is regulated by the length of time it is stored and the temperature of the water in which it is stored. After a hot pack has been used, 20 to 30 minutes is needed for the hot pack to reach the temperature of the water in the storage unit. This is an important consideration if hot packs are frequently used in a clinic.

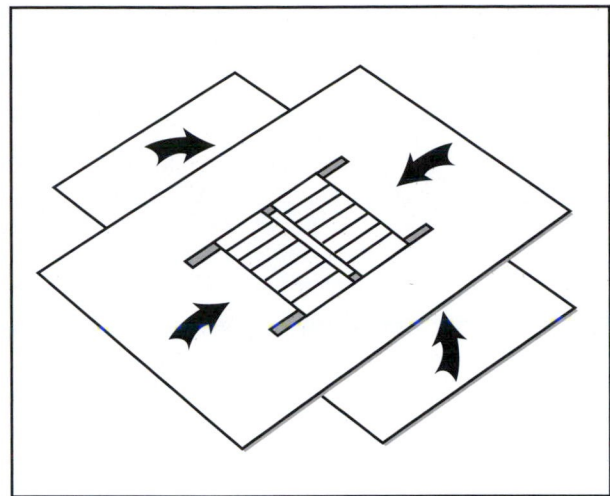

Figure 3-3 Hot pack that has been placed on two towels, folded in half to provide eight layers of toweling.

Before application to the patient, the hot pack is covered with six to eight layers of toweling that insulate the hot pack from heat loss and protect the patient from potential burn. Commercial terrycloth covers are also available and are equivalent to two to four layers of toweling (Fig. 3-3).

Thermal energy is conducted from hot packs to the skin surface, and heat is absorbed superficially. The resultant change in temperature depends on the thermal conductivity and the size of the area being treated, the temperature of the hot pack, the size of the hot pack, and the duration of the application.

Hot packs are manufactured in several sizes and shapes to better match the body part to which they are applied. The standard size of 10×12 inches is suitable for treating medium-sized flat surface areas. The oversize pack is approximately twice the size of the standard pack and is suited for larger flat surface areas. Cervical packs are designed to fit the contours of the neck and are also appropriate for use around peripheral joints (Fig. 3-4). Size and shape are important because the mechanism of heat transfer is conduction, so optimal contact with the skin surface ensures optimal heat absorption. The weight of the hot packs also helps to maintain contact with the body surface. Weight of the pack increases with the size and is a consideration when deciding to use this form of superficial heat. Patients may not tolerate the weight of the pack during treatment.

Preparing the patient for treatment includes proper positioning and draping of the patient, visual inspection of the area to be treated, and assessment of the patient's ability to report sensory changes. The area to be treated should be clear of clothing and jewelry to ensure even heating. Select and prepare the hot pack with the appropriate layers of toweling. Make sure the patient is in a comfortable position, and apply the hot pack. Instruct the patient in what to expect to experience from the heat, and ask him or her to report any abnormal or unusual sensations such as overheating or burning. Monitor the initial response to intervention during the first 5 to 10 minutes by asking the patient for feedback and by visually inspecting the skin, emphasizing that the sensation of heat should be "warm," not "hot." The old adage of "the hotter the better" should be dispelled. If necessary, adjust the layers of toweling, by adding more toweling to reduce heat delivery or

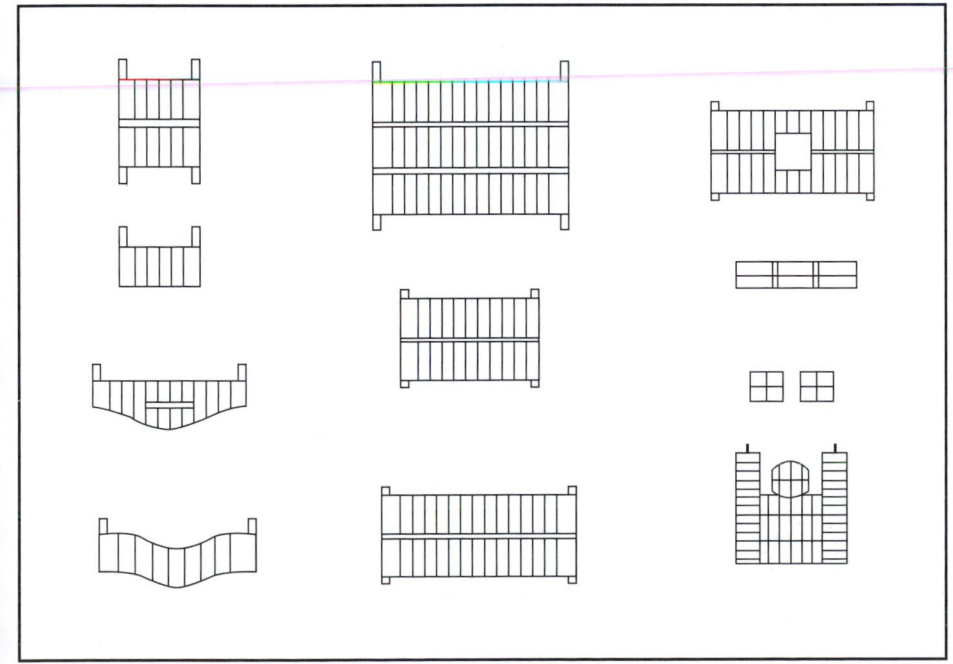

Figure 3-4 Variety of hot packs that are available. Variation in sizes allows for the selection of the appropriate size pack to fit the treatment area. Left column (top to bottom): standard size, half size, cervical packs. Middle column (top to bottom): oversize, "spinal" sizes. Right column (top to bottom): "knee or shoulder pack," obstetric size, others.

removing toweling to increase heat delivery. Maximum skin temperature change is achieved within the first 10 minutes of hot pack application and maintained for approximately an additional 10 minutes. Therefore, the application time is typically 20 minutes. Observe the skin again after the hot pack is removed and assess the patient's response to the intervention.

Commercial hot packs are also available for home use. In addition to hydrocollator packs, there are reusable, microwavable products that deliver heat in a similar manner to hydrocollator packs. Detailed instruction to patients and care providers regarding safe and appropriate use is essential, and a demonstration on use is recommended. Use of superficial heating agents at home, as part of an established home program, may be beneficial to the patient in maintaining range of motion, managing pain, and alleviating joint stiffness.

Paraffin

Paraffin is another superficial heating agent in which conduction is the method of heat transfer. Paraffin baths contain a mixture of paraffin wax and mineral oil, which are combined to lower the melting point and the specific heat in comparison to water.[2] Paraffin is stored in double-walled, thermostatically controlled, stainless steel tanks, and temperatures are maintained in the range of 47.0° to 54.4°C. The low specific heat of paraffin allows patients to tolerate the higher temperatures.

Paraffin is best suited for distal extremity joints, such as the wrist, hand, and foot, because of the primary methods of application: "dip and wrap" and "dip and immerse." The former is far more popular, more practical, and probably safer than the latter. The dip-and-wrap method involves dipping and removing the body part from the paraffin bath for 8 to 10 repetitions. A solid glove is formed that serves to insulate the body part against heat loss. It is common to place a plastic bag over the glove and to wrap a towel around the extremity to further assist in heat retention. The wrapped extremity is then positioned in elevation to minimize edema formation (Figs. 3-5 and 3-6). Intervention duration is 15 to 20 minutes, after which time the glove is removed, and the wax is discarded or returned to the unit to be reused.

The dip-and-immerse method is similar to the above method in that the patient is asked to dip and reimmerse the body part, allowing the glove to form. Rather than wrapping the hand or foot, the part is reimmersed and left in the paraffin bath for the duration of the intervention. This method is more effective in raising tissue temperature but places the patient at greater risk for burn. This method also does not allow for elevation of the body part being treated and an increase in edema may result. As with any therapeutic heat application, careful monitoring of the patient during and after intervention is essential to safe practice. It is this author's opinion (S.M.) that for reasons of practicality and safety, other techniques of heat should be selected rather than the paraffin dip and immerse.

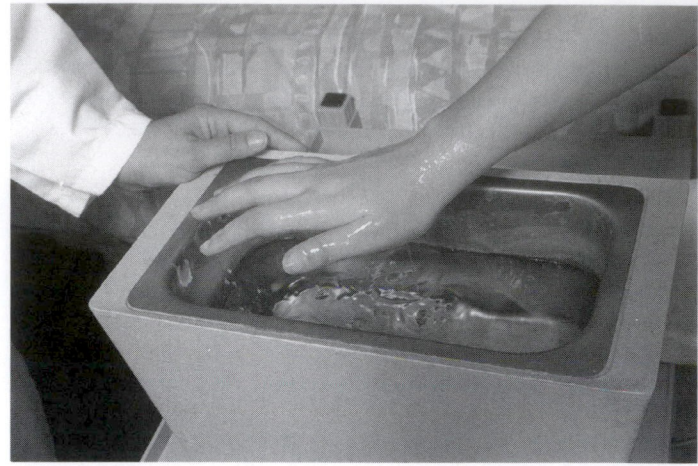

Figure 3-5 Paraffin unit with an application of paraffin to the hand.

Before intervention, the patient should be instructed to remove clothing and jewelry from the area and to thoroughly wash and dry the area to be treated. The skin should be visually inspected and sensation and heat tolerance assessed. The patient should be instructed in what to expect during the paraffin application and to report any abnormal sensations. Care should be taken by the patient to avoid touching the sides or bottom of the unit to minimize the risk of skin burn.

Paraffin has advantages over hydrocollator packs in that it conforms to the body part and may provide more evenly

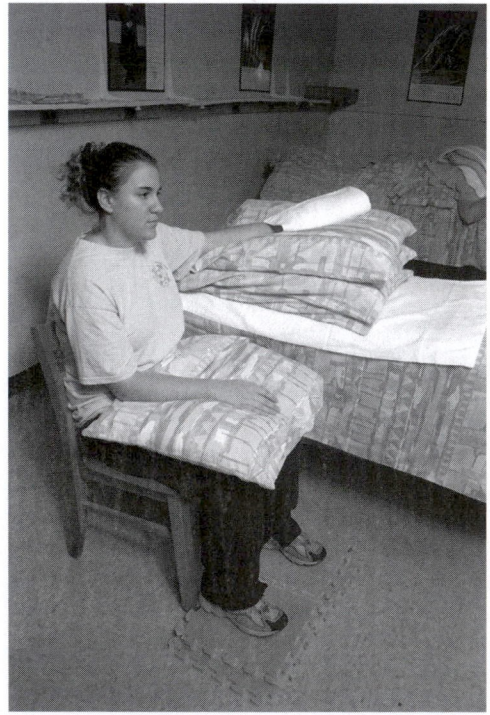

Figure 3-6 Hand with the paraffin glove is wrapped in a towel and positioned in an elevated position.

distributed and intense heat. However, the higher temperatures may not be as easily tolerated, and there is no way of adjusting the level of heat delivery to the patient, as is the case with hot packs. Home units are available but are more expensive than commercial hot packs. For in-clinic use, the paraffin "glove" should be disposed when removed from the patient's hand or foot. If only one person is using the paraffin, such as in the case of home use, the paraffin can be returned to the bath after each use. If too much sediment builds up in the unit, then the paraffin wax should be disposed and replaced.

Fluidotherapy

Fluidotherapy allows stimulation of both thermoreceptors and mechanoreceptors and therefore can serve for the simultaneous uses of enhancing motion and reduction pain and hypersensitivity. Fluidotherapy units contain particles of natural cellulose enclosed in a cabinet, through which dry, warm air is circulated. The method of heat exchange, which occurs with Fluidotherapy, is convection. The units are thermostatically controlled, and specific temperatures can be selected. The turbulence level has a separate control. The moving suspended particles create a medium similar to that of a liquid, and stretching and exercise can be performed during the heat application.

Fluidotherapy units have been manufactured to accommodate the distal upper extremity (Fig. 3-7) and the distal lower extremity (Fig. 3-8). Fluidotherapy is used for pain relief, tissue healing, and increasing range of motion. It is also indicated to promote desensitization of hypersensitive tissues. The effects of Fluidotherapy are the result of the combination of heat and the movement of the natural cellulose particles.

Unlike paraffin and hydrocollator packs, there is no loss of heat over time. The temperature is selected and maintained for the duration of the intervention when using Fluidotherapy. The constant temperature may result in greater heating, and elevated temperatures in joint capsules of the hand and foot have been reported.[32] Unlike paraffin and hot packs, Fluidotherapy allows movement of the extremity during heat application.

Preparation for Fluidotherapy interventions is similar to that for paraffin intervention. The area to be treated should be thoroughly washed and dried, and jewelry and clothing should be removed from the area. Sensation and heat toler-

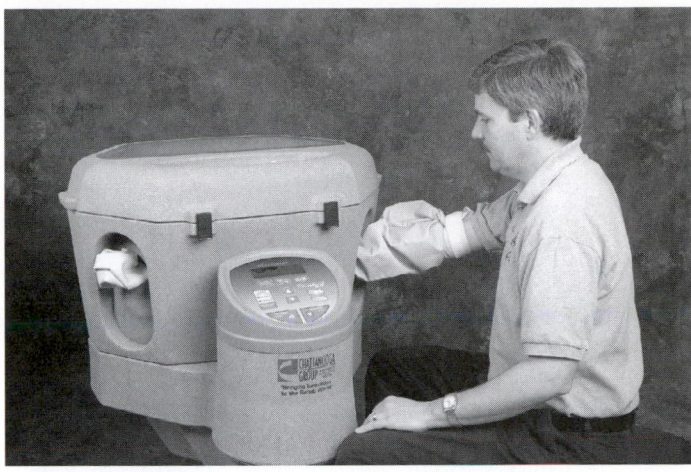

Figure 3-7 Fluidotherapy treatment for the hand and wrist. (From Michlovitz, SL, and Nolan, TP, eds. Modalities for Therapeutic Intervention, ed 4. FA Davis, Philadelphia, 2005, with permission.)

ance should be assessed, and the skin carefully inspected. Open lesions should be covered with a plastic barrier before intervention to prevent the cellulose particles from entering the wound. The plastic barrier contributes to a moist wound environment.

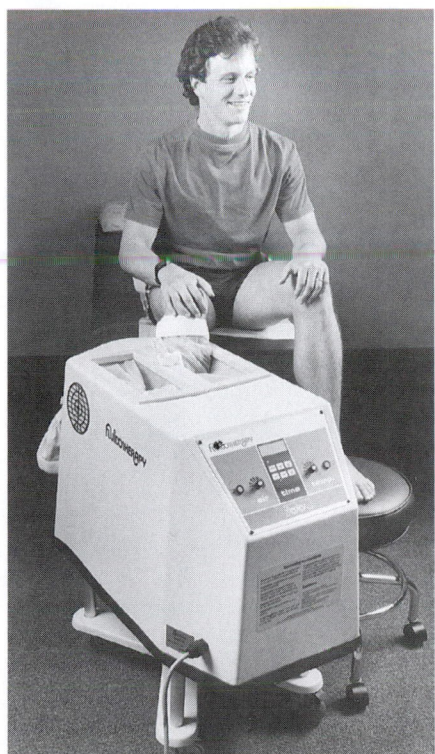

Figure 3-8 Fluidotherapy for the foot and ankle. (From Michlovitz, SL: Biophysical principles of heating and superficial heat agents. In Michlovitz, SL, ed. Thermal Agents in Rehabilitation, ed 2. FA Davis, Philadelphia, 1990, p 99, with permission.)

● **Why Do I Need to Know About...**

Status of Circulation and Skin Integrity

If there is an impaired (e.g., reduced) circulation, heat cannot dissipate from the area and you risk burning the patient. If there is an open area of skin, the paraffin can get into that area and cause an irritation or a burn.

Fluidotherapy has been reported to be safe when used in the presence of splints, bandages, tape, metal implants, plastic joint replacements, and artificial tendons.[32] Splints that are designed to apply a stretch to joints can be applied before intervention in the Fluidotherapy unit, such that the stretch can be applied during the heat application to the joint. Exercise equipment, such as small balls, can also be used by patients during intervention.

Air-Activated Heat Wraps Continuous low-level heat can be delivered via air-activated heat wraps. These heat wraps are comfortable and provide a low-profile low-level heat source that can be worn during activity and sleep for up to 8 hours at a time. These wearable heat wraps maintain a temperature of about 40°C (104°F) and elevate tissue temperature, and can be worn by the patient during activities of daily living and work and during sleep.

These wraps are available in different sizes and shapes to accommodate body size and contour (Figs. 3-9 and 3-10).

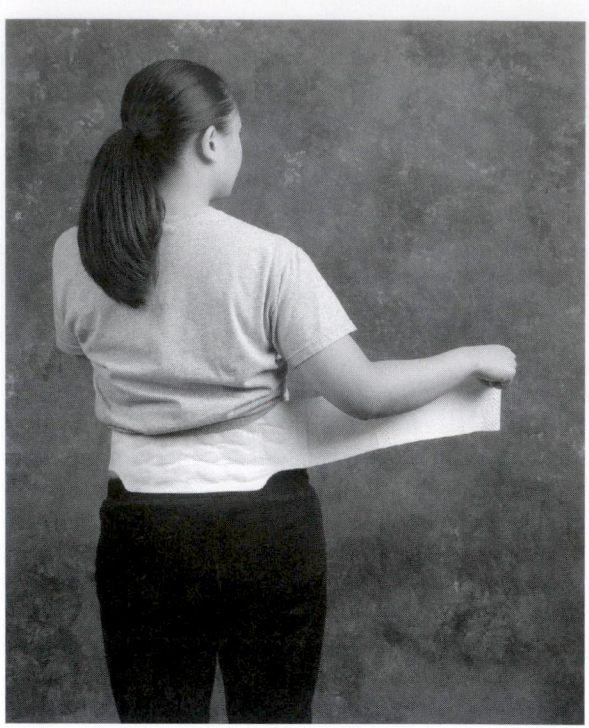

Figure 3-10 Air-activated heat wrap (Thermacare; Procter & Gamble, Cincinnati, OH) being applied to the low back.

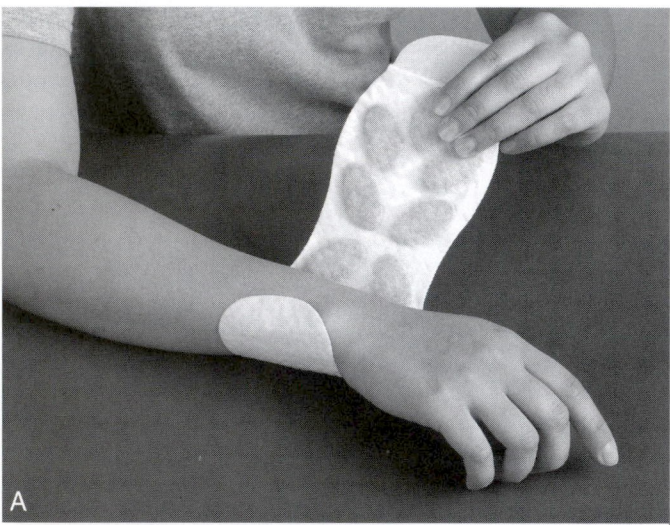

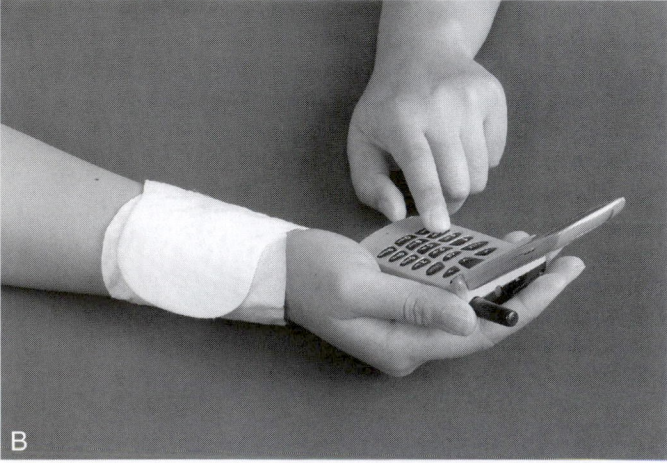

Figure 3-9 Air-activated heat wrap (Thermacare; Procter & Gamble, Cincinnati, OH) (a) applied to the wrist and (b) worn during activity.

The concept of applying low-level heat over a long time (e.g., hours) has been the concept of the use of electric heating pads. With an electric heating pad, the patient must be at the site of an electrical outlet. Also, some of the pads may heat up enough to produce superficial burns, particularly if the person falls asleep while the electric heat pad is plugged in and turned on. Studies have been done that show these air-activated heat wraps are effective in controlling pain, improving muscle flexibility, and improving function in patients with acute and chronic low back pain.[14,15] In addition, pain is improved, stiffness is reduced, and hand grip strength is increased when wearing these wraps on the wrist in those with tendonitis, arthritis, and symptoms consistent with carpal tunnel syndrome.[33]

Shortwave Diathermy

Shortwave diathermy can be used as a deep heating agent because it can produce increases in tissue temperature at depths of 3 to 5 cm below the skin surface,[33] without overheating the skin and subcutaneous tissues. The literal meaning of diathermy is "to heat through." Electromagnetic radiation, the energy of diathermy, in a nonionizing form is within the range of radiofrequency waves. As the high-frequency waves pass into the body, the internal kinetic energy of the tissue is increased. Heat is generated from the conversion of electromagnetic energy emitted from the diathermy electrode to mechanical energy within the body.

The benefits of diathermy are the same as those associated with conductive heating agents and include the following:

- Increased blood flow
- Decreased pain
- Increased tissue extensibility

The primary difference lies in the depth of penetration, thus allowing for heating of deeper tissues. Selected tissues may be targeted depending on the method of energy transfer associated with the type of diathermy used.[2]

Two types of diathermy are described: microwave (MWD) and shortwave (SWD). Both use electromagnetic energy that falls within the radiofrequency portion of the electromagnetic spectrum. The Federal Communications Commission has assigned specific frequencies for shortwave and microwave diathermies. The most widely used frequency associated with SWD is 27.12 MHz. MWD is rarely used in contemporary physical therapy practice. There are two methods of application for SWD: capacitance and inductance. Electrical fields (capacitance) and magnetic fields (inductance) are generated by the SWD unit, with the latter being more prevalent The body part being treated is placed between two electrodes and essentially becomes part of the circuit. As energy passes through the tissue, more heat is generated in tissues of low conductivity or high resistance, such as fat, ligaments, tendons, and cartilage. The ratio of the electrical field to the magnetic field is higher for capacitance SWD.

Inductance SWD primarily utilizes the magnetic field. The body part is not part of the circuit, and heat is generated as eddy currents generated by the magnetic field pass into the tissue (Fig. 3-11). Tissues with high conductivity, such as blood, muscle, and sweat, are most affected because they allow greater current flow.

Selection of the method of SWD depends on the tissue characteristics of the area being treated. If the goal of intervention is to increase tissue extensibility and the limitation is primarily to capsular tightness, then capacitance SWD is the more appropriate choice. If the intervention goal is to increase blood flow to aid healing of a muscle injury, then inductance diathermy should be chosen.

SWD is not commonly used in clinical practice, in part because of the variety and portability of other therapeutic heating agents. The amount of heat generated in the tissues is not easily quantified, and there are more contraindications associated with diathermy than with other heat agents.

Intervention Considerations

The selection of the appropriate heat agent is based on the size and location of the area to be treated, the depth of tissue targeted for intervention, the intervention goals, and the contraindications and precautions associated with the intervention and the heat agent. Table 3-2 lists the contraindications and precautions for superficial heating agents and diathermy. For example, use of a hot pack is appropriate for intervention of a patient with low back pain if the goals of the intervention are to decrease pain and muscle spasm. Diathermy may also be appropriate, especially if deeper muscles are to be heated. However, diathermy would not be considered appropriate if the patient had low back pain after a surgical procedure for the spine in which a metal rod was used as a fixation device.

Intervention and the response to intervention should be carefully monitored, regardless of the heat agent used. Before intervention, the area should be carefully inspected; the patient's sensation, heat tolerance, cognitive status, and ability to communicate should also be determined, because deficits in any of these areas require more careful monitoring during intervention.

Cryotherapy

Cryo means "cold" or "freezing," and *cryotherapy* refers to the practice of using cold to achieve therapeutic goals. Cooling agents, such as cold packs, cool whirlpool, and ice massage, are used in the management of pain and edema and are effective in decreasing muscle guarding and spasm. The primary methods of heat transfer, or in this case heat abstraction or cooling, are conduction and convection.

Physiologic Effects of Cold

When cold is applied to the surface of the skin, the initial response is vasoconstriction of superficial blood vessels. If skin temperature is sufficiently lowered, the cooler temperature stimulates free nerve endings, which in turn causes reflex vasoconstriction. Local blood flow is also decreased.

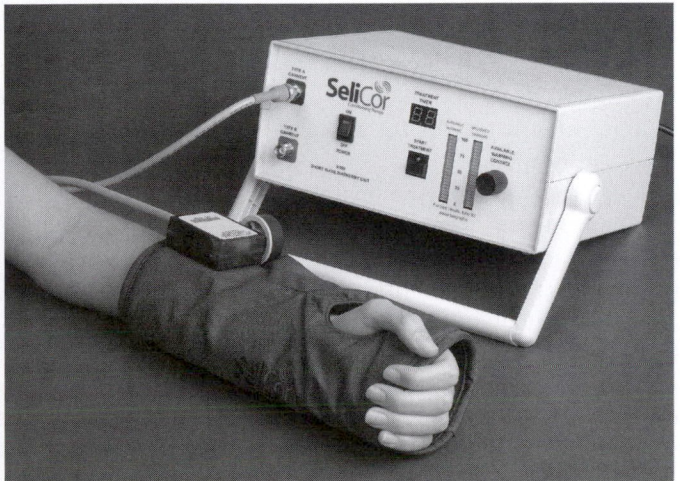

Figure 3-11 Inductance shortwave diathermy applied to the hand and wrist. (Seli-Cor shortwave diathermy unit courtesy of Seli-Cor, 7000 North Mopac Expressway, Austin, TX 78731.)

TABLE 3-2 Contraindications to and Precautions for the Use of Superficial Heating Agents and Diathermy

GENERAL CONTRAINDICATIONS FOR HEATING AGENTS	RATIONALE
Acute inflammation	Local heat application may exacerbate the inflammatory response.
Existing fever	Heat application may further elevate body temperature.
Malignancies	The increased blood flow that results from localized heat application may promote a metastasis.
Acute hemorrage	Hemorrhage may be prolonged if heat is applied after an acute injury.
Peripheral vascular disease	Heat increases metabolic demands and a patient with peripheral vascular disease has a diminished capacity to meet the increase in metabolic demands of heated tissue.
Radiation (x-ray therapy)	Tissue that is devitalized by x-ray therapy should not be heated.
SPECIFIC CONTRAINDICATIONS FOR DIATHERMY*	
Metal implants or any metal within the treatment area (snaps, zippers, hair pins)	Metal will alter the flow of electromagnetic energy and may result in a burn.
Cardiac pacemakers	Pacemaker function may be altered.
PRECAUTIONS TO THE USE OF HEAT	
During menses	May have an increase in blood flow if heat is applied to the low back.
In the presence of sensory deficit	There is an increased potential for a burn; need to be monitored closely.
During pregnancy	The effect on the fetus has not been established; heat application to peripheral joints may be given with caution.

*Diathermy equipment should not be operated within close proximity to cardiac pacemakers or other equipment that may be adversely affected by electromagnetic radiation (traction, electrical stimulation equipment).

However, when a sufficient amount of cooled blood flows through the general circulation, the hypothalamus may be stimulated, resulting in further reflex vasoconstriction. The vasoconstriction and the resultant reduction in blood flow are a means for the body to retain heat by restricting the volume of cooled blood in systemic circulation. Shivering is also a heat-retaining mechanism and may result if a large area of the body is exposed to cooler temperatures.

Vasodilation has been reported to occur in response to extended exposure to cold.[34,35] Lewis[35] postulated that cycles of vasodilation followed periods of vasoconstriction to increase the flow of relatively warmer blood to the body areas affected by cold. He termed this phenomenon the "hunting response" and proposed that it occurred as a result of an axon reflex. Cold vasodilation was also reported to occur without the cycling component and was attributed to local responses in deeper tissues.[36] Responses have included the following: (1) skin vessels were shown to maximally constrict at 15°C followed by vasodilation at temperatures below 15°C, reaching maximal vasodilation at 0°C,[36] and (2) cold-induced vascular responses, to which the prevention of local tissue injury is ascribed.[34,37,38] The hunting response is described as cycles of vasoconstriction-vasodilation lasting approximately 12 to 30 minutes during cold exposure.[39–47] Vasodilation occurs before the vasoconstrictive phase of the hunting response, and changes in sensation accompany the cycles. Cold vasodilation was also reported to occur without the cycling component and was attributed to local responses in deeper tissues.[37]

Tissue temperature changes in response to cold applications have been reported at depths of 1 to 4 cm,[48] depending on the temperature gradient and the duration of the exposure. More intense cold and longer durations result in greater decreases in tissue temperature. The presence of adipose tissue also affects the depth of cold penetration because it acts as insulation. It may not be possible to lower temperatures of deeper structures if the intensity of the cooling agent and the duration of the application are not adequate, and if the area of the body being treated has low conductivity. However, cooling of muscles and joints is possible when these structures are located more superficially without the presence of excessive adipose tissue. For tissue temperature changes at greater depths to be noted, longer application times are needed.

Decreases in tissue temperature to 10°C or below may result in thermal damage to tissues.[48] Thermal damage may trigger an inflammatory response and result in an increase in edema. This may account, in part, for somewhat conflicting results in animal studies of the effect of cryotherapy on posttraumatic edema.[49–52]

The viscoelastic properties of tissue are also affected by cold application. Just as heat increases elasticity and decreases viscosity, cold has the opposite effect. Tissues that are cooled may not respond as favorably to length changes, and range of motion measures after cold application may not be accurate.

Therapeutic cold reduces the metabolic rate and slows the production of metabolites, resulting in less metabolically generated heat production. The reduction in the metabolic rate also decreases the oxygen demand for tissues, such that tissues can accommodate the decreased blood flow.

Intervention Goals

Knowledge of the physiologic effects of cold helps to identify the benefits of the use of therapeutic cold as an adjunctive intervention in physical therapy. The rationale for using cold is similar to that of the use of therapeutic heat. Addressing impairments, such as edema, pain, muscle guarding and spasm, and abnormal muscle tone, helps in attaining meaningful therapeutic goals related to mobility and function (see Tables 3-2 and 3-3).

Edema Reduction

Cold is commonly used in the management of acute inflammation and edema. Vascular responses to cold affect cell wall permeability, thus inhibiting fluid accumulation in the interstitium. In a recent study of microcirculatory changes in response to cold, Smith and colleagues[54] suggested that the amount of interstitial fluid is controlled by an increase in the reabsorption rate. They reported that there was an increase in the diameter of venules, but no change in arteriolar diameter in response to cold.

The decrease in blood flow associated with vasoconstriction and the decrease in metabolic rate with cold application may result in less accumulation of metabolites and chemical irritants in the injured area. The presence of chemical irritants may themselves trigger an inflammatory and pain response. By minimizing the presence of these irritants, a decrease in the rate of the inflammatory response may be possible, resulting in less edema formation.

Cold applications in combination with compression have been reported to be more effective than compression alone for the management of edema. Basur and associates[55] compared the use of cold and compression to the use of compression alone in the management of acute ankle sprains. They reported that edema was better controlled when using combined cold and compression rather than compression alone. Levy and Marmar[56] reported similar findings in their study of the postoperative management of patients with total knee arthroplasties. In addition to improved edema control with

TABLE 3-3 Treatment Goals for Therapeutic Cold

INDICATION	RATIONALE
Pain reduction	A-beta and C fiber stimulation
Muscle spasm reduction	Decreased muscle spindle activity
Inflammation reduction	Decreased vascular responses
Edema reduction	Vasoconstriction
Hemorrhage containment	Decreased by minimizing effects of active bleeding

cold and compression, they also reported less pain and a greater increase in range of motion. The intensity and duration of cold application appear to influence the effect on edema. More intense cold applied for longer durations may have an adverse effect. Therefore, less intense cold applied for durations of 20 to 30 minutes is recommended. To maximize edema reduction, concomitant compression is also advised. A recent review concluded that more evidence is needed to determine if cold positively affects the consequences of acute soft tissue injury.[56]

Pain Reduction

Cryotherapy is commonly used to decrease pain. The proposed mechanisms by which cold influences pain are similar to those for heat. Cooling agents applied to the skin surface may elevate the pain threshold. Cold is also a counterirritant and may lessen pain sensation by stimulating thermal receptors.

Pain associated with edema and inflammation is both directly and indirectly mediated with cryotherapy. Analgesia is a direct effect of therapeutic cold. Further pain reduction may result from the decrease in chemical irritant response to the decrease in metabolic rate. There may be a decrease in stimulation of mechanoreceptors in the area of injury as swelling is reduced.

Reduction of Muscle Spasm

Muscle guarding or spasm is a local reaction to injury, in which a tonic contraction is sustained in an attempt to "guard" or protect the tissue from further injury. It is also a component of the pain-spasm-pain cycle, and as such may be reflexively affected by a decrease in pain. Muscle tightness may be reduced following cryotherapy if sufficient analgesia is induced to allow stretch of the muscle.

Reduction of Muscle Spasticity

Spasticity is differentiated from muscle spasm in that it is associated with increased resistance to passive stretch, an increase in deep tendon reflexes (DTRs), and clonus. Clonus is defined as the spasmodic alteration of contractions between antagonistic muscle groups because of a hyperactive stretch reflex from an upper motor neuron lesion. Several studies indicate that spasticity can be reduced by cryotherapy.[57–62] Cold application temporarily decreases the amplitude of DTRs. The reduction may be a result of direct cooling of the muscle and can be attributed to stimulation of skin receptors.

Miglietta[60] investigated the effects of cold on sustained ankle clonus and reported that clonus was either decreased or eliminated after cold whirlpool at 18.3°C for 15 minutes. The changes were maintained for several hours.

The decrease in spasticity associated with cryotherapy may have a positive effect on mobility and may allow an increased level of participation in a therapy program. Because the reduction in spasticity can be sustained for several hours, the exercise or activity should be initiated within that time frame. This becomes especially important when establishing a home

Before You Begin

Ask the patient if he or she has a known hypersensitivity to cold. You may choose not to use cold because you do not want to cause an adverse response.

program and instructing the patient, family members, and other care providers in carrying out the program.

Methods of Cold Application

Ice Massage

Ice massage is the application of ice directly onto the skin surface. Because it is an intense cold application, it is usually applied to small areas, such as a muscle belly or trigger point. To cover an area 10 cm by 15 cm, 5 to 10 minutes is needed.[63] Intervention time for ice massage can also be determined by the amount of time needed to numb the area. Before numbness or analgesia occurs, a patient experiences stages of cold, burning, and aching. It is important for the patient to understand that these sensations are normal responses, so that the patient may better tolerate the intervention. The ability to produce numbness depends on the size of the area treated. Smaller areas are recommended because the intensity and localization of the cold application do not allow for effective local temperature regulation, and tissue cooling is achieved.

Paper or Styrofoam cups are filled with water and placed in a freezer. The use of paper or Styrofoam cups provides insulation to the therapist handling the ice cup. The skin surface to be treated should be exposed and the surrounding area draped with a towel to absorb the water as the ice melts.

Cold Packs

Cold packs are a simple and effective method for cooling tissue. There are commercially available cold packs, as well as cold packs that can easily be made a means of delivering very cold temperatures to the intervention area and are considered a good choice for cold interventions. Commercial cold packs contain a semigelled substance, covered in durable plastic. They are manufactured in sizes similar to those of hydrocollator packs. The cold packs are stored in freezer units and remain cold for up to 10 minutes after removal from the cooling unit. They may be applied either directly to the skin or can be used with a wet or dry interface, depending on the desired intensity of the cold application. These cold packs conform to irregular surface areas, but maintaining a constant cold temperature is problematic. Commercial cold packs are reusable and self-contained.

Ice packs can be made using a plastic bag or towel and crushed ice or ice cubes. The use of crushed ice allows for better conformity when applying the ice pack to the body part. The pack can be applied directly to the surface of the skin or it may be applied using a wet or dry towel as an inter-

face. An Ace wrap or second towel may be used to secure the cold or ice pack and to absorb water as the ice melts. Ice packs can be easily made at home and are inexpensive.

The patients should be positioned comfortably and draped appropriately for the duration of the ice application. Average intervention time for a cold or ice pack application is 10 to 15 minutes.

Cold or Ice Baths

Immersion in water that contains partially melted ice cubes is primarily used for distal extremities or larger body parts. Immersion of the body part allows complete conformity of the cooling agent to the skin. Therapeutic temperature ranges for cold baths are between 13° and 18°C, and lower temperatures within this range are tolerated for shorter durations. This method of cryotherapy is easily applied in the home setting.

Controlled cold units   Controlled cold units that apply a simultaneous compression are available as portable home model units and can be effective in controlling postoperative pain and edema. One of these units is pictured in Figure 3-12. Different sleeves and cuffs are available for different areas of the extremity.

Intervention Guidelines

Patient preparation and proper positioning are primary considerations for any method of cold application. The intervention should be explained prior to its initiation. Encourage the patient to ask questions, and stress the importance of verbalizing the response to intervention. Patients should be positioned for comfort, and the area to be treated should be clear of clothing and jewelry. Proper body mechanics for both patient and clinicians is also an important consideration in intervention preparation and patient positioning.

Visual inspection includes an assessment of skin integrity

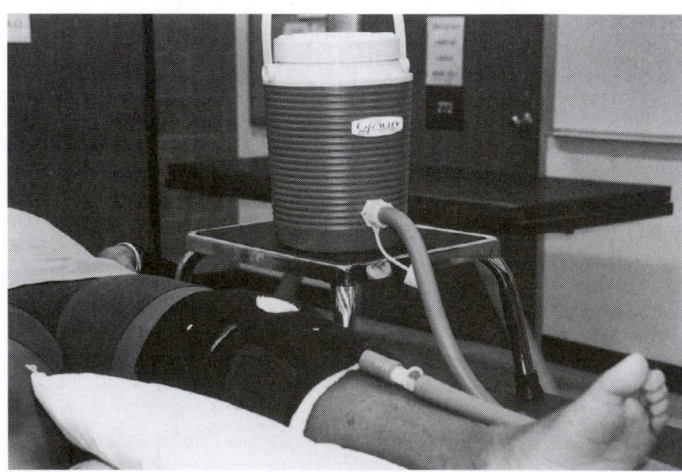

Figure 3-12   Controlled cold unit. (From Michlovitz, SL, and Nolan, TP, eds. Modalities for Therapeutic Intervention, ed 4. FA Davis, Philadelphia, 2005, with permission.)

and appearance and tissue response before, during, and after cryotherapy interventions. In addition to visual inspection, the patient's subjective response should be checked periodically throughout the duration of the intervention.

Safety Considerations with the Application of Cold Intervention

Precautions

Cryotherapy should be used with caution on patients with thermoregulatory problems, sensory deficits, hypersensitivity to cold, and impaired circulation. If cryotherapy is to be used, careful monitoring is essential. Appropriate adjustments of the treatment parameters may be necessary to decrease stress to body systems. For example, if a patient reports an abnormal level of discomfort in response to ice massage, perhaps a method involving less intense cold could be substituted. Cold should not be applied directly over an area of compromised circulation.

Cold applications can cause a transient increase in blood pressure.[64,65] Careful monitoring of blood pressure should be performed before, during, and after cold application if the patient is hypertensive. Intervention should be discontinued if an excessive elevation in blood pressure occurs.

Contraindications

Cryotherapy is contraindicated for patients with particular cold sensitivities. Cold urticaria may include both local and systemic reactions. The local response is characterized by wheals, or raised, reddened areas, that appear in direct response to a local cold application.[66,67] The systemic response may include facial flushing, a drop in blood pressure, an increase in heart rate, and syncope.[68]

Patients with cryoglobulinemia are at risk for developing ischemia or gangrene because of an abnormal blood protein. This protein forms a gel when exposed to cold. This condition is seen in patients with multiple myeloma, chronic liver disease, and several rheumatic diseases.[69]

Patients with Raynaud's disease exhibit cycles of pallor, cyanosis, rubor, and normal color in the hands and feet in response to cold. Numbness, tingling, or burning may also occur. These sensations are similar to the normal stages of sensation experienced with cold, so it is important to pay attention to visual cues as well as subjective responses from the patient.

Paroxysmal cold hemoglobinuria is characterized by the presence of blood in the urine. It can result from either local or systemic exposure to cold. It may not be possible to observe this response in the clinic, but a complete and thorough patient history will help in identifying those individuals at risk.

Clinical Decision Making: Heat or Cold?

Responses to both therapeutic heat application and cryotherapy may be similar. Both heat and cold are effective pain management techniques and both are beneficial in reducing muscle guarding or spasm. Some guidelines apply when making recommendations for the use of heat or cold. The benefits of cold in the management of acute injuries are well documented. For painful conditions associated with acute injuries, cryotherapy is the intervention of choice. Neither heat nor cold provides lasting benefit in the management of chronic pain,[70] but heat may aid in promoting relaxation and could be recommended for home use. Either heat or cold could be used for relief of joint stiffness. Heat enhances the viscoelastic properties of connective tissue and may result in increased motion and decreased pain. Although cold has the opposite effect on connective tissue, it may provide greater pain relief for a given patient. An increase in motion may result, because pain no longer limits the motion.

For pain associated with muscle guarding, either heat or cold may be effective. If a patient has received heat interventions and there is no documented change in the pain level or in range of motion, then a trial of therapeutic cold may be indicated.

Acute injuries are treated with cold because the rates of the inflammation and edema formation are reduced. Heat is contraindicated for acute injuries because it may exacerbate the inflammatory process. However, an increase in blood flow may promote the reabsorption of exudates and may be appropriate in the management of chronic edema and inflammation.

Precautions and contraindications may guide the intervention choice when the intervention goal could be achieved with either heat or cold. Patient tolerance of the thermal agent should not be discounted. If either heat or cold produces discomfort, and if the intervention goal can be achieved with either heat or cold, then patient preference may be the primary determinant.

Documentation

The goals of documentation are to provide an accurate and complete description of the intervention and the patient's response to intervention. Documentation should include all the necessary parameters and components, such that the intervention could be easily reproduced by another clinician. Documentation of the use of any thermal agent should include a description of the type of agent used, the method of application, the area treated, and the position of the patient. For example, report that a "cervical" hot pack was applied to a patient's shoulder using eight layers of toweling. Also, report the position of the patient and the involved extremity if it was supported in a particular position.

Documentation of the patient's response to intervention is important, because it provides a means for evaluating the effectiveness of the intervention and the patient's readiness to progress in the intervention plan. Both subjective and objective responses should be documented. Subjective statements by the patient regarding pain and activity levels are indications of how effective the use of thermal agents is for pain management. Pain levels can be better quantified by using a visual analog scale or verbal rating scale. Objective measures are essential in determining intervention efficacy. Girth and volume measures should be reported to reflect changes in edema and can be used to determine whether changes have been maintained over time. The same is true for goniometric measurements, which are useful in assessing changes in range of motion in response to intervention. Improvement in function is the ultimate therapeutic goal. Although the use of heat or cold may not have a direct effect on function, the functional status of the patient reflects the overall effectiveness of the intervention plan.

 Summary

Throughout this chapter, the safe and effective clinical application techniques for a variety of thermal agents have been presented. Goals of heat or cold intervention, mechanisms of thermal exchange, patient positioning, general health and the age of the patient all play an important part in the clinical decision making involved in the selection and use of thermal agents. Every patient is an individual with a specific set of symptoms and previous or co-existing medical conditions. Clinicians must fully understand not only the benefits of thermal agents application, but also the potential adverse effects that they may cause.

Discussion Questions

1. When would ice or cryotherapy be contraindicated and heat be indicated?
2. When would heat be contraindicated and cryotherapy potentially be indicated?
3. How would you explain the sensations that a patient should expect to feel during an application of superficial heat?
4. How would you explain the sensations that a patient should feel during cryotherapy?

CASE STUDY

Diagnosis: Ankle fracture with loss of range of motion of the ankle in all planes.

Henry is a 45-year-old van driver who has been referred to physical therapy for treatment to relieve pain and stiffness in his left ankle. He has a healed bimalleollar fracture of the ankle. He is 8 weeks postfracture, had surgery to reduce the fracture, and has been out of his cast for 2 days. He is permitted weight-bearing to tolerance and is using crutches for ambulation. The goal of intervention is to reduce pain and stiffness prior to using techniques to restore range of motion.

- What heat agent could you use to reduce pain and stiffness?

Response: If swelling in the ankle were under control, the other options would include Fluidotherapy or warm whirlpool. The advantage to using either Fluidotherapy or whirlpool is that exercise can be performed during heat application. Moist heat packs are another option.

- How would you carry out this intervention? What patient position would you use? Duration of application?

Response: Fluidotherapy could be applied between 106° and 108°F, or whirlpool at about 102°F, with the foot and ankle immersed in the cellulose medium or water, respectively. The agitation for either modality would provide a desensitization and pain control. Henry would be positioned supine with his leg elevated on a pillow. Moist heat could be applied for 15 to 20 minutes; then range-of-motion exercises would follow. (The physical therapist may determine that between heat and range-of-motion exercises, joint mobilization techniques on Henry's ankle should be performed by the physical therapist.)

- Can you give an example where heat would be contraindicated?

Response: Is circulation intact? Does he have a dorsal pedis pulse? Does he have any disease like diabetes or peripheral vascular disease that may impede circulation and prevent dissipation of heat? You do not want to risk a burn as a result of heat application.

- How would you determine if heat was appropriate in accomplishing the intervention goal?

Response: In part, you could determine if pain and stiffness were relieved before exercise (patient self-report).

References

1. Scanlon, VC, and Sanders T: Essentials of Anatomy and Physiology, ed 4. FA Davis, Philadelphia, 2003, pp 376–379.
2. Lehmann, JF, and de Lateur, BJ: Therapeutic heat. In Lehman, JF (ed): Therapeutic Heat and Cold, ed 4. Williams and Wilkins, Baltimore, 1990.
3. Moritz, AR, and Henriques, FC, Jr: Studies in thermal injury. II. The relative importance of time and surface temperature in causation of cutaneous burns. Am J Pathol 23:695, 1947.
4. Henriques, FC, Jr: Studies in thermal injury. V. The predictability and the significance of thermally induced rate processes leading to irreversible epidermal injury. Am J Pathol 23:489, 1947.

5. Abramson, DI, et al: Changes in blood flow, oxygen uptake and tissue temperatures produced by the topical application of wet heat. Arch Phys Med Rehabil 42:305, 1961.

6. Abramson, DI, et al: Indirect vasodilation in thermotherapy. Arch Phys Med Rehabil 46:412–420, 1965.

7. Rabkin, JM, and Hunt, TK. Local heat increases blood flow and oxygen tension in wounds. Arch Surg 122:221, 1987.

8. Melzack, R, and Wall, PD: Pain mechanisms: A new theory. Science 150:971, 1965.

9. Gammon, GD, and Starr, I: Studies on the relief of pain by counter imitation. J Clin Invest 20:13, 1941.

10. Benson, TB, and Copp EP: The effects of therapeutic forms of heat and ice on the pain threshold of the normal shoulder. Rheumatol Rehabil 13:101, 1974.

11. Coseutino, AB, et al: Ultrasound effects on electroneuromyographic measures in sensory fibers in the median nerve. Phys Ther 63:1789, 1983.

12. DeVries, H: Quantitative electromyographic investigation of the spasms theory of muscle pain. Am J Phys Med 45:119, 1966.

13. Harris, R: Physical methods in the management of rheumatoid arthritis. Med Clin North Am 52:707, 1968.

14. Nadler, SF, Steiner, DJ, Erasala, GN, et al: Continuous low-level heat wrap provides more efficacy than ibuprofen and acetaminophen for acute low back pain. Spine 27(10):1012, 2002.

15. Nadler, SF, Steiner, DJ, Petty, SR, et al: Overnight use of continuous low-level heat wrap therapy for relief of low back pain. Arch Phys Med Rehabil 84:335–342, 2003.

16. Mense, S: Effects of temperature on the discharges of muscle spindles and tendon organs. Pflugers Arch 374:159, 1978.

17. LeBann, MM: Collagen tissue: Implications of its response to stress in vitro. Arch Phys Med Rehabil 47:345, 1966.

18. Enneking, WF, and Horowitz, M: The intra-articular effects of immobilization on the human knee. J Bone Joint Surg <AM> 5:973, 1972.

19. Kottke, FJ, Pauley, DL, and Ptok RA: The rationale for prolonged stretching for correction of shortening of connective tissues. Arch Phys Med Rehabil 47:345, 1966.

20. Warren, GC, Lehmann, JF, and Koblanski, JN: Heat and stretch procedures: An evaluation using rat tail tendon. Arch Phys Med Rehabil 57:122, 1976.

21. Light, KE, et al: Low-load prolonged stretch vs high-load brief stretch in treating knee contractures. Phys Ther 664:330, 1984.

22. Backlund, L, and Tiselius, P: Objective measurement of joint stiffness in rheumatoid arthritis. Acta Rheum Scand 13:275, 1967.

23. Greenberg, RS: The effects of hot packs and exercise on local blood flow. Phys Ther 52:273, 1972.

24. Chastain, PB: The effect of deep heat on isometric strength. Phys Ther 58:543, 1978.

25. Edwards, HT, et al: Effect of temperature on muscle energy metabolism and endurance during successive isometric contractions, sustained to fatigue of the quadriceps muscle in man. J Phys 220:335, 1972.

26. Wickstrom, R, and Polk, C: Effect of whirlpool on the strength endurance of the quadriceps muscle in trained male adolescents. Am J Phys Med 40:91, 1961.

27. Abramson, DI, et al: Changes in blood flow, oxygen uptake and tissue temperatures produced by the topical application of wet heat. Arch Phys Med Rehabil 42:305, 1961.

28. Greenberg, RS: The effects of hot packs and exercise on local blood flow. Phys Ther 52:273, 1972.

29. Lehmann, JF, et al: Temperature distributions in the human thigh produced by infrared, hot packs and microwave applications. Arch Phys Med Rehabil 47:291, 1966.

30. Whyte, HM, and Reader, SB: Effectiveness of different forms of heating. Ann Rheum Dis 10:449, 1951.

31. Borrell, RM, et al: Comparison of in vivo temperatures produced by hydrotherapy, paraffin wax treatment and Fluidotherapy. Phys Ther 60:1273, 1980.

32. Borrell, RM, et al: Fluidotherapy: Evaluation of a new heat modality. Arch Phys Med Rehabil 58:69, 1977.

33. Kloth, LC, and Ziskin, MC: Diathermy and pulsed electromagnetic field. In Michlovitz, SL (ed): Thermal Agents in Rehabilitation, ed 2. FA Davis, Philadelphia, 1990.

34. Michlovitz, S, Hun, L, Erasala, GN, Henehold, DA, and Weingand, KW: Continuous low-level heat wrap therapy is effective in treating wrist pain. Arch Phys Med Rehabil 85:1409, 2004.

35. Lewis, T: Observations upon the reactions of the vessels of the human skin to cold. Heart 15:177, 1930.

36. Fox, RH, and Whyatt, HT: Cold-induced vasodilatation in various areas of the body surface in man. J Physiol 162:289, 1962.

37. Downey, JA: Physiologic effects of heat and cold. J Am Phys Ther Assoc 44:713, 1964.

38. Clarke, RSJ, Hellon, RF, and Lind, AR: Vascular reactions of the human forearm to cold. Clin Sci 17:165, 1958.

39. Clarke, RSJ, and Hellon, RF: Hyperemia following sustained and rhythmic exercise in the human forearm at various temperatures. J Physiol 145:447, 1959.

40. Behnke, R: Cold therapy. Athletic Train 9:178, 1974.

41. Behnke, R: Cryotherapy and vasodilation. Athletic Train 8:106, 1973.

42. Grant, AE: Massage with ice (cryokinetics) in the treatment of painful conditions of the musculoskeletal system. Arch Phys Med Rehabil 45:233, 1964.

43. Hayden, C: Cryokinetics in an early treatment program. J Am Phys Ther Assoc 44:11, 1964.

44. Knight, KL, Aquino, J, Johannes, SM, and Urbano, CD: Reexamination of Lewis cold induced vasodilation in the finger and the ankle. Athletic Train 15:248–250, 1980.

45. Moore, R, Nicolette, R, and Behnke, R: The therapeutic use of cold (cryotherapy) in the care of athletic injuries. Athletic Train 2:6, 1967.

46. Moore, R: Uses of cold therapy in the rehabilitation of athletes, recent advances, Proceedings of the 19th American Medical Association National Conference on the Medical Aspects of Sports. San Francisco, June 1977.

47. Murphy, AJ: The physiological effects of cold application. Phys Ther Rev 40:1112, 1960.

48. Olson, JE, and Stravino, U: A review of cryotherapy. Phys Ther 52:840, 1972.

49. Michlovitz, SL: Cryotherapy. In Michlovitz, SL (ed): Thermal Agents in Rehabilitation, ed 2. FA Davis, Philadelphia, 1990.

50. Matsen, FA, Questad, K, and Matsen, AL: The effect of local cooling on post fracture swelling. Clin Orthop 109:201, 1975.

51. Jezdinsky, J, Marek, J, and Ochonsky, P: Effects of local cold and heat therapy on traumatic oedema of the rat hind paw. I: Effects of cooling on the course of traumatic oedema. Acta

Universitatis Palackianae Olomucensis Facultatis Medicae 66:185, 1973.

52. Marek, J, Jezdinsky, J, and Ochonsky, P: Effects of local cold and heat therapy on traumatic oedema of the rat hind paw. II: Effects of various kinds of compresses on the course of traumatic oedema. Acta Universitatis Palackinanae Olomucensis Facultatis Medicae 66:203, 1973.

53. McMaster, WC, and Liddle, S: Cryotherapy influence on post traumatic limb edema. Clin Orthop 150:283, 1980.

54. Smith, TL, et al: New skeletal muscle model for the longitudinal study of alterations in microcirculation following contusion and cryotherapy. Microsurgery 14:487, 1993.

55. Basur, R, Shephard, E, and Mouzos, G: A cooling method in the treatment of ankle sprains. Practitioner 216:708, 1976.

56. Levy, AS, and Marmar, E: The role of cold compression dressings in the postoperative treatment of total knee arthroplasty. Clin Orthop Rel Res 297:174, 1993.

57. Bleakley, C, McDonough, S, and MacAuley, D. The use of ice in the treatment of acute soft-tissue injury: A systematic review of randomized controlled trials. Am J Sports Med 32(1) 251, 2004.

58. Knuttsson, E, and Mattsson, E: Effects of local cooling on monosynaptic reflexes in man. Scand J Rehabil Med 1:126, 1969.

59. Newton, M, and Lehmkuhl, D: Muscle spindle response to body heating and localized muscle cooling: Implications for relief of spasticity. Phys Ther 45:91, 1965.

60. Miglietta, O: Electromyographic characteristics of clonus and influence of cold. Arch Phys Med Rehabil 45:508, 1964.

61. Miglietta, O: Action of cold on spasticity. Am J Phys Med 52:198, 1973.

62. Eldred, E, Lindsley, DF, and Buchwald, JS: The effect of cooling on mammalian muscle spindles. Exp Neurol 2:144, 1960.

63. Hartvikksen, K: Ice therapy in spasticity. Acta Neurol Scand 38:79, 1962.

64. Waylonis, GW: The physiologic effect of ice massage. Arch Phys Med Rehabil 48:37, 1967.

65. Boyer, JT, Fraser, JRE, and Doyle, AE: The haemodynamic effects of cold immersion. Clin Sci 19:539, 1980.

66. Claus-Walker, J, et al: Physiological responses to cold stress in healthy subjects and in subjects with cervical cord injuries. Arch Phys Med Rehabil 55:485, 1974.

67. Austin, KD: Diseases of immediate type hypersensitivity. In Isselbacher, KJ, et al (eds): Harrison's Principles of Internal Medicine, ed 9. McGraw-Hill, New York, 1980.

68. Nadler, SF, Prybicien, M, Malanga, GA, and Sicher, D. Complications from therapeutic modalities: Results of a national survey of athletic trainers. Arch Phys Med Rehabil 84(6):849–853, 2003.

69. Horton, BT, Brown, GE, and Roth, GM: Hypersensitiveness to cold with local and systemic manifestations of a histamine-like character: Its amenability to treatment. JAMA 107:1263, 1936.

70. Schumacher, HR (ed): Cryoglobulinemia. In Primer on Rheumatic Diseases, ed 9. Arthritis Foundation, Atlanta, GA, 1988, p 82.

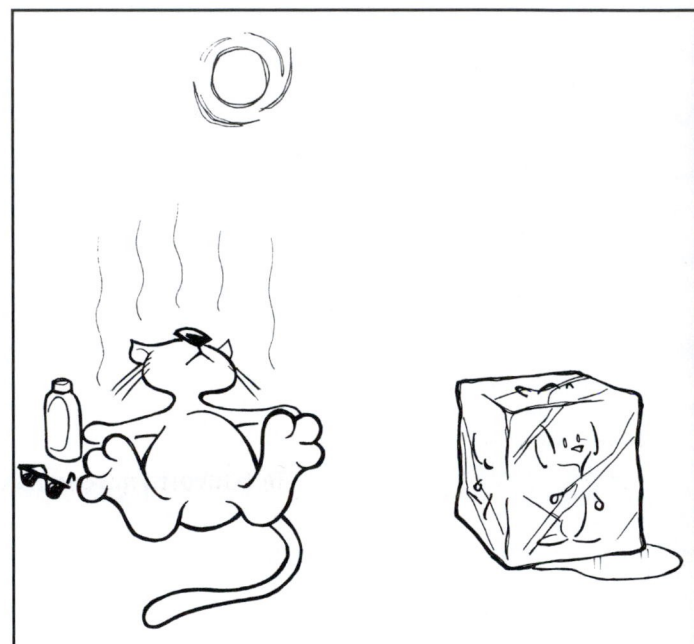

Appendix
Temperature Conversions for Fahrenheit and Centigrade*

To convert Centigrade to Fahrenheit: $\frac{9}{5}\,°C + 32$

°C	°F	°C	°F	°C	°F	°C	°F
46	114.8	22	71.6	34	93.2	10	50.0
45	113.0	21	69.8	33	91.4	9	48.2
44	111.2	20	68.0	32	89.6	8	46.4
43	109.4	19	66.2	31	87.8	7	44.6
42	107.6	18	64.4	30	86.0	6	42.8
41	105.8	17	62.6	29	84.2	5	41.0
40	104.0	16	60.8	28	82.4	4	39.2
39	102.2	15	59.0	27	80.6	3	37.4
38	100.4	14	57.2	26	78.8	2	35.6
37	98.6	13	55.4	25	77.0	1	33.8
36	96.8	12	53.6	24	75.2	0	32.0
35	95.0	11	51.8	23	73.4		

To convert Fahrenheit to Centigrade: $\frac{5}{9}\,(°F - 32)$

°F	°C	°F	°C	°F	°C	°F	°C
120	48.9	76	24.4	98	36.7	54	12.2
119	48.3	75	23.9	97	36.1	53	11.7
118	47.8	74	23.3	96	35.5	52	11.1
117	47.2	73	22.7	95	35.0	51	10.6
116	46.7	72	22.2	94	34.4	50	10.0
115	46.1	71	21.7	93	33.9	49	9.4
114	45.6	70	21.1	92	33.3	48	8.9
113	45.0	69	20.6	91	32.8	47	8.3
112	44.4	68	20.0	90	32.2	46	7.8
111	43.9	67	19.4	89	31.7	45	7.2
110	43.3	66	18.9	88	31.1	44	6.6
109	42.8	65	18.3	87	30.6	43	6.1
108	42.2	64	17.8	86	30.0	42	5.6
107	41.7	63	17.2	85	29.4	41	5.0
106	41.1	62	16.7	84	28.9	40	4.4
105	40.5	61	16.1	83	28.3	39	3.9
104	40.0	60	15.5	82	27.8	38	3.3
103	39.4	59	15.0	81	27.2	37	2.8
102	38.8	58	14.4	80	26.7	36	2.2
101	38.3	57	13.9	79	26.1	35	1.7
100	37.8	56	13.3	78	25.6	34	1.1
99	37.2	55	12.8	77	25.0	33	0.6
						32	0

*From Michlovitz, SL (ed): Thermal Agents in Rehabilitation, ed 3. FA Davis, Philadelphia, 1996, pp 381–383, with permission.

4

Objectives

- Define the parameters and terminology used in therapeutic ultrasound.
- Discuss the effects of varying the parameters in therapeutic ultrasound.
- Describe the clinical applications of therapeutic ultrasound.
- Discuss the theory and rationale for the application of therapeutic ultrasound.
- Discuss the clinical decision-making process for determining treatment parameters when using therapeutic ultrasound.
- Outline current clinical and research trends in the utilization of ultrasound.
- Describe safety factors in the use of therapeutic ultrasound including contraindications., precautions, and equipment considerations.

Key Terms

Absorption
Acoustic
Beam nonuniform
  ratio
Cavitation
Couplant
Dosage

Effective radiating
  area
Frequency
Intensity
Longitudinal
  wave
Megahertz

Nonuniformity
  ratio
Penetration
Phonophoresis
Propagation
Reflection

Refraction
Sound
Standing wave
Transverse wave
Ultrasound
Vibration

Ethne L. Nussbaum, PT, PhD   *Barbara J. Behrens, PTA, MS*

Therapeutic Ultrasound

Outline

> *"Ultrasound, isn't that what they used to take a picture
> of my baby when I was pregnant?"*

Acoustic principles have been used for detection since early in the twentieth century. During the development of underwater detection apparatus in the 1920s, it was observed that extremely high pressure waves were damaging to living tissues. As early as the 1930s, low intensities of ultrasound were used for the first time in physical medicine to treat soft tissue conditions with mild heating. Today therapeutic ultrasound is a commonly used modality in therapy clinics, being used for its deep heating properties. However, the therapeutic ultrasound that is available in the twenty-first century is capable of many more applications than just deep heat. Some of the research that is discussed in this chapter outlines the potential benefits of ultrasound for nonthermal applications.

 ## Physical Principles

Sound is produced by vibration of a medium. If a column of air is vibrated, the human ear may be able to perceive the disturbance. However, ultrasound has a pitch that is too high for the human ear to perceive; that is, its frequency is beyond audible sound, hence the term *ultra*sound. A sound wave exerts pressure on the medium it travels through, alternately compressing, or "squeezing," and then releasing pressure on the particles of the medium. During the release phase, which is referred to as rarefaction, molecules are spread out more than during the compression phase (Fig. 4-1). Sound can be transmitted through liquid, gas, or solid media, but not through a vacuum.

Beating a drum is an example of transmitting a sound wave through air. We hear the disturbance of the air particles because the frequency or pitch of the sound is within our audible range of 30 up to 20,000 cycles per second. Therapeutic ultrasound is typically applied at either 1 million cycles per second (megahertz) or 3 MHz. Why?

Because sound energy is transmitted as a wave, there are a number of principles from wave theory that are valid for sound and ultrasound. A principle common to all wave formation is that matter in a wave does not itself travel; only the wave energy is transmitted. Each vibrating particle collides with and displaces its nearest neighbor, transferring momentum in a chain reaction. A desk ornament, sometimes called Newton's Balls of Motion, illustrates some principles of this type of energy transfer. This mobile consists of a frame with five metal balls suspended on thin rods from a horizontal bar so that they touch each other at rest. A person lifts and releases the first ball to set the mobile in motion. When the first ball swings back into place it bumps into the next ball, which in turn bumps into the one after it. In this way, the energy is transferred from ball to ball. Because the last ball is unopposed it swings out into space. However, when it drops back into line, a new cycle is set in motion (Fig. 4-2). The mobile will continue to oscillate until it runs out of energy and the balls then come to rest. And how does this relate to ultrasound in the body?

Waves travel through media in three modes: longitudinal, transverse, and standing waves. When the particles of a medium are compressed and decompressed in the direction that the wave travels, it is termed a *longitudinal wave*. When the particle movement is at right angles to the direction of travel, it is termed a *shear* or *transverse wave*. Shear waves propagate more readily in solids, and longitudinal waves, in liquids and gases. Note that a wave traveling on the surface of water is a shear wave, which means that it is an exception to the rule. Sound travels in longitudinal mode in human tissues. However, a shear wave may be propagated when a pressure wave reaches bone, at which point a wave is transmitted along the periosteum, the outer covering of the bone.

 ### Patient Perspective

Remember that your patient does not understand what you are doing. It is important to explain ultrasound to him or her in terms that can easily be understood. Many patients are accustomed to feeling something with treatment interventions. This may or may not be the case with ultrasound. It is important for you to explain this before, during, and after your session with the patient.

Palpation of the area if appropriate, before and after treatment, can provide valuable information regarding soft tissue response to the treatment intervention as well as instill a more human touch to treatment.

PATIENTS' FREQUENTLY ASKED QUESTIONS

1. Will I feel anything from this?
2. Is this like what they use for babies?
3. Would a dog be able to hear ultrasound?
4. How does that work?
5. Why do you use that gel?
6. Why do you move that "thing" on me during a treatment?
7. If it is doing something, why don't I feel anything?
8. Is there a maximum number of treatments you can have with ultrasound?
   a. If yes, what is it?

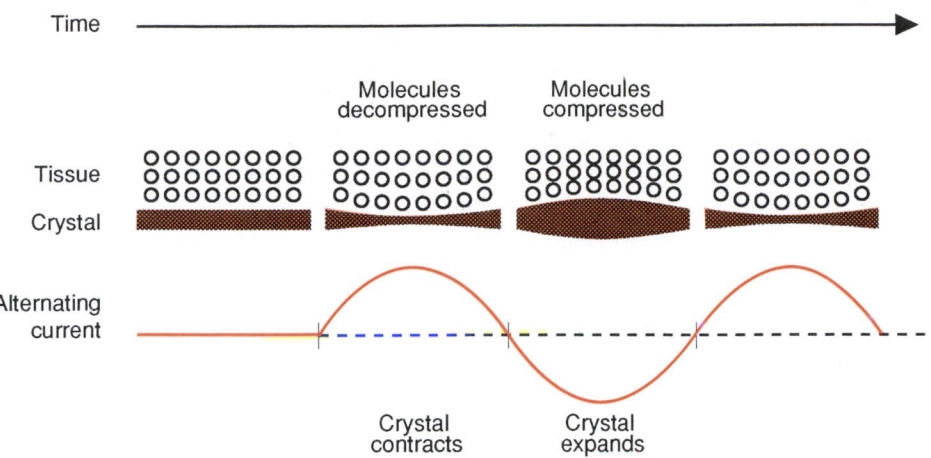

Figure 4–1 Schematic diagram showing the effect of a changing electrical field on crystal size and the effect of changing pressure on tissue molecules in the sound field.

If the source of a wave is kept stationary opposite a boundary and the path of the incident and reflected waves coincide, the resultant energy along the path is the algebraic sum of the two waves. If the waves are also exactly in phase so that the high and low peaks of the inbound wave reinforce the high and low peaks of the returning wave, very intense peaks and lows of power result and the position of the wave is stationary. This is called a standing wave. To prevent the formation of standing waves during a treatment intervention with ultrasound, the transducer must be continuously moved.

Therapeutic Ultrasound

With therapeutic ultrasound, the wave transmitted to the tissues cannot be perceived as audible sound, by either the patient or the clinician. However, if sufficient energy is delivered to the tissues, the patient will experience a sensation of mild warmth. Two characteristics of audible sound, pitch and volume, which describe (or quantify) the frequency and power of sound, respectively, are important parameters in therapeutic ultrasound.

Another important characteristic in ultrasound is whether emission is in a continuous or an interrupted mode.

The role of these and other parameters in the effects of ultrasound will be discussed in this chapter (Box 4-1).

Characteristics of Ultrasound Emission and Relevance to Intervention Outcome

Characteristics discussed in this section include the following: frequency, pulsed- as opposed to continuous-wave delivery, absorption and penetration, attenuation, reflection and refraction, power, intensity and dosage, and beam profile. Understanding the clinical implications of these factors will assist the clinician in providing effective and safe applications using ultrasound (Table 4-1).

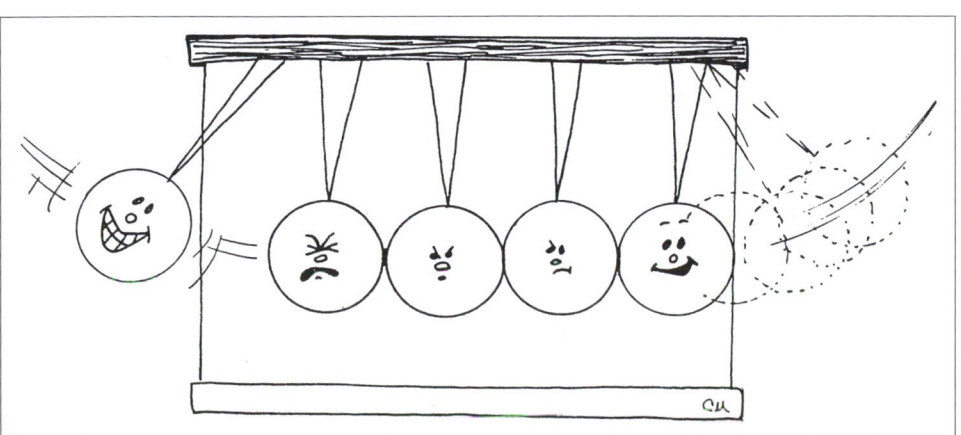

Figure 4–2 Illustration of Newton's Balls of Motion desk mobile. Movement of the first ball is translated into movement of the second ball just as compression force applied to soft tissues would be transferred to the underlying soft tissues during the application of ultrasound. Energy is lost as the distance from the source is increased and a rebound effect occurs, which can result in a cancellation of energy, or implosion.

Before You Begin

PARAMETER SELECTION QUESTION

1. Is the tissue I am treating superficial (use 3 MHz) or deep (use 1 MHz)?

Operational definitions

Superficial: something that can be easily palpated, 1 to 3 cm deep

Deep: 3 to 5 cm deep within the tissue

Frequency

Frequency describes the number of events that take place within a set time frame. In sound waves, frequency refers to the number of completed wave cycles that pass a fixed point in 1 second. The higher the frequency, the greater is the number of cycles per second; conversely, lower frequency means fewer cycles per second. Previously, the concept of pitch was mentioned in relation to the frequency of sound. Higher pitch sounds have higher frequency than lower pitch sounds. High-frequency sound waves vibrate air molecules more rapidly and thus expend their energy sooner, which means over a shorter distance, than do lower-frequency sounds. In contrast, lower-pitch sounds vibrate air molecules more slowly, thus expending their energy more slowly, and consequently have a greater capacity to travel distances than do higher-frequency waves. Consider which pitch sounds you would most likely hear if your neighbors were having a noisy party—higher- or lower-pitch sounds? It is often the pounding of the bass speaker that alerts uninvited neighbors to the fact that someone is hosting a party. The fact that bass tones or lower-frequency sound waves travel a greater distance than higher-frequency sound waves is a physical characteristic of sound that will apply in determining whether to use a 1-MHz (1 million cycles per second) or a 3-MHz sound wave for ultrasound therapy. The decision should depend on whether the target tissue lies in deep (1 MHz) or superficial (3 MHz) tissue layers.

Pulsed or Continuous Ultrasound

Continuous ultrasound refers to an uninterrupted flow of sound waves. Pulsed ultrasound is produced by intermittently interrupting the supply of electrical energy to the ultrasound head, which causes the acoustical energy, or sound waves, to be discontinuous. The effects of ultrasound depend partly on duration of application; hence, there is a different effect when the output of the device is pulsed.

The percentage of "on" time of ultrasound output is known as the duty factor, which can be expressed as a percentage or as a ratio. Clearly, when output is continuous, the duty factor is 100%; the output must have an "off" time for it to be considered pulsed. For example, if an ultrasound unit was programmed to emit for equal on and off periods, that is output for half the time, the duty factor could be expressed as either 50% or a ratio of 1:1. Commonly used duty factors are shown in Table 4-2.

The intensity registered on an ultrasound unit during delivery of pulsed ultrasound signifies the intensity delivered *during* each pulse (i.e., the "on" period). This should be made clear in documentation by using the term "temporal peak intensity," or sometimes just I_{SATP}, to describe the intensity of pulsed ultrasound treatment. The average intensity delivered during pulsed ultrasound is not shown on the unit. Average intensity of a treatment would depend on the duration of the "off" periods: the lower the duty cycle, the longer are the "off" periods and therefore the lower is the average intensity. "Temporal average intensity" is sometimes abbreviated as the term I_{SATA}.

Practice varies with respect to documentation of pulsed ultrasound. Some clinicians describe intensity delivered during the pulse (I_{SATP}), yet others describe intensity averaged over the on and off pulse periods (I_{SATA}). The manner of reporting in textbooks and journals is similarly confusing. Thus, it is important that clinicians understand when using pulsed ultrasound that the unit controls always refer to the intensity delivered during the pulse. Appropriately, it is

TABLE 4-1 Sound Terminology		
SOUND	**ULTRASOUND PARAMETERS**	
Pitch	Frequency	3 MHz to 1 MHz
Volume	Power	Watts (W)
Temporal quality	Mode of energy delivery	Continuous wave or pulsed wave

TABLE 4-2 Common Duty Factors for Ultrasound		
Continuous	Duty factor	100%
1:1 Ratio	Duty factor	50%
1:4 Ratio	Duty factor	20%

Before You Begin

PARAMETER SELECTION QUESTIONS

1. Is the tissue I am treating superficial (use 3 MHz) or deep (use 1 MHz)?

2. Are the signs and symptoms suggestive of acute inflammation? (Use a 20% duty factor, i.e., a ratio of 1:4, when treating acute inflammation.).

becoming the norm in current literature to define the terminology used for pulsed ultrasound intensity. In this chapter, intensity of pulsed ultrasound signifies the intensity delivered during the pulse, that is, the intensity registered on the ultrasound unit (W/cm^2).

When ultrasound is applied continuously (100% duty factor), the mechanical vibrations transmitted to the tissue molecules may cause heating of the underlying tissues. Thus, it is important to consider the underlying processes or metabolic state of the tissues when planning to use ultrasound. The five cardinal signs of acute inflammation are pain, erythema, edema, heat, and loss of function. If a heightened level of inflammatory activity were already present in the tissues, it would not be prudent to use continuous ultrasound because it might make the condition worse by adding more heat to the area. A pulsed form of ultrasound, which would not likely generate additional heat in already hot tissues, might be more prudent. The relative acuteness of the patient's problem presents the second question that a clinician must consider when

determining the parameters for ultrasound: Are the signs and symptoms suggestive of acute inflammation? Acute inflammation should be treated using a 20% duty factor and low intensity of ultrasound, delivered for periods of 10 to 20 minutes depending on the size of the treatment area and the transducer.

Absorption and Penetration

To absorb is to "take something in." Penetrate means to "enter into." Penetration in ultrasound is the term used to describe the distance from the sound source at which 50% of the original energy remains. As tissues absorb energy from a sound wave, a reduced amount of energy remains to be carried forward by the wave, which lessens its penetration; hence there is an inverse relationship between absorption and penetration. If energy penetrates deeply into the tissues, then it means it was not absorbed. Conversely, if energy does not penetrate deeply, then the tissues must have absorbed it (Fig. 4-3).

Ultrasound energy is absorbed differently by different types of tissue depending on the compactness of the tissues. Acoustic impedance is the term that denotes the relative resistance of a medium to wave energy: the more dense or compact the molecules and the less compliant they are when squeezed, the greater is the impedance. More work has to be done to transmit a wave against high impedance. Thus, it follows that over any given distance that a wave travels, the denser is the medium, the greater is the amount of energy absorbed from the wave, and the greater is the decrease in distance that the wave travels.

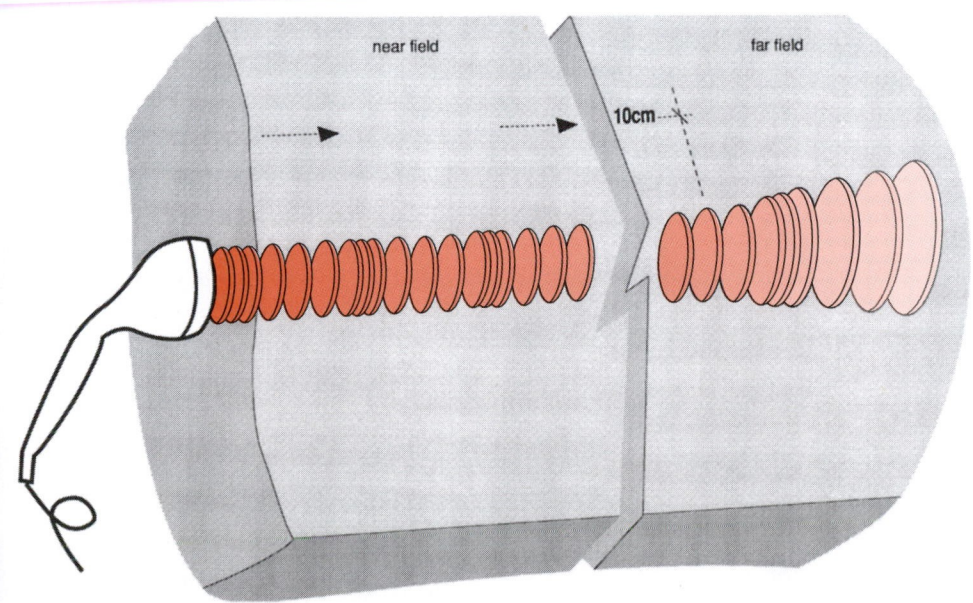

Figure 4-3 Schematic diagram showing transmission of ultrasound through a large homogeneous tissue with beam divergence in the far field.

The density of a medium similarly affects the distance that audible sound travels. The rate of absorption of sound in air is relatively low because gas molecules are easily compressed; this explains the great distance that sound travels through air. In contrast, through a dense medium such as brick, energy is rapidly consumed because the molecules resist compression. Unfortunately, there are few materials that completely absorb sound. However, the volume that you hear from your neighbor's party is not as high as the volume that you would hear if you were at your neighbor's party. Clearly, walls absorb some acoustical energy!

Tissue is a medium that is more dense than air but less dense than brick. Tissue, however, is not a homogeneous medium; it consists of many layers and compartments of quite different densities. Each tissue layer transmits and absorbs ultrasound according to its specific acoustical properties. Fluid elements, such as blood and water, have the lowest impedance values and lowest acoustic absorption coefficients. This means that these elements are poor absorbers of ultrasound. Bone, the densest of all tissues, has the highest impedance value and highest acoustic absorption coefficient. This implies that bone is a good absorber of ultrasound. This is an important factor to consider when selecting the appropriate frequency of ultrasound, because the frequency controls the depth of penetration.

Reflection and Refraction

To reflect, according to *Webster's*, is "to bend or cast back (as light, heat, or sound)." Sound waves may be partially reflected from boundaries or obstacles that they encounter (Fig. 4-4). The reflected portion of the wave continues to be subject to the effects of absorption, transmission, or further reflection on the original side of the boundary. The portion of the wave transmitted across the boundary is reduced in power as a result of reflection. Within biologic tissues, such boundaries may be formed by any two heterogeneous tissue surfaces, such as bone and nerve, or muscle and adipose tissue, and many other examples.

In human tissues, ultrasound repeatedly encounters boundaries. The acoustic properties of skin, fat, blood vessels, and muscle are similar. When ultrasound encounters boundaries between acoustically similar tissues, such as adipose and muscle, the amount of reflection is insignificant to treatment outcome. However, reflection increases in proportion to the difference in acoustic impedance of the two boundary materials.

Because the impedance characteristics of metal and air are so different, the amount of reflection at a metal-air interface is about 99%, which means that the amount of ultrasound transmitted from a metal transducer to air is negligible. This is the reason for using a coupling medium between the transducer and the skin during ultrasound treatment. At a tissue-bone interface, about 25% of incident energy is reflected (see Fig. 4-4). If a wave meets a boundary at an angle, the reflected wave is directed away from the boundary on a new path that has the same angle but is a mirror image of the inward-bound wave.

The wave portion that is transmitted across a boundary is also subject to "bending" if the wave meets the boundary at an angle. This is known as refraction. As children, many of us played with a prism that split, or refracted, white light into the colors, or wavelengths, of the rainbow. The light was bent, that is, refracted at the glass-air interface because the prism walls were at an angle to the light source. Refraction is proportional to the difference in acoustic impedance of the boundary materials and to the incident angle of the wave. Refraction at boundaries formed by touching layers of skin, fat, blood, or muscle is very small. At tissue-air boundaries, however, because the impedance characteristics of tissue and air are so different, the transmitted wave changes direction by 90°. This means the wave travels along the boundary of the original side instead of crossing it, which is known as total internal reflection. The clinical relevance is that ultrasound energy cannot be transmitted from the skin surface to air. For example, ultrasound applied to one surface of the hand would penetrate the tissue and at the opposite skin surface of the hand the beam would be "bent" back into the tissues, where an additional amount of the remaining energy would be absorbed.

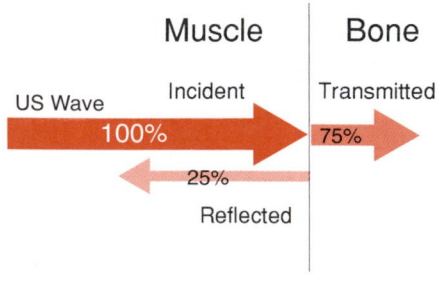

A.

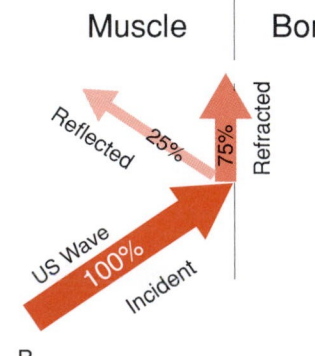

B.

Figure 4-4 Schematic diagram showing reflection and refraction of ultrasound at a muscle-bone interface. (*A*) A wave arriving perpendicular to the boundary. (*B*) A wave arriving at an angle of 34° from the perpendicular.

When a wave is stationary opposite a boundary and the paths of the inward bound and reflected waves coincide, the resultant energy along the path is the algebraic sum of the two waves. If the waves are also exactly in phase so that the high and low peaks of the inbound waves reinforce the high and low peaks of the reflected waves, very intense changes occur in pressure. This is known as a standing wave. Standing waves may result in unstable cavitation at high ultrasound intensity, which could cause tissue damage. To prevent standing wave formation, the ultrasound transducer should be continuously moved during treatment.

Cavitation

Cavitation is the term for the stimulated behavior of micron-sized gas bubbles in the fluids in a sound field. These bubbles alternately shrink and expand as they lose and gain air during the compression and rarefaction phases, respectively, of a sound wave. Cavitation can be potentially helpful or harmful to human tissues depending upon the type of cavitation. During stable cavitation the ebb and flow of gasses causes small changes in bubble radius. It is thought that these effects may contribute to the increased cell membrane permeability that is observed following ultrasound application.

Cavitation activity increases as wave intensity increases. Under more intense pressure fluctuations, gas bubbles in an ultrasound field gradually increase in size, because they take in more air than they lose. During unstable cavitation, gas bubbles that have grown relatively large collapse violently under pressure. This event might have a parallel in the implosion of a building, which is a sight that most people find fascinating for a building but not for living tissues. Explosive devices are set off in a highly orchestrated pattern so that the building loses its structural integrity and literally falls into itself. Although bubble collapse occurs on a microscopic scale in living tissue under the influence of ultrasound, it, too, can be highly destructive. However, a number of conditions must coexist for unstable cavitation to occur: ultrasound intensity must be high, the duration for bubble expansion must be relatively long, and there needs to be sufficient repetition of cycles for bubbles to reach a critical size. Frequency and cycle duration are inversely related; therefore, the duration for bubble growth is longer for lower-frequency waves. This explains why unstable cavitation occurs more readily at 1-MHz ultrasound rather than at 3 MHz.[10]

Unstable cavitation is more likely to occur during therapeutic ultrasound when improper technique is used, such as *not* moving the transducer during treatment, and may occur during pulsed or continuous modes of ultrasound.

Beam Qualities

The importance of being aware of the characteristics of the beam of one's ultrasound device is often not fully appre-

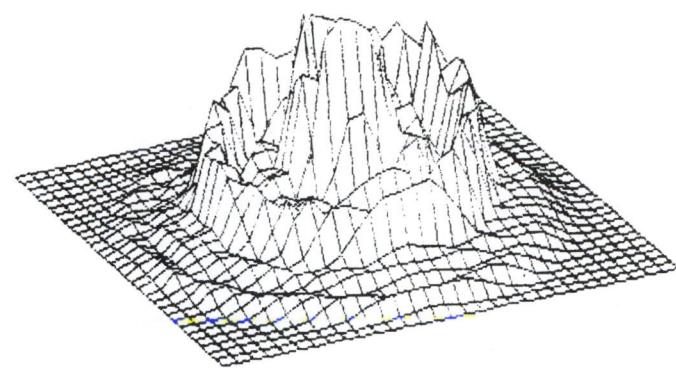

Figure 4-5 Hydrophone scan of an ultrasound beam in water showing uneven spatial distribution of energy. Characteristics: frequency 1 MHz; distance from transducer 0.5 cm; ERA 5.2 cm^2; BRN 4.2. (Courtesy of Excel Tech Ltd., Mississauga, Canada.)

ciated. Two characteristics are of particular importance: the beam nonuniformity ratio (BNR) and the effective radiating area (ERA).

Beam Nonuniformity Ratio

The BNR is the ratio of the peak power to the average power in the ultrasound beam measured in any cross-sectional plane. BNR is measured using an underwater microphone known as an acoustical hydrophone. The ultrasound applicator is mounted in a tank of degassed water, and the hydrophone moves over the surface of the applicator measuring the output. A plot of the energy values is produced. BNR varies with distance from the transducer face. The BNR measured at point of manufacture of a device usually refers to

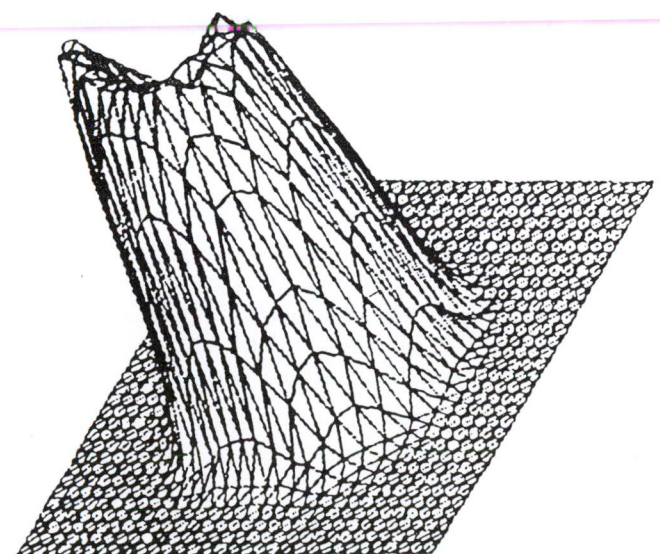

Figure 4-6 Hydrophone scan in water of an ultrasound beam of 1 MHz taken at a distance 10.0 cm from the transducer face. (Courtesy of Excel Tech Ltd., Mississauga, Canada.)

the values measured at a distance of 0.5 cm from the transducer surface (Figs. 4-5 and 4-6).

A beam ratio of 1:1 would mean that intensity would be unvarying over the entire cross-sectional area of the beam. However, this is not possible because of the physical phenomenon of wave interference, which occurs when waves meet in a medium. An acceptable BNR for ultrasound devices in the United States is approximately 6:1 or lower. This means that as the transducer is moved over the skin, there is a "spot" in the tissues receiving ultrasound at an intensity of up to six times higher than the set dose (W/cm^2). This "hot spot" occurs whether the applicator is moved or held stationary. It is disturbing to find evidence in the literature that some devices operate with much higher BNR values than 6 because there is substantial evidence that very high doses of ultrasound can be hazardous to regenerating tissue.[7,8]

Effective Radiating Area

The ERA (cm^2) describes the radiating area of the ultrasound applicator. This area is usually determined at a distance of 0.5 cm from the transducer face using the same underwater hydrophone mentioned previously. As a rule the ERA signifies the area of the beam that transmits clinically effective radiation power (5% or more of the maximum intensity in that plane). By this rule, the very low pressure area around the perimeter of the ultrasound beam is not considered part of the ERA. The ERA is less than the geometric area of the crystal. Accurate measurement of the transducer ERA is important because this value is incorporated into the intensity value registered on the device during ultrasound treatment (W/cm^2).

If the crystal is in some way defective and the actual ERA is not equal to the ERA measured at point of manufacture, then the registered dose is not an accurate reflection of the actual dose being received by the patient. The finding of discrepancies between actual and nominal ERA in supposedly functioning units is reported in the literature.[5,6] Furthermore, poor-quality crystals are inefficient and are capable of operating with only a fraction of the surface area transmitting a sound wave. In the event of using a severely damaged crystal to deliver ultrasound, it would be hit and miss whether the target area actually received treatment.

To ensure that the intended dose of ultrasound can be delivered safely and reliably to the tissues, clinicians are encouraged to have the BNR and ERA of their ultrasound devices characterized on an annual basis, or more often if damage is suspected.

Biophysical Effects

The effects of ultrasound vary depending on whether the intensity delivered is high enough to cause heating of the tissues or whether heating is minimized or eliminated by using low-intensity, pulsed-mode delivery.

Thermal Ultrasound

The ultrasound beam does not itself transmit heat; however, heat is generated within the tissues as a result of increased molecular vibration due to absorption of ultrasound energy. Unstable cavitation may also contribute to tissue heating: gas bubble "implosion" sends shock waves through the tissues, which releases energy that increases tissue temperature.

More heat is generated using ultrasound at a frequency of 3 MHz than at 1 MHz because more energy is delivered at the higher frequency. You can crudely mimic this effect by rubbing back and forth with a fingertip over a small area of your skin. The skin becomes heated. Note that rubbing faster will produce greater heat. However, when energy is absorbed, penetration is reduced. Thus, although heating is greater using 3-MHz ultrasound, the effect is more superficial when compared with 1-MHz ultrasound. Ultrasound at 3 MHz is too superficial for heating deep-seated lesions, such as plantar fasciitis or adhesive capsulitis of the shoulder.

Energy is absorbed from an ultrasound beam in proportion to the density of the tissue. Different tissues will therefore become heated in proportion to their density. This is the basis of the statement often seen in the literature that protein structures "selectively" absorb ultrasound. It is probably more correct to state that ultrasound provides clinicians with an opportunity to deliver heat selectively to dense tissues, such as scar tissue, joint capsule, ligament, and tendon.

General principles of heat transfer also apply to heating with ultrasound. This means that the temperature produced in the tissues will be the net effect of absorbed mechanical energy that is converted to heat, and heat transfer to or from the tissues by conduction and convection. It was noted previously that ultrasound is rapidly absorbed by periosteum, which becomes significantly heated. As a result, structures adjacent to bone gain additional heat in an ultrasound treatment by conduction of heat from the periosteum. Convection currents exist both within tissues, via circulating blood and lymph, and external to tissues, via circulating air or water acting on the skin. Clinically this means that relatively dense, less-vascular structures, such as branches of peripheral nerves, scar tissue, capsule, ligament, tendon, and bone, that rapidly absorb ultrasound and therefore heat well also retain heat better than more vascular structures. Muscles, on the other hand, especially large, "red" postural muscles, have an abundant capillary network, with the result that they rapidly lose heat to adjacent cooler tissue through convection and conduction.

It is important to note that heating effectiveness of ultrasound is reduced when treatment is applied under water. There are two reasons for this. First, some energy "escapes" from the skin surface to the water as a result of reflection. Second, some heat is transferred from the skin surface to the water by conduction. To compensate for the above, the intensity of ultrasound should be increased by at least 50% when treatment is applied under water. For example, if you typically apply ultrasound directly to the skin with gel coupling using an intensity of 1.0 W/cm², you would deliver 1.5 W/cm² to achieve similar thermal effects under water.

Effects of tissue heating generally depend on the the temperature produced rather than on the modality used. Effects of ultrasound in the temperature range of 40° to 45°C include reduced pain due to decreased nerve conduction velocity, increased metabolic rate, increased blood flow to assist in resolution of swelling, enhanced immune system response, increased extensibility of soft tissue, and decreased viscosity of tissue fluids.[11] Temperatures above 45°C are noxious to tissues and can cause nonreversible tissue changes. However, pain is normally felt before dangerous temperatures are reached.

Nonthermal Ultrasound

When heating effects of ultrasound are reduced, either by application of very low intensity or by pulsing the ultrasound, changes in cell function are noted. Mechanical vibration and acoustic streaming are possible mechanisms underlying the nonthermal changes.

Mechanical Vibration Effects and Acoustic Streaming

Cell membranes may become destabilized as a result of the deformation and distortion to which cells are subjected during ultrasound.[12] Radiation force is the proper term to describe this mechanism, but it is sometimes referred to by the slang term "micromassage." Stable cavitation is thought to contribute to these effects.[10] Cavitation produces eddy currents in the fluid surrounding a vibrating bubble; eddy currents in turn subject cell membranes and intracellular organelles in the vicinity of vibrating gas bubbles to additional rotational forces and stresses.[13] This fluid movement in a sound field is generally known as acoustic streaming, but in an ultrasound field in living tissue, the scale of the events is microscopic, so it is sometimes called microstreaming.

To summarize the role of bubble activity (cavitation) in ultrasound mechanisms, it appears that gas bubbles are readily generated in an ultrasound field in living tissue even at low intensities.[14] Bubble activity augments the mechanical effect of a pressure wave. The scale of cavitation depends on the ultrasound characteristics; bubble growth is limited when ultrasound is pulsed, intensity is low, and frequency is high. Higher frequency means shorter cycle duration, so that the time for bubble growth is restricted. Pulsed ultrasound restricts the number of successive cycles for growth, which allows the bubble to regain its initial size during the off period. The likelihood of unstable cavitation during ultrasound is very low when using 3 MHz, 20% duty cycle, and low inten-

sity. Cavitation is a phenomenon, however, that must be considered in both thermal and nonthermal ultrasound.

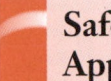

Safety Considerations with the Application of Ultrasound

Precautions

Precautions are necessary to protect patients and equipment. Discomfort should not be experienced during treatment. Pain is usually a sign of too much periosteal heating, and treatment settings must be adjusted by decreasing intensity or moving the transducer more quickly. It is possible to cause a burn with ultrasound,[53] and this is the reason why some national radiation councils have regulated output limits for ultrasound.[23]

A stationary transducer technique is not safe for most clinical applications; there is a great risk of overheating at "hot spots" in the field and there is an added risk of standing wave formation. This caution especially applies when there are implanted materials in the tissues.[98,99] Metal reflects about 90% of incident ultrasound,[5] and therefore the chance of standing wave formation is increased. Plastic responds like periosteum and it absorbs a large percentage of ultrasound.[98,100] Generally, treatment over implanted materials is safe provided proper technique is used. It should be noted that a stationary transducer technique (20 minutes daily at intensity of 0.15 W/cm² I_{SATP}, pulsed 1:4) is used in treatment of fractures; however, the intensity is very low compared with most other clinical applications.

Skin integrity is not essential for ultrasound treatment, but direct contact with gel may be inappropriate over some skin lesions or in conditions such as dermatitis. A water-immersion technique can be used provided infection control procedures are followed. Clinicians should protect themselves by wearing loose-fitting gloves when applying ultrasound under water. A glove traps air, which reflects ultrasound, and thus prevents self-treatment at the same time as preventing the risk of cross-infection.

Transducer crystals are fragile and transducers should be handled with care. Intensity should be increased only when the transducer is in contact with a suitable medium, because a metal-air interface prevents transmission of the pressure wave. When energy cannot flow from the transducer, the metal cap itself becomes heated. Heat may affect the bonding of the crystal within the transducer. Repeated careless use of the transducer will eventually damage the crystal.

Contraindications

Ultrasound promotes cell proliferation and cell activity. Abnormal cell division occurs in many serious medical conditions, including cancer and tuberculosis, and in non–life-threatening diseases such as psoriasis. Ultrasound is contraindicated over or close to the site of any abnormal growth. The clinician should be extraordinarily cautious in treating undiagnosed pain in patients with a past history of malignancy.[101] Tissue being treated with radiation therapy should not be treated with ultrasound.

Rapid cell division is also a feature of fetal development and, as yet, the effect of therapeutic ultrasound on the human fetus is unknown.[102,103] For safety, ultrasound treatment should never be applied over the lower back or abdomen of a pregnant woman. It should be noted that diagnostic ultrasound, at 2.5 MHz, is used at significantly lower doses than therapeutic ultrasound (less than 0.1 W/cm^2).

The contraindication to treatment over epiphyseal plates in children has been passed on as part of the tradition of ultrasound. These plates give rise to new bone cells. The original work that gave rise to concern was done on legs of anesthetized dogs at very low frequency (0.8 MHz) and high intensity (0.5–3.0 W/cm^2) using a stationary transducer. These characteristics would have caused high absorption and intense heating of bone. Subsequent work on animal bone by Dyson[104] and others[76] suggests that healing fractures in fact benefit from ultrasound at low doses. In view of the adverse treatment characteristics of the early work and advantages found in recent work, treatment over epiphyseal plates in children is not considered a contraindication at the present time. However, it is suggested that low treatment intensity should be used.

Treatment of the orbits of the eyes and directly over the gonads is contraindicated. Ultrasound should not be applied over the area of a thrombus.[105] Treatment of the calf after a deep vein thrombosis is also contraindicated: it is thought that ultrasound might dislodge a thrombus, which could have catastrophic consequences.

Pain and temperature awareness must be checked before treatment with continuous-mode ultrasound. Sensation must be intact to proceed with heating dosages.

Infection that is enclosed under tension, that is, abscesses, should not be treated with ultrasound. Infection with open drainage can be treated using very low pulsed dosages but should be discontinued if there are any signs of increased redness, heat, or pain.

Ultrasound vibration may interfere with operation of any implanted medical device, such as a pacemaker, and should be avoided directly over the device. Ultrasound should not be applied below the ribs directed toward the heart.[106]

Ultrasound should not be used when there is uncontrolled bleeding. It is ideal for enhancing resorption of fluid, but treatment should begin after bleeding has ceased or after replacement factor has been administered in conditions such as hemophilia.

Second-Order Effects of Nonthermal Ultrasound

The primary site of ultrasound interaction is the cell membrane.[12] Destabilization of membranes leads to increased permeability, which allows various ions and molecules to diffuse into cells, where they precipitate a series of secondary events. Research on ultrasound has particularly focused on influx of calcium ions because calcium is a known second messenger for other cell functions, including protein synthesis. Histamine has also attracted interest because of its influence on circulation and stimulating effect on protein synthesis. Clinically, it has been demonstrated that ultrasound facilitates tissue repair, and researchers are exploring various events that could explain the clinical benefits.[15] Some of the observed effects are discussed later.

Histamine and other vasoactive substances are released from granules in mast cells and from circulating platelets during ultrasound.[16] The extent of mast cell degranulation is in proportion to the ultrasound intensity. It is important to keep treatment intensity low as there is some indication from animal research that high-intensity ultrasound could produce too much histamine, which could potentially prolong inflammation rather than producing the desired stimulus to healing. Prolonged inflammation can potentially occur with any heat treatment given during the acute inflammatory stage of an injury.

Increased plasma and cells for repair appear in the extravascular tissues following ultrasound. The result is an enhanced inflammatory response. Inflammation is an essential step in tissue repair because it brings cells that are normally in the circulation into the injury site. It is hypothesized that ultrasound may enhance the normal response. For example, monocytes arrive at the wound site and are turned into macrophages, which cleanse the wound. The macrophages also release growth factors that attract fibroblasts.

Phagocytic activity of macrophages is increased during ultrasound. Accompanying this is an increase in the concentration and activity of lysosomes; lysosomes are the enzymes that break down foreign material. Clearing of tissue debris and bacteria is essential for tissue regeneration to begin.

Fibroblasts increase in number and show increased motility following ultrasound, a response that has been linked to macrophage release factors.[18] An increase in early fibroblast activity may provide a better basis for the subsequent step of fibroblast attachment and proliferation. Ultrasound also increases protein synthesis by fibroblasts. Protein synthesis is the basis of collagen production.

Angiogenesis is enhanced following ultrasound.[18] This is the process of endothelial cell "budding" and formation of new blood vessels. The mechanism by which ultrasound stimulates this process is not clearly identified. It may be secondary to enhanced macrophage activity.

Capillary density is increased in ischemic tissue after repeated treatment with ultrasound. The effect, though, is only evident after repeated doses. The same effect has not been demonstrated in nonischemic tissue.[19]

Ultrasound enhances wound contraction.[18] During contraction, healthy collagen fibers at the edge of the lesion exert a centralizing pull on the wound edges, which assists in closing the wound. Accelerated contraction is an advantage in tissue repair because less scar tissue is required to fill the wound gap. Ultrasound has been shown to increase myofibroblast activity, which may be the mechanism through which ultrasound enhances wound contraction.

In summary, the effects of ultrasound have been examined during different stages of tissue repair. Benefits have been demonstrated for various components of inflammation, proliferation, and maturation processes. Research is ongoing to identify the mechanisms and interactions that occur.

Sequence of Ultrasound in a Treatment Plan

Stimulation of tissue healing by pulsed ultrasound is effected through a cascade of events triggered by the treatment and the benefit is not immediately evident. Pulsed ultrasound may be sequenced prior to any other activities in a treatment plan to take advantage of possible pain-relieving effects of the modality.[107-109]

The purpose of thermal treatment with ultrasound is to increase tissue temperature and subsequent length; therefore, stretch must be imposed on the tissue immediately after ultrasound. Without proper sequencing, thermal doses of ultrasound are pointless. There are numerous methods of stretching tissues, and clinicians generally have individual approaches they prefer.[38] The important point is not how the stretch is achieved but that heated tissues should be stretched through the full available range of motion, without increasing pain levels. Independent or assisted exercise using static stretch techniques, mechanical devices, proprioceptive neuromuscular facilitation techniques, or end-of-range mobilization techniques are all appropriate methods of applying stretch.

Some research suggests that optimum results are achieved if the stretch is maintained until tissue temperature returns to baseline.[110-112] Based on studies that investigated the time it takes for human tissues to cool after heating with ultrasound,[31,113] full-range stretching activities should continue for a duration of 8 to 10 minutes post-ultrasound. Strengthening and other activities that do not fully stretch the shortened tissue should be postponed until after the cool-down period.

It is the practice of some clinicians to apply ice in combination with ultrasound. The reason for applying ice is not clear. Cooling changes the depth at which ultrasound is absorbed because attenuation increases as temperature decreases.[114] Thus prior cooling results in more superficial absorption of ultrasound. In fact, ice and ultrasound appear to have contradictory effects. Ice causes vasoconstriction, decreases cell metabolism, and overall has an anti-inflammatory effect. Low-dose ultrasound is a proinflammatory agent. Ice effectively restricts bleeding and swelling in acute tissue trauma; low-dose ultrasound should be initiated 24 hours after injury to promote resolution of the swelling and repair of tissue. Application of ice immediately before or after ultrasound would likely inhibit the beneficial effects of the ultrasound treatment.

The use of ice and thermal doses of ultrasound also appears to be contradictory.[115] Decreasing tissue temperature, and thereby increasing stiffness, prior to or after using ultrasound to heat the tissues in order to resolve the stiffness appears to be indefensible! Moreover, there is no advantage to rapid cooling of tissues during or after stretch.[116] Applying any heating modality when sensory nerves have been numbed is a dangerous practice, and for this reason ice should not be applied before ultrasound.

The use of ice for pain control at the end of a treatment session that initially included thermal ultrasound may be seen clinically. There seems to be no conflict in this practice, as long as the ice application is of brief duration. Research shows that for an application of less than 8 minutes, the effect of ice is very superficial (less than $1/_2$ inch or 1 to 2 cm).[117] Therefore, a 5-minute ice pack will relieve post-treatment pain without ounteracting the benefit achieved from deep heating ultrasound, stretch, and exercise.[118]

Ultrasound Treatment Procedures

A minimum amount of preparation is required for ultrasound treatment, which probably accounts for its high favor among clinicians. No discomfort is experienced during treatment with ultrasound, which no doubt explains why it is well accepted by patients.

1. Preparation for Treatment Before uncovering the body part to be treated and positioning the patient, all accessory items should be collected.

Treatment in a whirlpool, or in water that has been vigorously stirred, is not recommended because air interferes with ultrasound transmission. Air bubbles on the patient's skin should be gently smoothed away before underwater treatments administered using a basin of water.

Air bubbles are also trapped on the skin under gel: they are just less obvious and thus get overlooked. When skin is generously covered in hair, trapped air can be a problem. Modern ultrasound devices, with electronic coupling indicators, confirm this by switching off power. Transmission improves if air is removed by smoothing down hair with a wet cloth before applying the gel.

2. *Patient Education and Consent to Treat*   Patient consent implies that the patient has been advised of the benefits and risks of the procedure, as well as the sensation they should experience during the procedure.

In the case of pulsed ultrasound, there should be no sensation other than the gliding of the transducer on the skin. When ultrasound is administered in a continuous mode, mild skin heating occurs, usually at doses above $0.8 \, W/cm^2$. Pain is a sign of excess periosteal heating. Patients should be instructed that the appropriate sensation is mild warmth and that excess heat, or pain, should be reported immediately.

For patient safety, and to ensure delivery of effective treatment, inability to report skin warmth should be an exclusion criterion for continuous-mode ultrasound. Potential to cooperate should be considered when patients are very young or very old or have limited understanding.

3. *Preparation of Equipment*   The treatment space must be organized for safety, comfort, and access. Clinicians should be seated with back support, and positioned so that the tissues being treated and device controls are simultaneously visible and within easy reach.

Time and intensity controls should be at zero before the main power is switched on and returned to zero after treatment. A reminder is appropriate at this point that the clinician checks on the ultrasound unit that the intensity meter is set at W/cm^2 (not total watts).

4. *Patient Position*   Patient comfort is basic to treatment with any modality. Support is required for trunk and limbs, whether the patient is lying or sitting. Injured limbs need the additional support of pillows or rolled towels and should be positioned in elevation when there is swelling, even though treatment periods are relatively short.

Specific positioning must be considered in addition to general principles. For example, the supraspinatus tendon lies partly under the acromion. If the arm is passively extended, the humeral head rotates forward from underneath the acromion, and the tendon can be reached where it inserts into the posterior aspect of the greater tubercle; in other positions, this tendon is not accessible. The patient can be seated in a high-backed chair with his or her arm resting on padding over the chair back to achieve the required position.

5. *Technique*   Gel is applied to the skin. There should be a 1- to 2-mm layer that would be sufficient to allow gliding of the soundhead without creating a mess. The soundhead is moved in overlapping circles or linear paths from the moment power is increased. Overlap ensures even distribution of energy to the treated tissue (recall that maximum intensity is distributed in the central one third of the ultrasound beam). The rate of transducer movement is slow, at a maximum of 3 to 4 cm/sec. If the transducer is "raced" over the skin, ultrasound effects may be reduced.

To ensure maximum penetration, the soundhead should be parallel to the tissue surface, which means adjusting the angle of the soundhead to the contours of the part being treated. In other words, the transducer is "pointed" toward the target tissue. This applies to treatment given in contact, when air gaps must not be allowed between the transducer and skin, and to water-immersion techniques, when treatment should be applied as close as possible to the skin.[10]

6. *Adjustment of Parameters During Treatment*   If a patient reports pain during a thermal mode treatment with ultrasound, the clinician must immediately lower intensity. There are two options for proceeding: the treatment can be delivered at a lower intensity, provided the patient still feels skin warmth, or the intensity can be delivered at a higher frequency, which will result in less periosteal heating and should eliminate pain. If pain persists despite the use of one of these steps or the patient complains of increased pain associated with the condition, treatment should be terminated.

7. *Repetition of Treatment*   There is no limit to the number of ultrasound treatments that can safely be applied, but treatment should continue only if measurable and sustained benefits are noted.

Observation and Documentation of Ultrasound Treatment

Assessment after treatment and prior to the next treatment is essential to demonstrate to the patient, as well as to satisfy the clinician and any third-party payer, that ultrasound is effective for the patient's problem.

Some immediate benefits can be expected. Ultrasound has a soothing effect on pain, possibly from stimulation of mechanoreceptors in the skin acting via a gate control mechanism, or from the sedative effect of heat. Another possible immediate benefit is a change in the "feel" of tissue as a result of heating effects. Palpation will provide the surest sign of such improvement. An example is the softening of an unresolved hematoma after ultrasound. However, the "feel" of tissues is a subjective measure, and as such is difficult to document.[119]

Incomplete documentation makes it difficult to repeat successful treatment or to determine how to modify treatment. Good documentation includes details of the patient's position; the treatment area; the technique; the transducer size; the machine settings for frequency, pulse ratio, intensity, and duration of treatment; and the nature and sequence of other activities.

Care of Therapeutic Ultrasound Equipment

Biomedical Department Inspection

Electrical safety checks should be left to technical experts who may be available through institutional biomedical departments or through manufacturers or distributors of

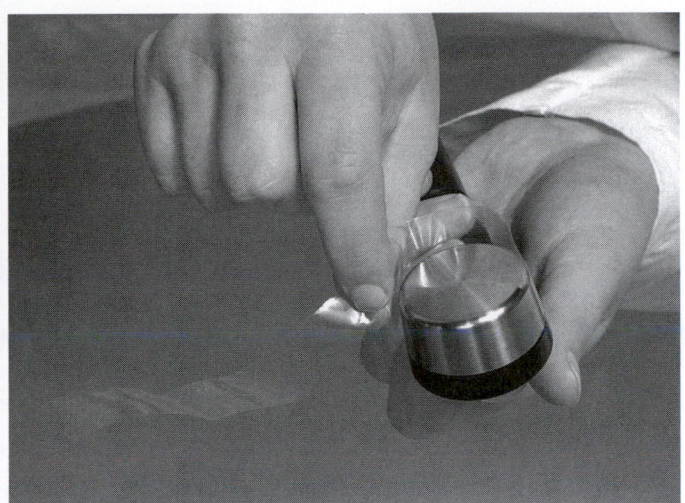

Figure 4-7 The transducer is being wrapped with a layer of cellophane tape. Once a "well" is created, then water can be added. Adjust the intensity to continuous and 1 W/cm². There should be movement of the water indicating that there is acoustical energy being emitted from the crystal. This simple exercise enables clinicians to test the transducer for output. It is recommended that this be performed frequently.

equipment. Specialized equipment is required to measure the total power, spatial distribution of power (BNR), and ERA of the ultrasound beam to recalibrate machines. In view of the fact that displayed dosage tends to be unreliable, recalibration every 6 months is advisable.

Clinical Monitoring

Clinicians should watch for signs of damaged or worn equipment. When the metal face of a transducer is old, it becomes dull or ridged and may not transmit ultrasound adequately. Undue heating of the transducer is a sign that energy is being lost within the transducer instead of being transmitted to the patient. The most common damage is inflicted by dropping the head. A dent in the transducer casing is a sign that the crystal might be damaged.

A water displacement test can be performed to see if the unit is emitting any sort of pressure wave. The ultrasound applicator is held under water with the transducer face angled upward but not parallel to the surface of the water. Tilting the face in this way will protect the crystal from a possible pressure wave being reflected from the water-air boundary back to the transducer face. Intensity is turned up to 1.0 W/cm². The beam should produce a cone-shaped displacement of water at the surface opposite the transducer face. The displacement should disappear as the intensity is reduced. Note that this simple test does not replace regular checks by qualified technicians (Fig. 4-7).

The conductivity of gels and medicated topical agents for phonophoresis can be tested in a similar manner. The height and shape of the water displacement are compared, using the method noted earlier, with and without a layer of the couplant (1 to 2 mm) spread over the transducer face.

Summary

Further research is essential in the field of therapeutic ultrasound. Randomized controlled clinical trials are needed to confirm the promising findings of preclinical studies and uncontrolled human trials.

An understanding of the physical properties and physiologic effects of ultrasound is fundamental for effective use of the modality. Distribution of energy in an ultrasound beam is dependent on frequency and beam characteristics. When the BNR is higher than 6, damaging "hot spots" might occur in the tissues. A moving head technique is required to distribute the points of maximum intensity evenly throughout the treated tissue. Absorption and penetration depend on frequency and the density of the tissue encountered.

Good clinical outcomes using ultrasound are achieved by careful treatment planning. Low-intensity pulsed ultrasound stimulates cellular activities that in turn trigger a chain of events leading to enhanced tissue repair. Benefit is obtained at dosages of about 1.0 W/cm² I_{SATP} (20% duty cycle) for about 5 minutes per 5 cm² of treatment area. Heating of tissue by ultrasound is for the treatment of chronic inflammatory conditions that restrict movement. Heating occurs with continuous-mode ultrasound using intensities between 0.8 and 1.5 W/cm² or higher. Tissue stretching should be performed immediately following heating. Appropriate timing is an important aspect of treatment.

Therapeutic Equipment

Generators and Transducers

Therapeutic ultrasound machines generate a pressure wave by causing a crystal to vibrate. The crystal, which is made of natural quartz or a synthetic material, contracts and expands in response to an applied alternating electric current (refer to Fig. 4-1). The crystal is housed inside an applicator called a transducer, which is the term used to describe a device that converts energy from one form into another. Current is delivered to the crystal via an insulated cable. As the current alternates in phase, the crystal changes its shape from concave to convex. In effect, the crystal vibrates; hence, electrical energy is converted to mechanical energy.

The treatment surface of the transducer consists of a metal plate that acts as an interface between the vibrating crystal and the patient's tissues. Continuity between the crystal, metal plate, and tissues is essential for transmission of the pressure wave to the tissues. Reflection at a metal-air boundary is about 99%. Therefore, an air gap between the transducer face and skin will prevent the pressure wave from leaving the transducer. This results in heating of the transducer, which is potentially damaging to the crystal.[4] An acoustically conductive couplant, oil or water based, is normally used between the transducer face and skin to ensure continuity. Ultrasound units may feature a light-emitting diode (LED) on the transducer head or some other type of signal to warn the operator when skin contact is inadequate. When contact is poor, power is interrupted and the unit timer pauses until good contact is resumed. This type of feature has been developed in an attempt to assist the clinician in improving the application technique: special attention has to be given to keeping in contact with the contours of the limbs and joints.

It has been noted that ultrasound treatment is applied at different frequencies. In older machines, a separate transducer had to be purchased for each frequency. Some devices offer 1 or 3 MHz on the same transducer head. Transducers are not interchangeable on ultrasound devices; you should not attempt to fit one transducer to another unrelated ultrasound unit. Transducer crystals are delicate and can be damaged by being dropped. This is a problem for clinicians because it is difficult without sophisticated measuring equipment to check the integrity of a crystal.

Therapeutic transducers are available in a variety of sizes from 1 cm^2 to 10 cm^2, with 5 cm^2 the most frequently used. The appropriate size, however, should be selected according to the anatomic area to be treated. For example, a 5-cm^2 or 10-cm^2 applicator may be suitable for use around the knee, whereas a 1-cm^2 applicator may be more appropriate to access the web space between the thumb and first digit of the hand.

Ultrasound units are produced with various options. Flexibility is an advantage because setting ultrasound characteristics specific to the tissue condition will lead to better treatment outcomes. Options should be available for the following characteristics:

- Frequency (1 or 3 MHz)
- Transducer size (various ERAs/external dimensions)
- Continuous or pulsed modes (with several options for pulsed modes)
- Dosage (intensity) from 0.1 to 3.0 W/cm^2

Features should include

- Intensity display (analogue or digital type)
- Treatment timer
- Electronic contact monitor (LED on the transducer head, or alert signal on the console)

 Intensity and Power of Ultrasound

The measured energy output of an ultrasound transducer should register on the device in two ways: as power and as intensity. Power, measured in Watts (W), refers to the electrical energy delivered to the crystal. Intensity, measured in

Before You Begin

PARAMETER SELECTION QUESTIONS

1. Is the tissue I am treating superficial (use 3 MHz) or deep (use 1 MHz)?

3. Are the signs and symptoms suggestive of acute inflammation?

   (Use a 20% duty factor, i.e., a ratio of 1:4, when treating acute inflammation.)

4. What is the transducer BNR? (Consider the potential for "hot spots" in the treatment field.)

5. What is the transducer ERA? (The treatment area should be approximately twice the size of the ERA of the transducer.)

Watts per square centimeter (W/cm^2), refers to the average power distributed over the ERA of the transducer. An intensity of 1 W/cm^2 would mean that 1 Watt of electrical energy was being delivered for each square centimeter of the ERA of the transducer. Intensity is the term used to describe clinical treatment.

The appropriate intensity of ultrasound to use in treatment is determined by the treatment goal—it depends on whether thermal or athermal effects are most wanted. Intensity of 3.0 W/cm^2 is often stated as the safe limit for treatment, based on the World Health Organization guidelines.[9] Lower intensities, however, are usually effective. A prudent approach to using any form of applied energy is to use the lowest dosage that achieves the desired effect.

In order to reproduce ultrasound treatment reliably and safely, it is important to document accurately and set treatment parameters correctly. It is critical for the reader to comprehend the difference between intensity (W/cm^2) and power (W).

Using faulty equipment forces the clinician into errors that he or she cannot detect and can make the difference between effective and noneffective treatment. For example, if the efficiency of the crystal or its housing is impaired, the electrical signal is not converted to ultrasound energy and the patient does not receive the dose registered on the meter. A discrepancy of 20% between the registered dosage and actual output is the limit of acceptability.[5]

Dosage of Ultrasound Treatment

Dosage incorporates the parameters previously discussed (frequency, intensity, and duty factor) as well as treatment time. Treatment time is based on the size of the treatment area relative to the ERA. The most recent evidence suggests that treatment time should be about 5 minutes per transducer ERA for treatments delivered in either pulsed or continuous mode. For example, for treatment of a 5-cm^2 area using a transducer with ERA of 5 cm^2, an effective treatment time would be approximately 5 minutes. For a treatment area of 10 cm², the treatment time using a transducer with ERA of 5 cm² would double (10 minutes). Areas larger than 10 cm² can be treated using pulsed ultrasound, but the time must be increased accordingly. With respect to thermal treatments, it is important to note that ultrasound does not produce clinically meaningful heating of deep tissues when the surface area treated exceeds 10 cm². Longer treatment times than 5 minutes per 5 cm² of surface area might be necessary to elevate deep tissue temperature if the patient is not capable of tolerating intensities greater than 1 W/cm². These examples are given as a starting point for the dosage of ultrasound.

Principles of Therapeutic Application

A Historical Perspective

Ultrasound was used therapeutically as early as 1930 using devices that produced only continuous-mode output.[9] During that early period, it was thought that treatment benefit was due entirely to heating effects. During the 1960s, although pulsed ultrasound was available, the common approach in rehabilitation was still to use continuous-wave output in the range of 0.5 to 1.5 W/cm². Then the development of focused ultrasound for medical diagnostics and continuing interest in ultrasound hyperthermia for treatment of cancer promoted intensive investigation into ultrasound effects. One finding of the early research was that ultrasound affected tissue growth using very low intensities. This knowledge, generated largely by medical biophysicists, filtered through to physical therapy literature in the early 1980s, leading to a gradual change in practice, in particular, a lowering of treatment dosage. The medical research also gave impetus to research activities led by physical therapists directed specifically toward therapeutic effects of ultrasound.

A Current Perspective: Research on Therapeutic Ultrasound

Research through the 1980s was most commonly conducted by scientists who were not themselves users of therapeutic ultrasound.[10,14,19] This trend has now been reversed. Also, the research in the early 1980s concentrated mainly on low-intensity pulsed ultrasound to promote tissue healing. However, current work also includes studies that evaluate heating doses of ultrasound.

Heating Tissues with Continuous-Wave Ultrasound

The literature on heating of human tissues using ultrasound is limited because invasive procedures are required to measure temperature at depth.[27,30,36] Some researchers have used a pig model to simulate heating in humans[23,24]; others

have used tissue specimens.[34] Heating effectiveness has been examined using ultrasound intensity in the range of 0.5 to 3.0 W/cm². It has been demonstrated that tissue temperature can be increased to 40°C or higher using ultrasound, as measured by thermistors inserted at various tissue depths.[27] However, some investigators evaluated effectiveness of thermal dosages of ultrasound by measuring tissue extensibility rather than temperature.[27,30,36] The research demonstrates that tendon heats at a faster rate than muscle.[30] It appears that the duration (10 minutes) and area (10 cm²) of ultrasound are both critical factors in effective heating because increased tissue extensibility was not produced when duration was decreased or treatment area increased.[33,36] However, further research on tissue heating with ultrasound is essential. It is not the purpose here to review all of the literature; the reader is encouraged to consult the reference list provided at the end of the chapter for additional information.

Interestingly, the literature demonstrates that ultrasound does not effectively heat large muscle bellies such as those of gastrocnemius or quadriceps. The likely explanation for this finding is that muscles have low capacity to absorb ultrasound and an excellent blood supply that dissipates any heat generated by ultrasound. Other modalities should be considered for heating large muscles: shortwave preferentially heats vascular tissue and may be a more effective approach to muscle heating than ultrasound. In contrast, ultrasound is effective for heating skin and subcutaneous tissue or high-protein content tissue such as tendon and ligament. Structures adjacent to bone, including the deep muscle layer, are also effectively heated by ultrasound because of conduction of heat from the periosteum.

Clinical Studies Using Ultrasound as a Heating Agent

There are a few controlled clinical studies that examine the effectiveness of ultrasound in chronic inflammatory connective tissue conditions, including lateral epicondylitis[26-28] and osteoarthritis.[29] The signs and symptoms of these conditions include soft tissue swelling, decreased range of movement, loss of strength, pain, and impaired function. The conditions have different etiology but there are some common underlying problems, including chronic inflammatory changes, with fibrosis, tissue contracture, and possibly adhesion development.[26-30]

Clinically, there is no good rationale for using ultrasound as a sole treatment in chronic conditions of the type noted earlier. When tissues are heated, the goal is usually to increase extensibility; thus, stretch must be applied and exercise through the range of motion must follow. What, then, can be learned from studies that treat chronic conditions with heating levels of ultrasound but without appropriate adjunctive treatment? Conversely, can ultrasound in combination with other treatment be properly evaluated? A dilemma is apparent for the researcher and clinician. For the reader it is clear: the literature must be approached critically. We need to be able to justify what we do with modalities. At the same time we do not want to discard treatments based on the negative findings of research when the research is problematic, the number of subjects in the study is small, and the treatment might yet be beneficial.

Clinical Studies Using Ultrasound to Facilitate Tissue Repair

The difficulty in studying effects of ultrasound on human tissue wounds is obvious, with the result that most of the research has been carried out on experimental animal wounds. Animal studies often draw criticism because loose-skinned animals, typically rats and guinea pigs, and to a lesser extent, pig skin, heal differently than human skin. While there are drawbacks to using animal models for ultrasound research, valuable information has emerged, which can and should be extrapolated to clinical practice, albeit with discretion.

Animal studies have been used to demonstrate the effects of ultrasound on wound contraction,[31] rate of wound healing,[32–36] rate and quality of tendon healing,[37–40] formation of new blood vessels,[41] activity of the phagocyte system,[42] and the role of calcium ions.[43] Pulsed ultrasound delivered at intensities of approximately 1.0 W/cm^2 I$_{SATP}$, using a 20% duty cycle, consistently appeared to accelerate healing in a variety of experimental wound models, including open wounds, tendon repair, and tissue damage induced by trauma or drug infiltration.

There are a number of clinical studies that have looked at the healing effects of ultrasound on venous ulcers[45–48] and pressure ulcers.[49] Treatments using ultrasound in continuous mode did not produce benefit.[46] Some treatments using low-intensity pulsed ultrasound (20% duty cycle) at a dosage of 1.0 W/cm^2 I$_{SATP}$ for 5 to 10 minutes were beneficial.[45,48] However, it should be noted that no benefit was seen when pulsed ultrasound was delivered at the same intensity (1.0 W/cm^2 I$_{SATP}$) but using a 10% duty cycle.[47] What is the optimum pulse ratio for stimulation of tissue healing? It has been shown that when the intensity is extremely high, even though the pulse is short (2 milliseconds), the occurrence of unstable cavitation is enhanced,[50] which may explain the lack of benefit using a 10% duty cycle.

Recent investigations have demonstrated that pulsed ultrasound (1.0 to 2.5 W/cm^2 I$_{SATP}$; 20% duty cycle) produced benefit when used in repetitive type of soft tissue injuries. In these studies, it is important to note the use of relatively long ultrasound duration (15 minutes) and increased treatment frequency (20 to 24 sessions over a 6-week period) compared with earlier studies.[24,25]

A new area of interest in ultrasound use has emerged, with the finding in large multicentered human trials that bone healing is enhanced with low-intensity ultrasound (0.15 W/cm^2 I$_{SATP}$, pulsed 1:4) applied for 20 minutes daily using a stationary transducer technique.[76,77]

In contrast to the facilitation of human tissue repair demonstrated by use of low-dose pulsed ultrasound, a study using high-intensity ultrasound to treat damaged tissues demonstrated a worsening of subjects' symptoms. Muscle inflammation and pain (delayed-onset muscle soreness) were induced in human volunteers and then ultrasound was applied to the muscle at 1 MHz, 1.5 W/cm^2 for 5 minutes using a 10-cm^2 transducer size.[51] Compared with controls, the treatment increased subjects' symptoms of pain. The results of this work suggest that such high-intensity ultrasound can aggravate tissue injury during the acute phase. Important points for treatment that can be deduced from the research include the following:

1. The area of tissue that can be realistically heated using ultrasound is an area equivalent to twice the size of the radiating area of the transducer, that is, 2 × ERA.

2. Water-immersion techniques considerably diminish skin and tissue heating. To compensate, treatment intensity should be increased by 50% or until the patient reports feeling warmth on the skin.

3. Using a frequency of 1 MHz, an intensity of 1.0 W/cm^2 and a stroking technique at a rate of 3 to 4 cm/sec, a change in temperature of 4° to 6°C can be expected in dense tissue close to bone.

4. Therapeutic temperatures (40°C) are achieved with 10 to 15 minutes of ultrasound treatment using intensities of 1 to 1.5 W/cm^2.[20,21]

Treatment techniques for the facilitation of tissue healing include the following:

1. Pulsed ultrasound is most likely to improve tissue healing using low intensity of 1.0 to 2.5 W/cm^2 I$_{SATP}$, with a 20% duty cycle.

2. Brief treatment duration, of about 2 minutes for each surface area equivalent to the ERA of the transducer, is sufficient to stimulate the healing process in chronic ulcers.

3. Soft tissue injuries, such as strains, sprains, subacute hematoma, and so on, should be treated for up to 5 minutes per ERA of the transducer.

4. Treatments should be repeated daily or every 48 hours to enhance healing.

Reliability and Efficiency of Ultrasound Equipment

A number of investigators have evaluated the accuracy of ultrasound equipment.[4–7] There appears to be agreement that equipment is not reliable and clinical units should be checked regularly. Researchers have found units with BNR values[7] and ERA characteristics[5] that do not agree with values reported by the manufacturer. The availability of suitable technology (since about 1980) and increasing awareness of the importance of accurate measurement of BNR and ERA have promoted this area of research.

Transmission Properties of Ultrasound Couplants

Some studies have compared transmission properties of ultrasound coupling media to determine their relative acoustic transmission efficiency.[52–54]

The comparator is usually degassed water. The results show that acoustic conductivity differs among products. The properties required of a couplant are that it lubricates the skin, absorbs very little ultrasound, has sufficient viscosity not to "run off," has no odor, does not stain clothing, and is not susceptible to bubble formation. A sterile, semisolid, 3.3-mm-thick gel dressing called Geliperm (Geltech Sons Ltd., Newton Bark, Chester, England) apparently transmits 95% of incident ultrasound power.[55] Testing of this product was carried out under water with the adhesive dressing applied directly to the transducer face. Although this product transmits well, it should be noted that it would be difficult to apply a dressing to skin without trapping air, which would significantly decrease its acoustic conductivity. The purpose of the dressing is to allow treatment directly over abrasions and wounds, using water or gel lubricant between the dressing and transducer. The authors who tested the product recommended using a syringe to fill shallow wounds with sterile saline before applying the dressing, to eliminate air gaps between the tissue and dressing. An adhesive transparent wound dressing available in North America (Opsite, Smith & Newphew, Inc., Lachne, Quebec, Canada) transmitted less than 10% of radiated ultrasound power when tested using similar procedures.[56]

Phonophoresis and Phonophoretic Products

Phonophoresis is the practice of applying ultrasound through a medicated couplant. The mechanism by which phonophoresis may enhance uptake of drugs is not known.[57] One theory is that ultrasound pressure drives the drug into the skin. An alternative theory is that heating of superficial tissue causes vasodilation of dermal capillaries, which speeds up the rate at which drugs are absorbed into the circulation. Another theory suggests that increased permeability of cell membranes enhances diffusion of the drug into the cell, which is the site of the chemical interactions. The studies on phonophoresis reflect all three theories.

The goal of some early studies[58,59] and some more recent work[60] was to determine the depth to which drugs were driven by ultrasound. Investigative procedures such as muscle sectioning in rabbits and joint aspirations in dogs were carried out as soon as 10 minutes after phonophoresis. Whereas drugs appeared in greater amounts at the depth of muscles, no benefit was found at the depth of the canine knee. It remains uncertain whether the drug needed more time to diffuse to greater depth or if in fact benefit is limited to the depth of muscle.

It is unclear from a review of the literature whether drugs that normally diffuse through the skin diffuse in greater amounts after ultrasound.[51,57,61] Early uncontrolled clinical trials[87,92,93] showed that patients with a variety of inflammatory conditions benefited from phonophoresis using hydrocortisone preparations; implying, as with the above in-depth studies, that the drug was successfully transmitted through skin by the ultrasound. However, in two recent controlled studies on epicondylitis,[65,66] hydrocortisone preparations of 10% and 1% were used without significant benefit compared with ultrasound alone. A topical nonsteroidal anti-inflammatory drug was rubbed on the skin in another study, and the same amount of drug was absorbed regardless of whether ultrasound was added.[67] In preliminary testing it was shown that less than 1% of ultrasound power was transmitted when 10% hydrocortisone acetate was mixed in gel and used as a couplant. Poor transmission qualities of some preparations may account for lack of benefit.[57]

The question of how much ultrasound is transmitted through phonophoretic preparations[54,68–70] was not examined until long after the early clinical trials. A variety of topical creams, ointments, and gels were generally found to be less efficient than regular gels and water for transmission. For most products tested, transmission was better at a frequency of 1.5 MHz and 3 MHz than at 0.75 MHz, and there was no difference in transmission between intensities of 0.3 W/cm^2 and 1.0 W/cm^2.[68] Preparations tested at 1.5 W/cm^2 suggested that drug-containing media that transmitted 80% ultrasound power could be considered good media. There was a choice of corticosteroids, local anesthetics, and nonsteroidal anti-inflammatory and salicylate drugs that met this criterion. The products tested included a variety of creams, ointments, gels, other media, and mixed media. Conflicting findings have been reported on some preparations.[70] Transmission through hydrocortisone cream has been reported as 47%.[57,69]

Neither level is satisfactory, and it makes it difficult to explain the earlier clinical successes of hydrocortisone phonophoresis.

The confusion in this field may be because of lack of uniformity in research methods. There are differences in the preparation of phonophoretic products, especially in concentration of active ingredients, in the type of base (gel, ointment, or cream), and in the dosage and number of ultrasound treatments. It seems that in preparation for phonophoretic treatment, a clinician should at the least perform a crude underwater test on the medicated product to see if it transmits any ultrasound.

Indications for Treatment

Apart from ultrasound, there are other modalities to stimulate tissue healing, such as pulsed shortwave diathermy, laser, and low-frequency transcutaneous electrical nerve stimulations (TENS). There are alternatives for heating tissues, such as continuous shortwave diathermy, hot packs, and other superficial agents. A series of questions may assist the inexperienced clinician in deciding whether ultrasound is indicated.

1. Is there a clinical diagnosis? Ultrasound is not a global treatment for undiagnosed pain or loss of function. Rather, ultrasound is indicated for treatment of well-defined localized tissue problems. The clinician should have clearly defined treatment goals when ultrasound is being considered.

2. Is stimulation of tissue repair indicated? Acute and subacute inflammation from strains and sprains, bruising, muscle tears, burns, superficial and deep skin wounds, crush injuries, and other similar types of conditions respond positively to low-intensity pulsed ultrasound.

3. Are heat and stretch indicated? Restriction of movement, with or without pain, because of muscle spasm, chronic edema, fibrosis, connective tissue contracture, adhesions, unresolved hematoma, and similar conditions of a chronic inflammatory nature are indications

for high-intensity continuous-mode thermal ultrasound.

4. Is ultrasound a time-effective approach to the problem? The clinician has to be with the patient for the duration of treatment. Ultrasound in excess of 15 minutes may not be efficient use of time. Shortwave diathermy is an alternative modality to consider.

5. Is the target tissue accessible? Ultrasound is preferentially absorbed by dense tissue; therefore, bone and joint structures should not lie between the target tissue and the path of the ultrasound beam. For example, this would mean selecting an alternative modality if swelling were inside a joint, whereas swelling outside a joint might be an indication for ultrasound. If the patient is unable to maintain a posture that makes the tissue accessible, another modality should be considered. For example, a contracture of the inferior portion of the shoulder joint capsule may be better heated with shortwave diathermy if a patient is unable to abduct the arm sufficiently for an ultrasound approach.

6. Is delivery of ultrasound practical? Either direct contact or a water-immersion technique has to be used. Skin breakdown, risk of infection, tenderness, and presence of dressings, casts, and splints may preclude the use of ultrasound.

7. Is the treatment goal to enhance delivery of topical medication? If difficult tissue contours preclude adequate transducer contact, phonophoresis, iontophoresis may be an alternative solution: for example, over the lateral epicondyle of the humerus or the calcaneal bursa in "bony" individuals.

8. Is ultrasound medically safe for the patient? There are some contraindications that would immediately preclude ultrasound as a choice of treatment. Screening of patients is essential.

Discussion Questions

1. The patient is a 50-year-old woman with chronic venous swelling of the lower legs. She has an ulcer 20 cm^2 in area and 2 cm deep on the anteromedial aspect of one leg. The ulcer has not healed in 10 months despite excellent wound cleansing by a visiting nurse and the use of moist dressings.
   a. Select ultrasound parameters that would be suitable to stimulate healing of the ulcer.
   b. Draw on paper a representative 20-cm^2 ulcer. Calculate the time it would take you to apply ultrasound around the perimeter of the ulcer at the rate of 2 minutes per 5 cm^2 of treatment area. If you have a 5-cm^2 transducer face, you can count exactly the number of 5-cm^2 areas that fit around the ulcer perimeter.
   c. The patient's skin circulation is also compromised in areas close to the ulcer because of severe tissue swelling. How can

---

 Before You Begin

PARAMETER SELECTION QUESTIONS

1. Is the tissue I am treating superficial (use 3 MHz) or deep (use 1 MHz)?

2. Are the signs and symptoms suggestive of acute inflammation?

   (Use a 20% duty factor, i.e., a ratio of 1:4, when treating acute inflammation.)

3. What is the transducer BNR?

   (Consider the potential for "hot spots" in the treatment field.)

4. What is the transducer ERA?

   (Consider contact between the transducer and tissue surface.)

5. How many areas equivalent to the ERA of the transducer fit into the treatment area?
   (Use a treatment time of about 5 minutes for each ERA, but remember that the treatment area must not be larger than twice the size of the transducer area for thermal effects.)

you use ultrasound to improve the condition of these other areas?

2. A 30-year-old patient suffered a whiplash injury 10 days ago. The present problems are painful muscle guarding of the upper trapezius, limited range of neck movement, and headache that the patient reports starts at the back of the head. As part of the current treatment session you plan to use ultrasound.

   a. Select ultrasound parameters that would be suitable for treating the muscle guarding.

   b. Would you also consider using ultrasound over the spinal joints at the level of the injury? If so, what parameters would you use?

CASE STUDY

Cindy is a 50-year-old amateur speed trial race car driver who has been referred to physical therapy for lower back pain and muscle guarding. The pain radiates into the buttocks and down to the left popliteal space. She has a history of lower back strains due to lifting injuries while working as a roofer when she was younger. She is 5 feet tall and weighs 90 pounds. Traction relieves her radiating pain, but heat relieves her muscle guarding.

- Is ultrasound potentially indicated for this patient?
- If yes, answer the following:

  Where would you apply it?

  What parameters would you use?

  What position should the patient be in during treatment?

  When in the treatment program would this potentially be indicated?

  Why?

  What would you expect to occur, and after how many treatments?

  How would you be able to determine whether or not it was effective?

  How would you document what you did?

References

1. Sternheim, MM, and Kane, JW: General Physics. Wiley and Sons, New York, 1991.
2. Barnett, SB, et al: Current status of research on biophysical effects of ultrasound. Ultrasound Med Biol 20:205, 1994.
3. Barnett, SB: Thresholds for nonthermal bioeffects: Theoretical and experimental basis for a threshold index. Ultrasound Med Biol 24:S41, 1998.
4. Apfel, RE: Acoustic cavitation: A possible consequence of biomedical uses of ultrasound. Br J Cancer 45(suppl V):140, 1989.
5. Williams, AR: Production and transmission of ultrasound. Physiotherapy 73:113, 1987.
6. Hekkenberg, RT, Reibold, R, and Zeqiri, B: Development of standard measurement methods for essential properties of ultrasound therapy equipment. Ultrasound Med Biol 20:83, 1994.
7. Pye, SD, and Milford, C: The performance of ultrasound physiotherapy machines in Lothian region, Scotland. Ultrasound Med Biol 20:347, 1994.
8. Hekkenberg, RT, Oosterbaan, WA, and van Beekum, WT: Evaluation of ultrasound therapy devices. Physiotherapy 72:390, 1986.
9. Fyfe, MC, and Bullock, MI: Acoustic output from therapeutic ultrasound units. Austral J Physiother 32:13, 1986.
10. Robertson, VJ, and Ward, AR: Limited interchangeability of methods of applying 1 MHz ultrasound. Arch Phys Med Rehabil 77:379, 1996.
11. Forrest, G, and Rosen, K: Ultrasound: effectiveness of treatments given under water. Arch Phys Med Rehabil 70:28, 1989.
12. Dinno, MA: The significance of membrane changes in the safe and effective use of therapeutic and diagnostic ultrasound. Phys Med Biol 34:1543, 1989.
13. Nyborg, WL: Ultrasonic microstreaming and related phenomena. Br J Cancer 45(suppl V):156, 1982.
14. ter Haar, GR: Ultrasonically induced cavitation in vivo. Br J Cancer 45(suppl V):151, 1982.
15. Maxwell, L: Therapeutic ultrasound: Its effect on the cellular and molecular mechanisms of inflammation and repair. Physiotherapy 79:421, 1992.
16. Al-Karmi, A, et al: Calcium and the effects of ultrasound on frog skin. Ultrasound Med Biol 20:73, 1994.
17. Harle, J, et al: Effects of ultrasound on the growth and function of bone and periodontal ligament cells *in vitro*. Ultrasound Med Biol 27:579, 2001.
18. Maxwell, L, et al: The augmentation of leucocyte adhesion to endothelium by therapeutic ultrasound. Ultrasound Med Biol 20:383, 1994.
19. De Deyne, PG, and Kirsch-Volders, M: In vitro effects of therapeutic ultrasound on the nucleus of human fibroblasts. Phys Ther 75:429, 1995.
20. Dyson, M, and Luke, DA: Induction of mast cell degranulation by ultrasound. IEEE Trans Ultrason Ferroelectr Freq Control UFFC-33 2:194, 1986.
21. Young, SR, and Dyson, M: Macrophage responsiveness to therapeutic ultrasound. Ultrasound Med Biol 16:809, 1990.
22. Reher, P, et al: Effect of ultrasound on the production of IL-8, basic FGF and VEGF. Cytokine 11:416, 1999.
23. Repacholi, MH: Standards and recommendations on ultrasound exposure. In Repacholi, MH, Grandolfo, M, and Rindi, A (eds): Ultrasound: Medical Applications, Biological Effects and Hazard Potential. Plenum Press, New York, 1987.
24. Ebenbichler, GR, et al: Ultrasound treatment for treating the carpal tunnel syndrome: Randomised sham controlled trial. BMJ 316:731, 1998.
25. Ebenbichler, GR, et al: Ultrasound therapy for calcific tendinitis of the shoulder. N Engl J Med 340:1533, 1999.
26. Draper, DO, et al: A comparison of temperature rise in human calf muscle following applications of underwater and topical gel ultrasound. J Orthop Sports Phys Ther 17:247, 1993.
27. Draper, DO, Castel, JC, and Castel, D: Rate of temperature increase in human muscle during 1 MHz and 3 MHz continuous ultrasound. J Orthop Sports Phys Ther 22:142, 1995.
28. Hasson, S, et al: Effect of pulsed ultrasound versus placebo on muscle soreness perception and muscular performance. Scand J Rehab Med 22:199, 1990.
29. Reed, BJ, and Ashikaga, T: The effects of heating with ultrasound on knee joint displacement. J Orthop Sports Phys Ther 26:131, 1997.
30. Chan, AK, et al: Temperature changes in human patellar tendon in response to therapeutic ultrasound. J Athl Train 22:130, 1998.
31. Lehmann, JF, DeLateur, BJ, and Silverman, DR: Selective heating effects of ultrasound in human beings. Arch Phys Med Rehabil 47:331, 1966.
32. Lehmann, JF, et al: Temperatures in human thighs after hot pack treatment followed by ultrasound. Arch Phys Med Rehabil 59:472, 1978.
33. Draper, DO, et al: Immediate and residual changes in dorsiflexion range of motion using an ultrasound heat and stretch routine. J Athl Train 33:141, 1998.
34. Robertson, VJ, and Ward, AR: Subaqueous ultrasound: 45 kHz and 1 MHz machines compared. Arch Phys Med Rehabil 76, 1995.
35. Kimura, IF, et al: Effects of two ultrasound devices and angles of application on the temperature of tissue phantom. J Orthop Sports Phys Ther 27:27, 1998.
36. Reed, BJ, et al: Effects of ultrasound and stretch on knee ligament extensibility. J Orthop Sports Phys Ther 30:341, 2000.
37. Wessling, KC, DeVane, DA, and Hylton, CR: Effects of static stretch versus static stretch and ultrasound combined on triceps surae muscle extensibility in healthy women. Phys Ther 67:674, 1987.
38. Knight, CA, et al: Effect of superficial heat, deep heat, and active exercise warm-up on the extensibility of the plantar flexors. Phys Ther 81:1206, 2001.
39. Robinson, SE, and Buono, MJ: Effect of continuous-wave ultrasound on blood flow in skeletal muscle. Phys Ther 75:145, 1994.
40. Lehmann, JF: Therapeutic temperature distribution produced by ultrasound as modified by dosage and volume of tissue exposed. Arch Phys Med Rehabil Dec:662, 1967.
41. Draper, DO, et al: Temperature change in human muscle during and after pulsed short-wave diathermy. J Orthop Sports Phys Ther 29:13, 1999.

42. Haker, E, and Lundeberg, T: Pulsed ultrasound treatment in lateral epicondylalgia. Scand J Rehab 23:115, 1991.

43. Binder, A, et al: Is therapeutic ultrasound effective in treating soft tissue lesions? BMJ 290:512, 1985.

44. Lundeberg, T, Abrahamsson, P, and Haker, E: A comparative study of continuous ultrasound, placebo ultrasound and rest in epicondylalgia. Scand J Rehab 20:99, 1988.

45. Stratford, P, et al: The evaluation of phonophoresis and friction massage as treatments for extensor carpi radialis tendinitis: A randomized controlled trial. Physiother Can 41:93, 1989.

46. Downing, DS, and Weinstein, A: Ultrasound therapy of subacromial bursitis. A double blind trial. Phys Ther 66:194, 1986.

47. Falconer, J, Hayes, K, and Chang, R: Therapeutic ultrasound in the treatment of musculoskeletal conditions. Arthritis Care Res 3:85, 1990.

48. Holdsworth, LK, and Anderson, DM: Effectiveness of ultrasound used with a hydrocortisone coupling medium or epicondylitis clasp to treat lateral epicondylitis: Pilot study. Physiotherapy 79:19, 1993.

49. Pienimaki, TT, et al: Progressive strengthening and stretching exercises and ultrasound for chronic lateral epicondylitis. Physiotherapy 82:522, 1996.

50. Falconer, J, Hayes, K, and Chang, R: Effect of ultrasound on mobility in osteoarthritis of the knee. Arthritis Care Res 5:29, 1992.

51. Dyson, M, and Smalley, DS: Effects of ultrasound on wound contraction. In Millner, R, Rosenfeld, E, and Cobet, U (eds): Ultrasound Interactions in Biology and Medicine. Plenum Press, New York, 1983.

52. Dyson, M, et al: The stimulation of tissue regeneration by means of ultrasound. Clin Sci 35:273, 1968.

53. Shamburger, RC, et al: The effect of ultrasonic and thermal treatment on wounds. Plast Reconstr Surg 68:860, 1981.

54. El-Batouty, MF: Comparative evaluation of the effects of ultrasonic and ultraviolet irradiation on tissue regeneration. Scand J Rheumatol 15:381, 1986.

55. Byl, N, et al: Incisional wound healing: A controlled study of low and high dose ultrasound. J Orthop Sports Phys Ther 18:619, 1993.

56. Young, SR, and Dyson, M: Effect of therapeutic ultrasound on the healing of full-thickness excised skin lesions. Ultrasonics 28:175, 1990.

57. Da Cunha, A, Parizotto, NA, and de Campos Vidal, B: The effect of therapeutic ultrasound on repair of the achilles tendon (tendo calcaneus) of the rat. Ultrasound Med Biol 27:1691, 2001.

58. Roberts, M, Rutherford, JH, and Harris, D: The effect of ultrasound on flexor tendon repairs in the rabbit. Hand 14:17, 1982.

59. Enwemeka, CS, Rodriguez, O, and Mendosa, S: The biomechanical effects of low-intensity ultrasound on healing tendons. Ultrasound Med Biol 16:801, 1990.

60. Turner, SM, Powell, ES, and Ng, CSS: The effect of ultrasound on the healing of repaired cockerel tendon: Is collagen cross-linkage a factor? J Hand Surg 14B:428, 1989.

61. Stevenson, JH, et al: Functional, mechanical, and biochemical assessment of ultrasound therapy on tendon healing in the chicken toe. Plast Reconstr Surg 77:965, 1986.

62. Jackson, BA, Schwane, JA, and Starcher, BC: Effect of ultrasound therapy on the repair of Achilles tendon injuries in rats. Med Sci Sports Exerc 23:171, 1991.

63. Gan, BS, et al: The effects of ultrasound treatment on flexor tendon healing in the chicken limb. J Hand Surg (Br) 20B:809, 1995.

64. Young, SR, and Dyson, M: The effect of therapeutic ultrasound on angiogenesis. Ultrasound Med Biol 16:261, 1990.

65. Mourad, PD, et al: Ultrasound accelerates functional recovery after peripheral nerve damage. Neurosurgery 48:1136, 2001.

66. Saad, AH, and Williams, AR: Effects of therapeutic ultrasound on the activity of the mononuclear phagocyte system in vivo. Ultrasound Med Biol 12:1986, 1986.

67. Dyson, M, Franks, C, and Suckling, J: Stimulation of healing of varicose ulcers by ultrasound. Ultrasonics Sep:232, 1976.

68. Eriksson, SV, Lundeberg, T, and Malm, M: A placebo controlled trial of ultrasound therapy in chronic leg ulceration. Scand J Rehab Med 23:211, 1991.

69. Lundeberg, T, et al: Pulsed ultrasound does not improve healing of venous ulcers. Scand J Rehab Med 22:195, 1990.

70. Callam, MJ, et al: A controlled trial of weekly ultrasound therapy in chronic leg ulceration. Lancet 2:204, 1987.

71. Nussbaum, EL, Biemann, I, and Mustard, B: Comparison of ultrasound/ultraviolet-C and laser for treatment of pressure ulcers in patients with spinal cord injury. Phys Ther 74:812, 1994.

72. ter Riet, G, Kessels, AGH, and Knipschild, P: A randomised clinical trial of ultrasound in the treatment of pressure ulcers. Phys Ther 76:1301, 1996.

73. Hashish, I, Harvey, W, and Harris, M: Anti-inflammatory effects of ultrasound in post operative morbidity: Evidence for a major placebo effect. Br J Rheumatol 25:77, 1986.

74. Crawford, F, and Snaith, M: How effective is therapeutic ultrasound in the treatment of heel pain? Ann Rheum Dis 55:265, 1996.

75. Oztas, O, et al: Ultrasound therapy effect in carpal tunnel syndrome. Arch Phys Med Rehabil 79:1540, 1998.

76. Heckman, JD, et al: Acceleration of tibial fracture-healing by non-invasive, low-intensity pulsed ultrasound. J Bone Joint Surg Am 76-A:26, 1994.

77. Kristiansen, TK, et al: Accelerated healing of distal radial fractures with the use of specific, low-intensity ultrasound. J Bone Joint Surg Am 79-A:961, 1997.

78. Rubin, C, et al: The use of low-intensity ultrasound to accelerate the healing of fractures. J Bone Joint Surg Am 83-A:259, 2001.

79. Warden, SJ, et al: Can conventional therapeutic ultrasound units be used to accelerate fracture repair? Phys Ther Rev 4:117, 1999.

80. Ciccone, CD, Leggin, BG, and Callamaro, JJ: Effects of ultrasound and trolamine salicylate phonophoresis on delayed-onset muscle soreness. Phys Ther 71:666, 1991.

81. Zeqiri, B: Calibration and safety of physiotherapy ultrasound equipment. Physiotherapy 83:559, 1997.

82. Balmaseda, MT: Ultrasound therapy: A comparative study of different coupling media. Arch Phys Med Rehabil 67:147, 1986.

83. Benson, HAE, and McElnay, JC: Transmission of ultrasound

through topical pharmaceutical products. Physiotherapy 74:587, 1988.

84. Docker, MF, Foulkes, DJ, and Patrick, MK: Ultrasound couplants for physiotherapy. Physiotherapy 68:124, 1982.

85. Klucinec, B, et al: Effectiveness of wound care products in the transmission of acoustic energy. Phys Ther 80:469, 2000.

86. Byl, N, et al: The effect of phonophoresis with corticosteroids: A controlled pilot study. J Orthop Sports Phys Ther 18:590, 1993.

87. Griffin, JE, and Touchstone, JC: Ultrasonic movement of cortisol into pig tissue: Movement into skeletal muscle. Am J Phys Med 42:77, 1963.

88. Novack, EJ: Experimental transmission of lidocaine through intact skin by ultrasound. Arch Phys Med Rehabil 45:231, 1964.

89. Muir, WS: Comparison of ultrasonically applied vs. intra-articular injected hydrocortisone levels in canine knees. Orthop Rev XIX:351, 1990.

90. Byl, N: The use of ultrasound as an enhancer for transcutaneous drug delivery: Phonophoresis. Phys Ther 75:539, 1995.

91. Davick, JP, Martin, RK, and Albright, JP: Distribution and deposition of tritiated cortisol using phonophoresis. Phys Ther 68:1673, 1988.

92. Kleinkort, JA, and Wood, F: Phonophoresis with 1% vs 10% hydrocortisone. Phys Ther 55:1321, 1975.

93. Wing, M: Phonophoresis with hydrocortisone in the treatment of temporomandibular joint dysfunction. Phys Ther 62:33, 1982.

94. Benson, HA, McElnay, JC, and Harland, R: Use of ultrasound to enhance percutaneous absorption of benzydamine. Phys Ther 69:114, 1989.

95. Warren, C: Ultrasound coupling media: Their relative transmission. Arch Phys Med Rehabil 57:218, 1976.

96. Cameron, MH, and Munroe, LG: Relative transmission of ultrasound by media customarily used for phonophoresis. Phys Ther 72:142, 1992.

97. Benson, HA, and McElnay, JC: Topical NSAID products as ultrasound couplants: Their potential in phonophoresis. Physiotherapy 80:74, 1994.

98. Lehmann, JF: Ultrasound: Considerations for use in the presence of prosthetic joints. Arch Phys Med Rehabil 61:502, 1980.

99. Skouba-Kristensen, E: Ultrasound influence on internal fixation with a rigid plate in dogs. Arch Phys Med Rehabil 63:371, 1982.

100. Krotenberg, R, Ambrose, L, and Mosher, R: Therapeutic ultrasound effect on high density polyethylene and polymethyl methacrylate (abstract). Arch Phys Med Rehabil 67:618, 1986.

101. Sicard-Rosenbaum, L, et al: Effects of continuous therapeutic ultrasound on growth and metastasis of subcutaneous murine tumors. Phys Ther 75:3, 1995.

102. Angles, JM, et al: Effects of pulsed ultrasound and temperature on the development of rat embryos in culture. Teratology 42:285, 1990.

103. Spadaro, JA, and Albanese, SA: Application of low-intensity ultrasound to growing bone in rats. Ultrasound Med Biol 24:567, 1998.

104 Dyson, M: Therapeutic applications of ultrasound. In Nyborg, W, and Ziskin, M (eds): Biological Effects of Ultrasound (Clinics in Diagnostic Ultrasound). Churchill Livingstone, New York, 1985.

105 Frizzel, LA, Miller, DL, and Nyborg, WL: Ultrasonically induced intravascular streaming and thrombus formation adjacent to a micropipette. Ultrasound Med Biol 12:217, 1986.

106. Williams, AR: Effects of ultrasound on blood and the circulation. In Nyborg, W, and Ziskin, M (eds): Biological Effects of Ultrasound. Churchill Livingstone, New York, 1985.

107. Williams, AR, et al: Effects of MHz ultrasound on electrical pain threshold perception in humans. Ultrasound Med Biol 13:249, 1987.

108. Gray, RJM, et al: Temporomandibular pain dysfunction: Can electrotherapy help? Physiotherapy 81:47, 1995.

109. Uygur, F, and Sener, G: Application of ultrasound in neuromas: Experience with seven below-knee stumps. Physiotherapy 81:758, 1995.

110. Lehmann, JF, et al: Effects of therapeutic temperatures on tissue extensibility. Arch Phys Med Rehabil 51:481, 1970.

111. Warren, CG, Lehmann, JF, and Koblanski, JN: Elongation of rat tail tendon: Effect of load and temperature. Arch Phys Med Rehabil 52:465, 1971.

112. Sapega, AA: Biophysical factors in range of motion exercise. Physician Sports Med 9:57, 1981.

113. Draper, DO, and Ricard, M: Rate of temperature decay in human muscle following 3 MHz ultrasound: The stretching window revealed. J Athl Train 30:304, 1995.

114. Gammell, PM, LeCroissette, DH, and Heyser, RC: Temperature and frequency dependence of ultrasonic attenuation in selected tissues. Ultrasound Med Biol 5:269, 1979.

115. Draper, DO, et al: Temperature changes in deep muscles of humans during ice and ultrasound therapies: An in vivo study. J Orthop Sports Phys Ther 21:153, 1995.

116. Lentell, G: The use of thermal agents to influence the effectiveness of a low-load prolonged stretch. J Orthop Sports Phys Ther 16:200, 1992.

117. Low, J, and Reed, A: Cold Therapy. Electrotherapy Explained: Principles and Practice. Heinemann Medical, Oxford, 1990, p 203.

118. Waylonis, GW: Physiologic effects of ice massage. Arch Phys Med Rehabil 43:38, 1967.

119. McLachlan, Z, et al: Ultrasound treatment for breast engorgement: A randomised double blind trial. Austral J Physiother 37:23, 1991.

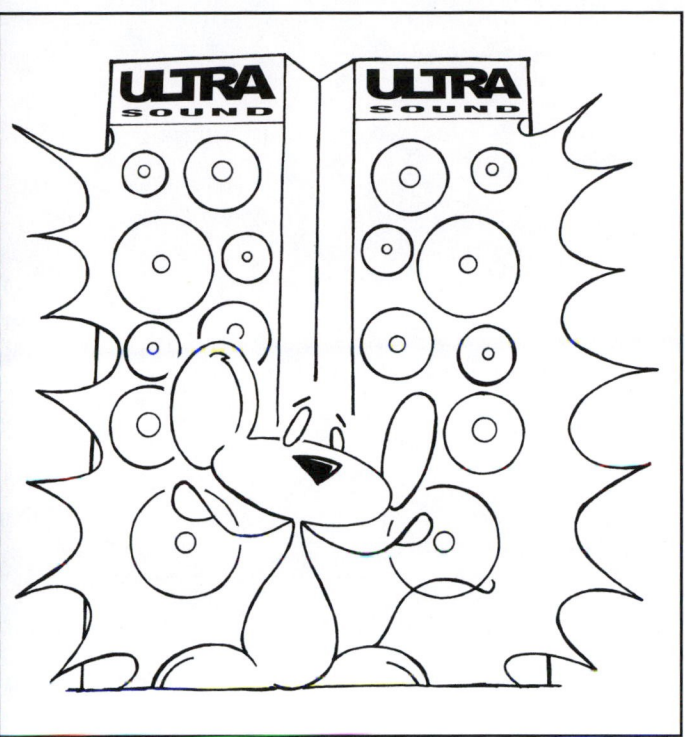

Objectives

- Describe the physical principles of water.
- Describe the therapeutic benefits of hydrotherapy.
- Describe the components and care for a whirlpool.
- Describe the benefits of aquatic exercise as a modality.
- Differentiate between the benefits of land and water activities.
- Describe the benefits of hydrotherapy for wound management.
- Describe the techniques for wound care with hydrotherapy.
- Differentiate between the benefits and potential problems of using hydrotherapy for wound care.

Key Terms

Aquatic pools	Debridement	Hydromechanics	Wound
Aquatic therapy	Hydrotherapy	Whirlpools	management
Buoyancy			

Russell Stowers, PTA, MS   *Robert Babb, PT*

Aquatics and Hydrotherapy

Outline

"Take a music bath once or twice a week for a few seasons, and you will find that it is to the soul what the water bath is to the body."
—*Oliver Wendell Holmes (1809–1894)*

Hydrotherapy has ancient roots and is one of the oldest forms of therapy. Hippocrates, the Greek father of medicine, used contrast baths of hot and cold water to treat various diseases. Europeans have been using warm-water spas for hundreds of years and developed a great deal of the original therapeutic water regimens that are used today. Exercise in water was popular in the polio era, and a resurgence of interest occurred in the 1990s as evidenced by the formation of the Aquatic Section of the American Physical Therapy Association, which defines *aquatic physical therapy* as "treatment time with therapeutic exercises in the water, utilizing supine, prone, vertical, or reclined positions."[1] Today, thousands of clinicians use water for therapeutic purposes every day in their practices. This use has evolved into two different areas: whirlpool treatments and aquatic therapy using aquatic pools. This chapter will define, discuss, and differentiate between the wide variety of therapeutic applications of water.

 ## Whirlpools Versus Aquatic Pools

Whirlpools use tanks of water such as a low boy or Hubbard tank. These tanks come in a variety of depths and sizes dependent on the amount of immersion required for the treatment.[2] Whirlpools involve the treatment of one patient at a time in an individual tank. Aquatic pools refer to the use of larger pools with more body immersion and potential treatment of more than one patient at a time. Individuals with a true phobia of the water would potentially be able to tolerate whirlpool treatment but not an aquatic pool (Tables 5-1 and 5-2).

 ## Physical Principles and Properties of Water

Buoyancy

Buoyancy is a force that works in the opposite direction to gravity. Gravity pulls downward; buoyancy pushes upward

TABLE 5-1 Indications for Use of Whirlpools and Aquatic Pools

INDICATIONS	WHIRLPOOLS	AQUATIC POOLS
Neuromuscular disorders		X
Musculoskeletal disorders	X	X
Cardiovascular disorders		X
Pulmonary disorders		X
Integumentary disorders	X	

TABLE 5-2 Contraindications for Use of Whirlpools and Aquatic Pools

CONTRAINDICATIONS	WHIRLPOOLS	AQUATIC POOLS
Edema	X	
Lethargy		X
Unresponsiveness	X	X
Maceration	X	X
Febrile	X	X
Compromised cardiovascular or pulmonary disorder	X	X
Acute phlebitis		X
Renal failure		X
Dry gangrene	X	X
Incontinence		X

from the bottom. When an object is placed in water, water displacement occurs because of the upward pressure of buoyancy. The amount of displacement has been described by Archimedes, who stated that an immersed body will experience an upward thrust equal to the weight of the liquid displaced.[3] Water is more supportive than air because of buoyancy. There will be greater buoyant forces acting on larger objects, creating more water displacement, than on smaller objects, which will experience less water displacement and less buoyancy. A relative "weightlessness" occurs when a body is immersed in water. The amount of weightlessness depends on the percentage of the body that is below the surface of the water (Fig. 5-1). Buoyant forces support the body, giving the sensation of weightlessness. This will also be affected by body density, postural alignment, and vital capacity of the lungs. When a patient fully inflates his or her lungs, he or she will be much more likely to float than if the lungs were not inflated. Buoyancy can offer enough support to the extremities, reducing the compressive forces that would be experienced out of the water. Buoyancy can provide opportunities for patients to perform assisted upper or lower extremity exercises or to run with reduced joint compression.

Center of Buoyancy

The center of buoyancy (COB) and center of gravity (COG) are functionally similar. COB refers to a point when a body is under water, and the COG refers to a point when a body is out of the water. They represent points or locations on the human body that need to be maintained within a base of support (BOS) to establish and maintain an upright and stable posture. The COG is located just anterior to the sacral vertebrae; the COB is located in the chest region. While a body is submersed in the water, the forces of buoyancy and gravity act in opposite directions to each other. Buoyancy devices or flotation devices can be used to help a patient maintain his or her COB within the BOS to maintain an upright position in the water. Anteriorly placed buoyancy

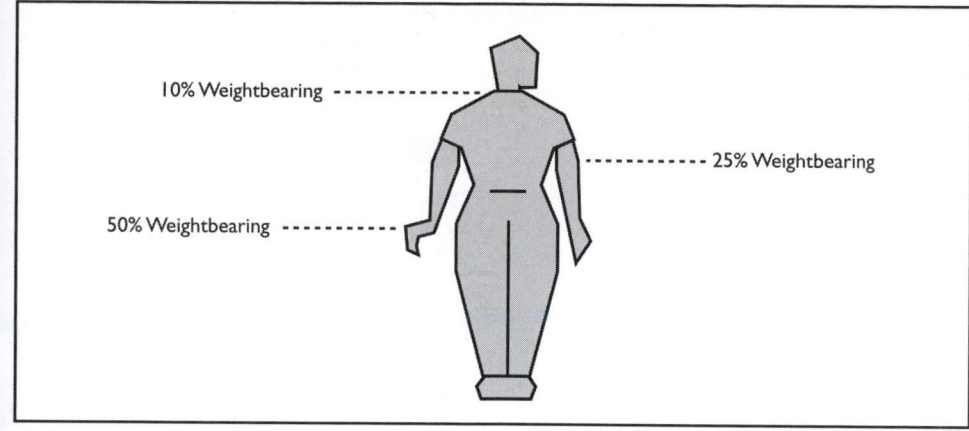

Figure 5-1 Percentage of weightbearing and immersion at three depths.

devices will tend to cause extension of the spine to assist in maintaining proper body alignment. For example, a patient who has had a total hip replacement needs to be able to perform buoyancy-supported hip abduction before he or she would be able to perform standing hip abduction.

Hydrostatic Pressure

Hydrostatic pressure is pressure exerted by water on an object immersed in the water. Pascal's law states that the pressure of a liquid is exerted equally on an object at a given depth, and the object will experience pressure that is proportional to the depth of immersion.[4] Pressure increases 0.433 lb/in^2 for each foot of depth. This pressure is thought to help control inflammation with water exercise. It will also assist in venous return, heart rate reduction, and a centralization of peripheral blood flow.[5] There is less inflammation when patients who have had anterior cruciate ligament repairs perform their exercises in the water than when performing their exercises out of the water.[6] Perhaps this is because of reduction of joint compression and shear forces.

Because hydrostatic pressure is proportional to the depth of immersion, exercises will be easier to perform closer to the surface of the water, where the pressure is less.

Specific Gravity

Specific gravity is the weight of a particular substance compared with the weight of an equal volume of water. It is related to the density of an object and therefore is also referred to as relative density. The specific gravity of a person increases when there is increased bone mass and muscle mass

and decreases when there are greater amounts of adipose tissue (body fat). An object with a low specific gravity or specific gravity of less than 1.0 will float; an object with a high specific gravity of greater than 1.0 will sink. Water has a specific gravity of 1.0. The human body has a specific gravity of 0.87 to 0.97; therefore, the human body will tend to float just beneath the surface of water. For example, children with chronic debilitating diseases do well in water therapy because they expend little energy to stay afloat and the buoyant forces assist in reducing weight-bearing. Men tend to have lower percentages of body fat than do women[7] and may require more buoyancy-assistive devices than do women to keep them afloat. The lower extremities will have larger bones than the upper extremities and therefore will tend to sink more than the upper extremities.

Viscosity and Resistance

Viscosity is a measure of the frictional resistance caused by cohesive or attractive forces between the molecules of a liquid.[5] *Resistance* is created by the viscosity of the liquid and is proportional to the velocity of movement through the liquid. Water has a higher viscosity than air but less than that of oil, so it would be easiest to move through air, then water, then oil. Exercise training in an aquatic environment can result in increased strength, improved cardiovascular responses, and improved VO_2 maximums.[8,9] The amount of resistance in water can be adjusted in several ways to vary the training regimen. Decreasing the length of the lever arm will decrease the resistance in a buoyancy-resisted movement, a movement down toward the bottom of the pool. Adding a "boot" or "paddle" will increase the resistance of an activity, because increasing the surface area of the part to be moved will also increase the resistance.

Specific Heat

Specific heat is defined as the amount of heat, in calories, required to raise the temperature of 1 gram of a substance by

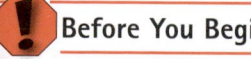

Before You Begin

Keep in mind that patients may be able to perform activities in the water that they would not be able to perform on land.

1° C (one degree). The specific heat of water is 1.0, and it is used as the standard for setting specific heat units of other substances. When heat is added to an object, the change in temperature depends on its mass and specific heat. The specific heat or thermal capacity of water is greater than that of air. This will cause more heat loss in the water compared with out of water at the same temperature. Cool or tepid water temperature is best for a long exercise session, whereas warm water is indicated for short-duration exercise and manual techniques. Patients diagnosed with multiple sclerosis will perform better in cooler water, which will assist in keeping their inner core body temperature low, preventing exacerbation of their symptoms, which might occur if the exercise were performed out of the water. Patients with arthritis will benefit from warmer water temperatures due to increased circulation and tissue elastcity. Warm-water exercise may increase the core body temperature of obese patients, because adipose tissue acts as an insulator, limiting proper heat exchange. Therefore, warmer water temperatures may be inappropriate for obese patients if they will also be exercising in the water, which would also increase the core body temperature.

Hydromechanics of Water

Hydromechanics is a term used to refer to movement through water. It is a function of velocity of movement, surface area of the moving object, and direction of the movement of the immersed object. *Turbulence* is a product of several forces acting on an object immersed in water. *Laminar flow*, *drag*, and *resistance* to forward movement all act on the body moving in the water (Fig. 5-2). *Frontal resistance* is encountered initially as a body moves through the water, creating a positive pressure. The resistance is proportional to the velocity. The faster the movement, the greater is the resistance.[3] Progressive resistance in aquatic exercise can be increased by increasing the velocity of movement, by increasing the surface area, or by moving closer to the surface of the water where the turbulence is greater.[10]

Frontal resistance, proportional to the surface area, will offer resistance to initiation of movement as inertial forces are overcome. The greater the surface area, the greater the

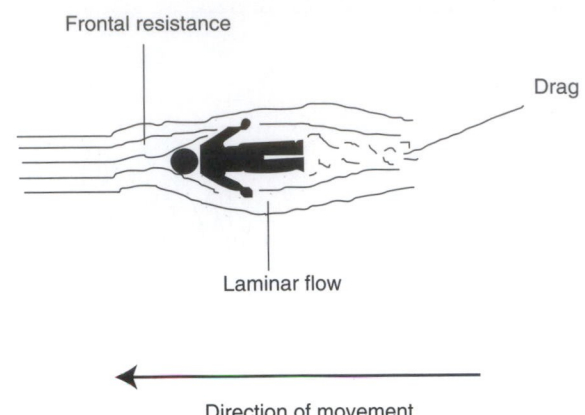

Frontal resistance

Drag

Laminar flow

Direction of movement

Figure 5-2 Various forces that will act on an object as it moves through the water.

amount of water is moved; therefore, more drag will be created. *Drag* inhibits movement by resisting forward motion. Quick changes in the direction of movement in water will also encounter greater resistance.

Laminar flow is the horizontal flow of water passing over a body part in motion that creates drag. The more irregular the laminar flow, the greater is the drag of a part. Irregular shapes will alter the laminar flow of the water. Increasing the velocity, surface area, and change in direction will raise the level of effort needed to accomplish a task in the water. Depending on the effort exerted, energy requirements in an aquatic environment have been reported to be 33% to 42% greater at any given workload when compared with land exercises (Table 5-3).

Water Temperature

Temperature regulation is more difficult in water in part because of diminished body surface area to lose heat. Conversely, cold water could produce a significant amount of heat loss because water conducts heat 25 times faster than air.[12] Therapeutic warmth is considered to be 94°F (34.4°C),

TABLE 5-3 Comparison of Treatment Goals for "Land" Versus Aquatic Exercise

	LAND	AQUATIC
Improving range of motion	Manual stretching	Manual stretching
Improving arthrokinematics	Joint mobilizations	Joint mobilizations
Improving strength	Open-chain manual resistive	Closed-chain manual resistance
	Resistive equipment	Paddles, boots, boards
Improving balance	Unilateral stance, mini-tramp	Unilateral stance, turbulence challenge
Improving endurance	Bike, treadmill	Deep water walk, run
Improving ambulation status	Parallel bars to crutches to cane	Deep water to shallow water to land

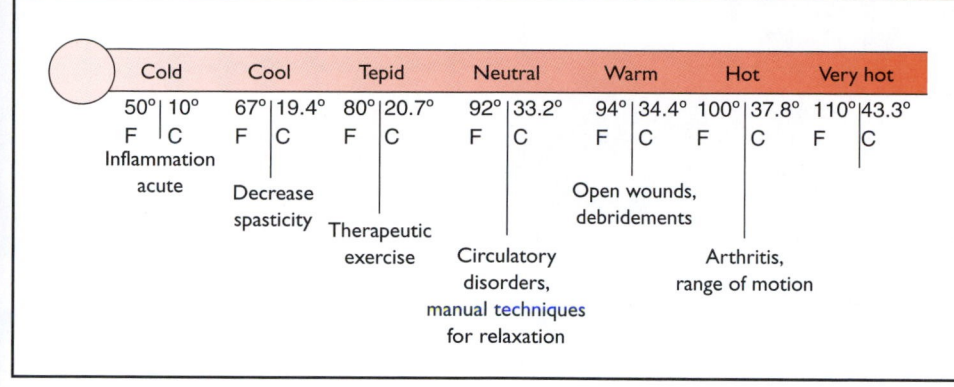

Cold		Cool		Tepid		Neutral		Warm		Hot		Very hot	
50°	10°	67°	19.4°	80°	20.7°	92°	33.2°	94°	34.4°	100°	37.8°	110°	43.3°
F	C	F	C	F	C	F	C	F	C	F	C	F	C

Inflammation acute
Decrease spasticity
Therapeutic exercise
Circulatory disorders, manual 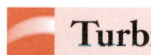 techniques for relaxation
Open wounds, debridements
Arthritis, range of motion

Figure 5-3   Water temperatures and potential applications for hydrotherapy.

which is appropriate for performing therapeutic exercises. Warm water may act as a superficial heating agent and has been reported to elevate pain threshold and decrease muscle spasm.[2] Inappropriate temperature selection could decrease the effectiveness of the therapeutic intervention and possibly cause adverse responses (Fig. 5-3).

Equipment

Equipment for hydrotherapy involves the use of whirlpools with stainless steel or fiberglass tanks that may be movable or stationary (depending on their size and configuration) and have a turbine, drain, and thermostatically controlled water supply. Whirlpools vary in size, and one is selected for treatment depending on the treatment goal and extremity or area to be treated. The smallest tanks are extremity tanks, which hold approximately 25 gallons of water depending on the manufacturer. They vary in depth from 20 to 25 inches and have one turbine. Full-body tanks are called "low boys," and they resemble a bathtub resting on the floor with enough room for patients to "long sit" in the tank with their legs outstretched in front of them. Low-boy tanks may hold as much as 200 gallons of water and they also have a turbine for aeration of the water. High-boy tanks are tall and are more appropriate for large body areas. They will hold up to 100 gallons of water. The extremity, low-boy, and high-boy tanks have been used in the treatment of open wounds, peripheral joint stiffness, sprain/strains, and postoperative joint replacements (Fig. 5-4).

Hubbard tanks are whirlpool tanks that were created to accommodate a patient in a supine position and allow range of movement in both the upper and lower extremities with support from the water (Fig. 5-5). These tanks may have a deep trough in the center of the tank with parallel bars for in-water ambulation. Patients who cannot be transferred into a low boy or who have too large a surface area for treatment in an extremity tank or low boy are candidates for the Hubbard tank. There are several turbines on Hubbard tanks that can be moved to different positions around the tank so that the turbulence can be directed to more than one area at a time. These tanks have a lifting device to transfer the patient from a gurney into the pool and then out. Often these lifts are hydraulically controlled and may be intimidating to certain patients. It is important to remember this when transferring a patient into any pool.

Turbines

Turbines mix air and water to provide agitation and turbulence to the water in a tank. The mechanical stimulation from the agitation to the skin receptors may promote an analgesic effect. The analgesic effect can be effective for pain reduction in sprains and strains, as well as other conditions. Turbines have several adjustable features, including height, direction of flow, and strength of the aerated flow. The more air that is mixed with the water, the more turbulence will be created in the water. Turbulence may assist in nonspecific debridement of an open wound if indicated. Wound management with hydrotherapy is discussed later in this chapter.

Therapeutic Aquatic Pools

Therapeutic aquatic pools vary in depth and size with water temperature ranges from 86° to 94°F (30° to 34.4°C). The therapeutic treatment goals for aquatic pools can be the same goals as those established for therapeutic exercise out of the water. Water immersion eliminates the effects of gravity, so water is an ideal environment for early interventions for many musculoskeletal and neurologic conditions. The initial assessment of the patient should be performed on land and then again in the water to ensure that the medium is capable of assisting the patient in meeting negotiated treatment goals. Aquatic rehabilitation should be combined with land techniques to progress the patient functionally, because the

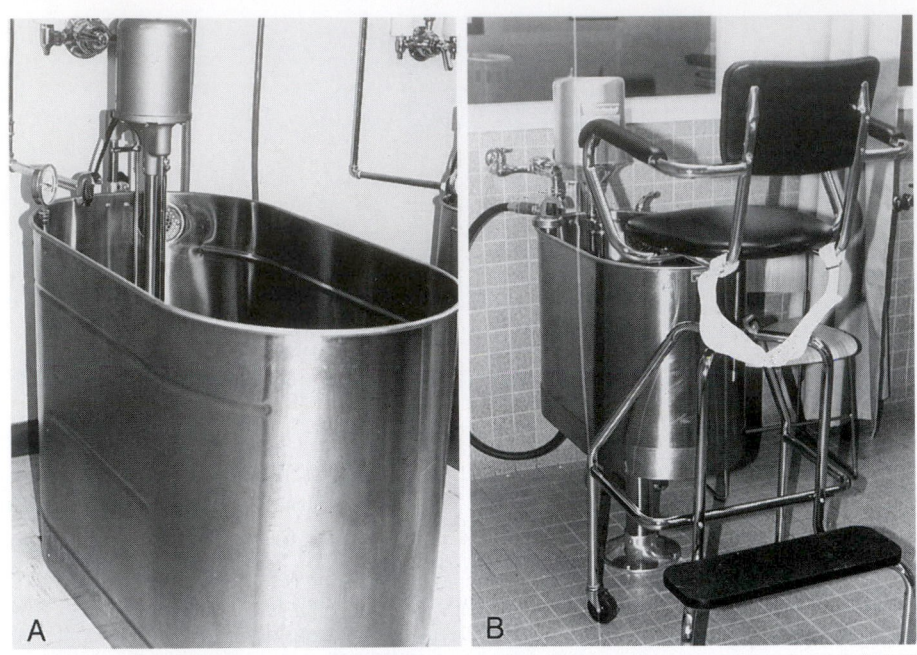
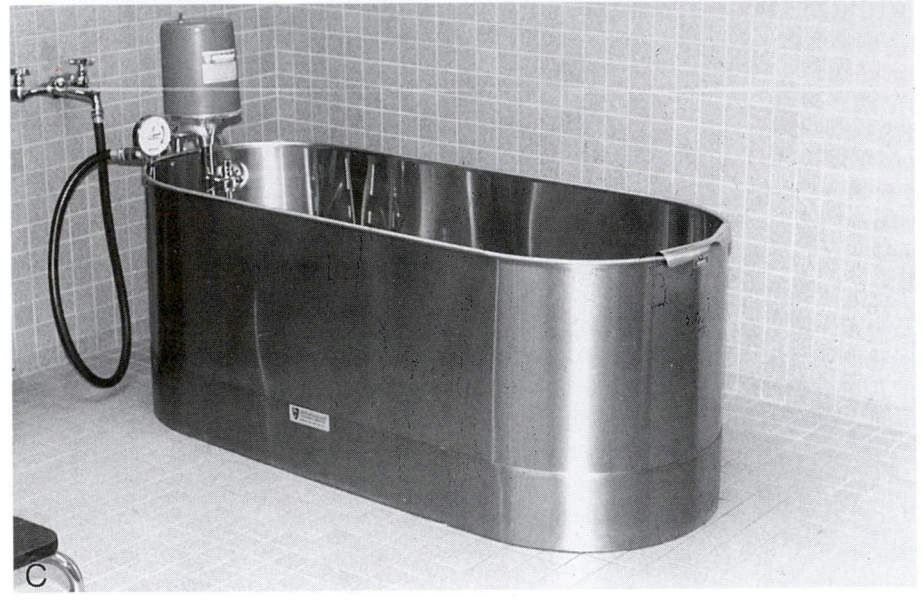

Figure 5-4   Various types and styles of whirlpools. (*A*) "High boy" for knees or hips. (*B*) Extremity tank for distal upper or lower extremities. (*C*) "Low boy." (From Walsh, MT: Hydrotherapy: The use of water as a therapeutic agent. In Michlovitz, SL, ed: Thermal Agents in Rehabilitation, ed 3. FA Davis, Philadelphia, 1996, p 144, with permission.)

land environment will ultimately be the goal (Table 5-4 and Fig. 5-6).

Hydrotherapy Techniques

Aquatic Pools

Aquatic Pools and Infection Control

Unlike whirlpool treatment, the water is not emptied for aquatic pools following every patient treatment. There are also situations where there will be more than one patient in the water at the same time. This presents some different considerations for infection control. First, it is recommended that patients shower to remove any excess soil from their skin before entering the aquatic pool. These pools have a filtration system that is either chlorinated or treated in some way to minimize the spread of organisms from one individual to another. It is not safe for a patient who is incontinent or who has an open wound to be immersed in an aquatic pool.

Aquatic Therapy Techniques

Aquatic therapy is a growing area of interest. The growth in commercial popularity is, unfortunately, not matched with

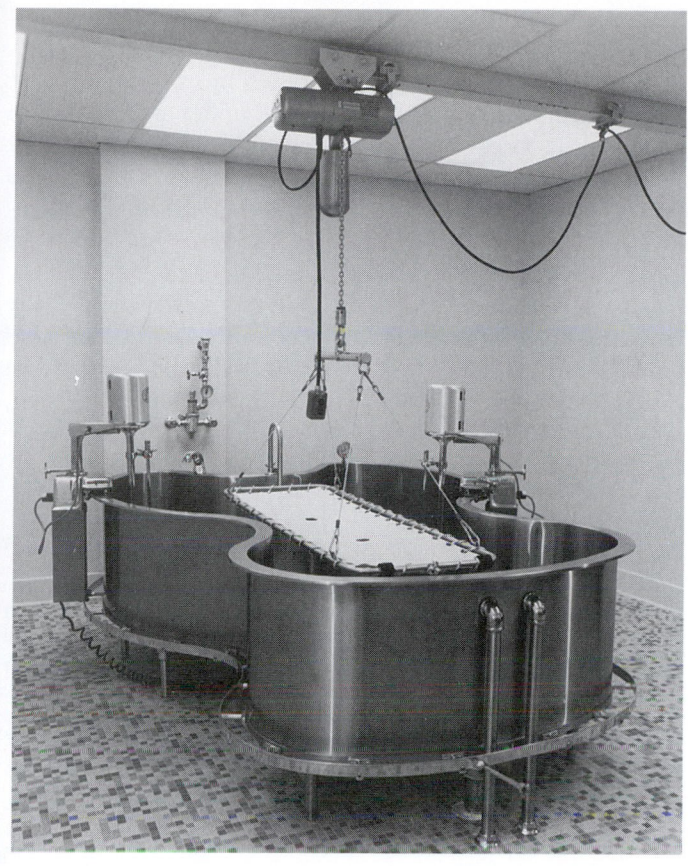

Figure 5-5   Hubbard tank for total body immersion. The shape enables full range of motion of both upper and lower extremities in a buoyant environment. (From Michlovitz, SL ed.: Thermal Agents in Rehabilitation, ed 3. FA Davis, Philadelphia, 1996, p 163, with permission.)

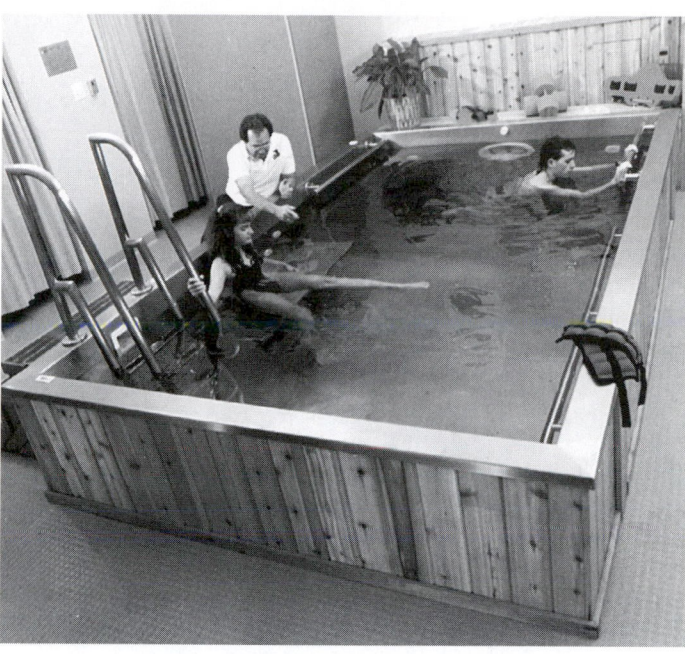

Figure 5-6   Patients performing aquatic exercises in a Therafit therapeutic pool. (Courtesy of Aqua Therapy Systems, Lafayette Hill, PA.)

effectiveness studies to determine the efficacy of the aquatic environment compared with a land program. Preliminary evidence and intuition lead many clinicians to believe that aquatic therapy is an effective tool for early intervention of acute injuries, for restoring function, for reducing the need for ambulatory assistive devices, for exercise, and for numerous other applications where gravity-resisted exercise and movement are difficult to perform. Therapeutic pools are sometimes equipped with underwater treadmills, stationary bikes, and various other exercise stations similar to what one would see in a therapeutic gym on land. Any of the strengthening or conditioning treatment goals that are worked on in a land environment can also be done in an aquatic environment. The difference between the two is that the aquatic environment will provide the patient with more support and will decrease compressive forces on weight-bearing joints because of the effects of buoyance. Despite this advantage, aquatic

TABLE 5-4 **The Relationship Between the Depth of Water in an Aquatic Pool and the Types of Activities That Would Be Possible in That Depth**		
DEEP WATER 5 FT OR > **(UNLOADED, OPEN CHAIN)**	**MIDLEVEL WATER, SHOULDER TO NIPPLE (MINIMAL LOAD, CLOSED CHAIN)**	**SHALLOW WATER, ILIAC CREST TO NIPPLE (MODERATE LOAD, CLOSED CHAIN)**
Cardiovascular with joint protection	Wall slides	Land-specific functional movements
Unloaded sport specific	Trunk PNF patterns	Progressive ambulation, balance/proprioceptive challenge
Ambulation without assistive devices	Progressive ambulation to wean from assistive devices	Sport-specific challenge
Unloaded exercises for spine/lower extermity injuries	Plyometrics	
	General flexibility	
	Sport progressive lateral challenge	
	Balance/proprioceptive challenge using turbulence	

PNF = proprioceptive neuromuscular facilitation.

> **Before You Begin**
>
> - Make sure that your patient feels comfortable in an aquatic environment.
> - Ask the patient if he or she knows how to swim or has any fear of the water.

therapy cannot completely meet all of the goals, because the ultimate goal of restoring function would be for a land environment. The patient must be able to return to a gravity environment in everyday life. Successive progressions from deep water to shallow water within the aquatic environment will enable patients to prepare for gravity as they recover.

Deep Water Exercise

Deep water exercises are those that take place in an aquatic pool that is deep enough so that the patient's feet do not touch the bottom. The feet are not "fixed" to the bottom; therefore, the exercises that are capable of being performed are termed "open chain." Depending on the height of the patient, the depth of the water should be at least 5 to 6 feet so that the patient is suspended in the water without touching the bottom. Buoyancy-assistive devices or tethering devices can be worn by the patient to maintain an upright posture in the water so that the lower extremities are free to move without having to try to maintain flotation. Deep ends of Olympic-size pools or public pools are effective for deep water unloaded exercise. The water temperature should be tepid (80° to 90°F) (26.7° to 32.2°C) because active and sometimes aggressive exercise is performed for treatment times that may approach 45 minutes. Deep water exercises can be successful and sometimes compare favorably with land exercise, particularly for patients recovering from stress fractures, because the weight-bearing load is decreased.[14]

"Unloaded" deep water exercises may also be an effective exercise medium during late pregnancy, because the pressure will be relieved from the lower back. Caution needs to be taken, though, regarding the length of immersion and water temperature. Generally, the resting heart rate is lowered when patients are immersed in water. This has an important implication when treating pregnant women with back pain, because exercise on land has been reported to increase fetal heart rates.[15] Results from some studies have indicated that there is an increase in oxygen consumption that occurs in the water compared with the same exercises on land.[10,16,17] This is a critical factor for maintaining levels of function and fitness when recovering from a spinal or an extremity injury. Athletes can perform the same amount of cardiovascular work with less strain to their joints because of the increased metabolic demands of exercise in the water, thus maintaining

their fitness levels of endurance and VO_2 maximums with "in-water running."[18] Conversely, the cardiac or pulmonary compromised patient may be unduly stressed by in-water exercise.

Full excursion of joints can occur under water without incurring the forces sometimes contraindicated with land or shallow water exercise. In a limited-space immersion deep water tank, tether cords are used to minimize forward movement in the tank. Full movement and forward progression are encouraged with deep water pool walking or running to facilitate normal movement patterns of the soft tissues. Many sizes and shapes of buoyancy belts or vests exist today to facilitate floating in an upright position. The devices can be adjusted to promote either lumbar extension or flexion, whichever is indicated for the patient.[19]

Midlevel to Shallow-Level Exercise

Midlevel (T-12 to chin) to shallow-level (knee to T-12) water depths permit the body to move over a fixed distal extremity, promoting some weight-bearing. Activities in these depths of water would be considered "closed-chain" activities, because there is weight-bearing on the distal extremities. Progression in weight-bearing is accomplished through the use of shallower water depths (see Table 5-4). When open-chain exercises are contraindicated, as with an unstable lower extremity or recent joint reconstruction where weight-bearing is desired, shallower depths can provide the closed-chain support that is necessary.[20] It has been reported that patients with intra-articular reconstructions had less joint effusion and faster return to perceived functional levels when performing water-based exercise compared with a similar group of patients performing the land exercises alone.[6]

Significant training effects have been reported with closed-chain water exercises. The findings included improved resting heart rates, improved VO_2 maximum measurements, and improved treadmill endurance tests.[16] Additional studies have reported improved VO_2 responses with water calisthenics and closed-chain exercise. Functionally, low-level patients can practice proper movement patterns of step climbing or upper-extremity reaching with the buoyant support of the water. To treat patients who have trunk weakness, dynamic stabilization of the trunk can be first addressed in midlevel water using buoyancy and hydrostatic pressure forces for support.[23] Pain with exercise can be minimized in an aquatic environment. For example, for a patient on land, pain can persist throughout a movement if weight is applied, whereas in the water the resistance to movement will stop once movement stops.

Bad Ragaz Techniques

Bad Ragaz techniques have been used and refined over the past 60 years. They were introduced at the Bad Ragaz Spa in Switzerland during the late 1950s. Bad Ragaz techniques use a buoyant ring to assist the patient in floating in the water. The ring may be placed around the trunk, under the extremities, or it may support the head and neck.[21] As knowledge of exercise and movement patterns increased, diagonal patterns of movement were developed using Voss's patterns of movement and applying them to a water environment.[22] These simple techniques are indicated for many musculoskeletal, neurologic, and arthritic conditions. Manual stretching is performed when there is a restriction in soft tissue movement. The patient's weight can be used to offer the overpressure needed to provide for an effective stretch. The patient is in effect lying supported by the buoyant force of the water, and his or her other body weight can act as resistance because of the drag that it creates to movement (Fig. 5-7). Positioning can be in supine buoyancy assisted, prone buoyancy assisted, or sidelying. Manual skills from massage such as soft tissue mobilization have sometimes been incorporated into buoyancy-supported movements. Aggressive stretching using techniques of Shiatsu massage have been incorporated into water techniques. Whatever the stretching technique performed, it should be based on a quantifiable dysfunction and have a desired specific outcome. For example, if the glenohumeral joint is hypomobile and the goal is to increase shoulder range of motion, stretching of the joint, long-axis distraction, and joint mobilization can all be applied by the clinician to the patient lying supine supported by the water. Bad Ragaz techniques also use isometric and isotonic exercises for the trunk or extremities. Trunk "pelvic neutral" exer-

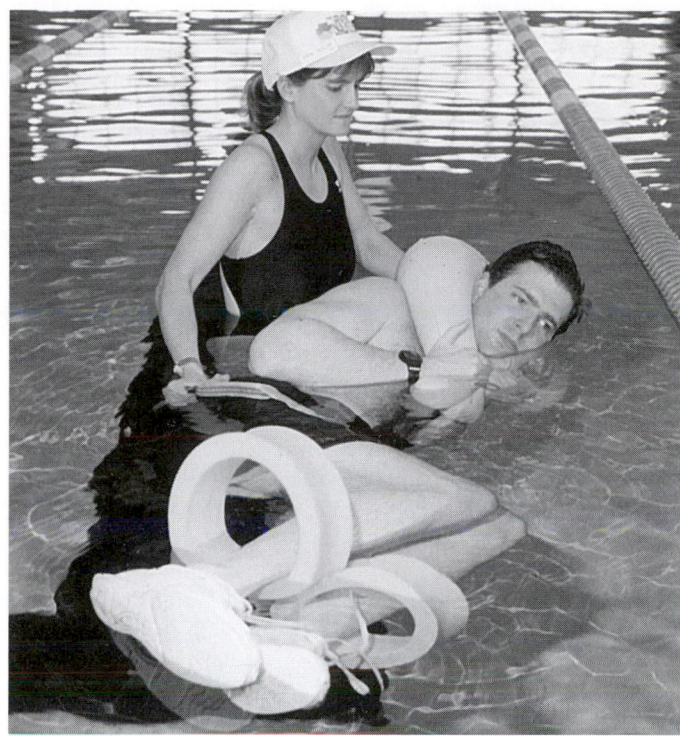

Figure 5-8   Patient performing buoyancy-assisted trunk flexion. He is supported by rings similar to Bad Ragaz rings as flotation devices.

cises have been described and studied developing proximal trunk stability (Fig. 5-8). Progression of exercise involves the addition of distal extremity mobility patterns.[23,24] The Bad Ragaz isometric techniques are often less painful to perform with an unloaded supine position compared with performance on land. For this reason, these exercises are an appropriate starting point for deconditioned patients, such as those with low back pain. The patient will progress appropriately to land activities for functional levels of activity or mobility to return.

Documentation

Functional rehabilitation should be carefully documented to record the parameters of care so that its efficacy can be established and the therapeutic program can be adjusted appropriately. A program with progression of exercises from buoyancy-assisted positions to buoyancy-resisted motion is illustrated in Table 5-5. Buoyancy-assisted motions use buoyancy devices to assist agonist muscle groups through the movement; buoyancy-resisted motions are the same motions without the device. These exercises are used to improve active motion and function. Buoyancy-resisted motions are

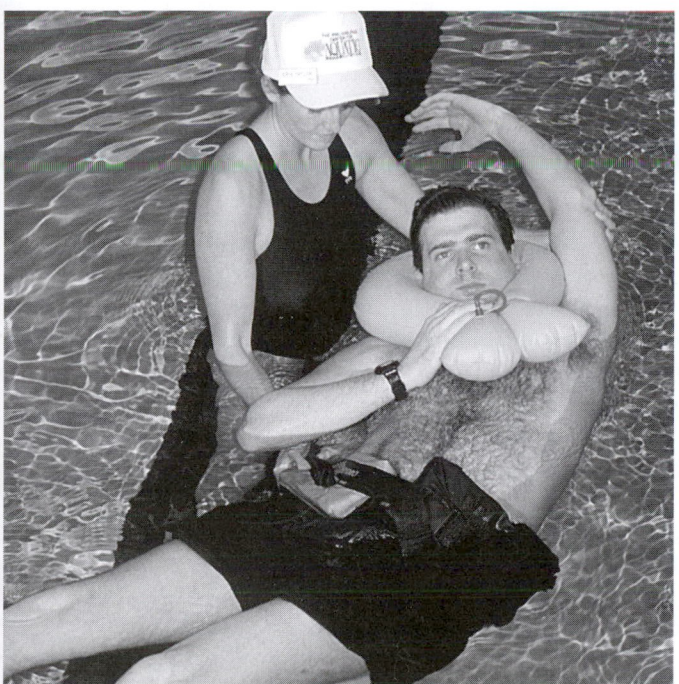

Figure 5-7   Patient supported by flotation devices while performing elongation of the left side of the trunk. Buoyancy is supporting the patient.

TABLE 5-5 Documentation and Progression of Hip Abduction in Aquatic Exercise

EXERCISE TYPE	ACTIVITY
Buoyancy-supported passive (supine in water)	Provider provides passive stretch.
Buoyancy-supported active assist (supine in water)	Provider assists movement of the motion while in buoyancy-supported position.
Buoyancy-supported active (supine in water)	Active range of motion.
Buoyancy supra assist	Standing, abduction with buoyancy-assist device on ankle.
Buoyancy-assisted	Standing, abduction.
Buoyancy resist	Standing, abduct with increasing speed against resistance.
Buoyancy supra resist	Standing, resistive boot secured, abduct against resistance.
Buoyancy-supported, manual resist (supine in water)	Closed chain, body moves over fixed extremity (fixed by provider)

performed with the agonistic muscle groups in a direction against the buoyancy of the water, with a supraresistive device added to increase the surface area and increase the resistance. It is imperative that the progression from buoyancy-assisted to buoyancy-resisted activities be documented clearly, as well as the depth and temperature of the water. Items that must be documented include the following:

- Equipment used
- Buoyancy-assisted devices
- Weights used
- Temperature
- Exercises
- How buoyancy-assisted devices were used
- Where weights were located and their purpose
- Depth of water

 Patient Safety

In an aquatic environment, it is important to remember that patients may not know how to swim. Many people have an innate fear of water and drowning. You will need to reassure the patient regarding safety precautions while in the aquatic environment.

- Check your surroundings and know what is going on at all times.
- Know your equipment.
- Know emergency evacuation procedures out of an aquatic environment.

Patient Education

The patient will need to be educated on the need to progress to a more functional type of exercises outside of an aquatic pool. There will need to be ongoing education to reassure and reinforce the patient of the aquatic environment, and

 Patient Perspective

Patients often say they have never felt better than when they are in an aquatic environment.

PATIENTS' FREQUENTLY ASKED QUESTIONS

1. What is the difference between aquatic exercise and aquatic physical therapy?

2. What is the range of pool temperatures for specific kinds of therapy and certain ailments?

3. Can patients with hepatitis B virus infection and other waterborne illnesses participate in aquatic therapy?

its purpose. Patients must be able to perform functional activities in a "land" environment to be considered functional.

Clinical Decisions for Hydrotherapy and Aquatic Therapy

Consideration should be given for what type of tank should be used to conserve water and optimally perform the treatment. If active wrist exercises are needed, a small extremity tank is well suited for this patient. If the patient is being treated for a decubitus ulcer on the ischial tuberosity, a low boy or Hubbard tank would be the most appropriate, because an aquatic pool would be contraindicated for this patient.

The water depth, temperature, and techniques are all important considerations for aquatic therapy. Deep water walking might be appropriate for a total hip replacement after the sutures have been removed, but it would be impossible as a land activity. Mid-level to shallow-level water exercises gradually increase the amount of weight-bearing for a patient; activities might include jumping, running, or walking, using the water to assist or resist the activity. Unilateral balance activities can be accomplished in midlevel water depths, and resistance can be increased by adding turbulence to perturb the balance.

Hydrotherapy for Wound Care

Whirlpools

The objective of therapeutic intervention for wound care is to provide an optimal wound healing environment. Based on knowledge of the expected progression of wound healing and on thorough assessment of intrinsic and extrinsic factors, treatment should facilitate normal cellular activity. Clinicians need to recognize how treatment will affect cellular function and provide care that will avoid wound trauma.

Additives to Prevent Infection

Whirlpools have been used for many years in the treatment of open wounds, fractures, and other orthopedic injuries.[13] To accomplish treatment goals without spreading infection, the tanks and their turbines must be thoroughly cleaned between patients. The most common agents used to prevent or reduce the chance of infection are povidone-iodine, chloramine-T, and sodium hypochlorite (household bleach). The size of the tank and the manufacturer's recommendations will guide the clinician toward the appropriate concentration of an additive. It is important to remember that the tank is not the only potential host for infections; the turbine is also a potential source. It is important to run the turbine with a disinfectant agent in the water so that the air intake valves of the turbine are also cleaned.

Whirlpool Cleaning Procedure

- Filling and emptying whirlpools
- Know where drain open/closure knob is
  - Open to drain
  - Close to fill
- Know where your water supply is
  - Hose
  - Wall mounted
- Cleaning of tank
- Spray/squirt disinfectant on all inside surfaces of tank (diluted solution)
  - Let set 5 minutes (while turbine is cleaning)
  - Wash with wet cloth
  - Rinse with water
- Spray stainless steel cleaner on outside surface of tank
  - Do once a day, usually at the end of the day
- Turbine cleaning
- Place turbine in bucket
  - Add one full squirt of full-strength disinfectant to each gallon of water.
  - Turn speed control/aerator to lowest speed or closed, so water filters up through turbine.

- Fill bucket with water sufficient to cover the air hole on the turbine.
- Run turbine for a minimum of 5 minutes.
- Empty cleaning bucket and refill with clean water. Place turbine in bucket and run for an additional 5 minutes to rinse.
- Small tanks into which buckets will not fit
  - Clean sides of tank as previously done.
  - Fill tank with water (sufficient to cover air hole on turbine).
  - Close aerator as previously done.
  - Run turbine for 5 minutes.
  - Drain tank and fill with clean water.
  - Run turbine for 5 additional minutes to rinse (Figs. 5-9 and 5-10).
- Cleaning of other tanks
  - Spray cleaner on all inside surfaces.
  - Wipe with wet cloth.
  - Let set 5 to 10 minutes.
  - Rinse with clean water.
- Types of cleaners (common)
  - Expose (full strength and diluted)
  - Stainless steel cleaner
  - Cenclean
  - Waxcide
- Exposure to chemicals
- Refer to Material Safety Data Sheet for all cleaners used.

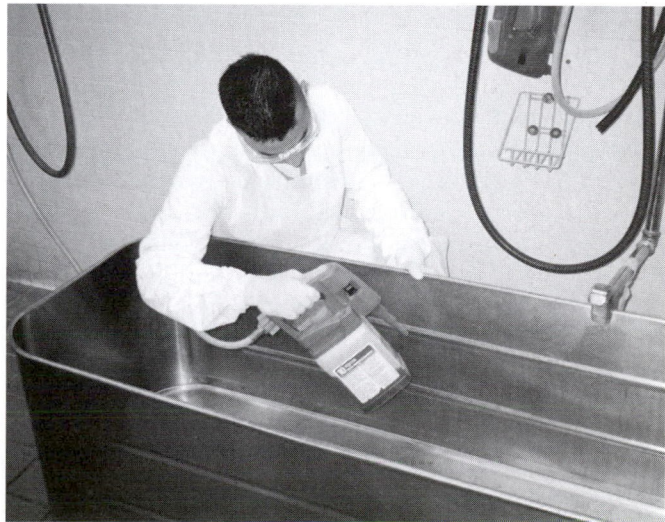

Figure 5–9 Gloved clinician has emptied the whirlpool to be cleaned and is spraying cleaner into the tank.

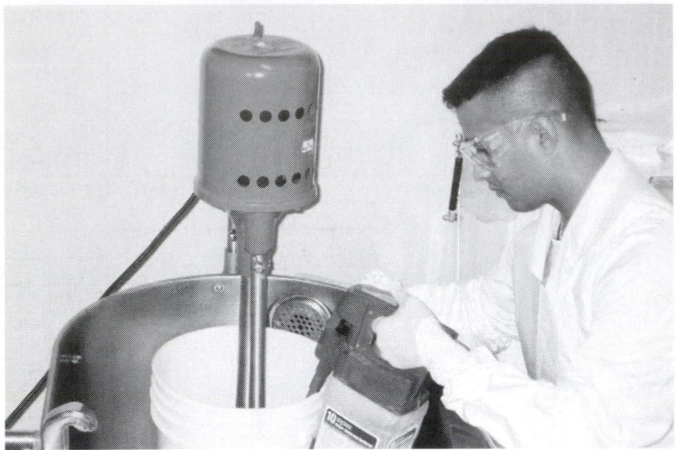

Figure 5-10 To clean the turbine, a bucket has been placed under the turbine, filled with enough water to cover the air intake hole. Then cleaner is being added before running the turbine in the bucket for at least 5 minutes.

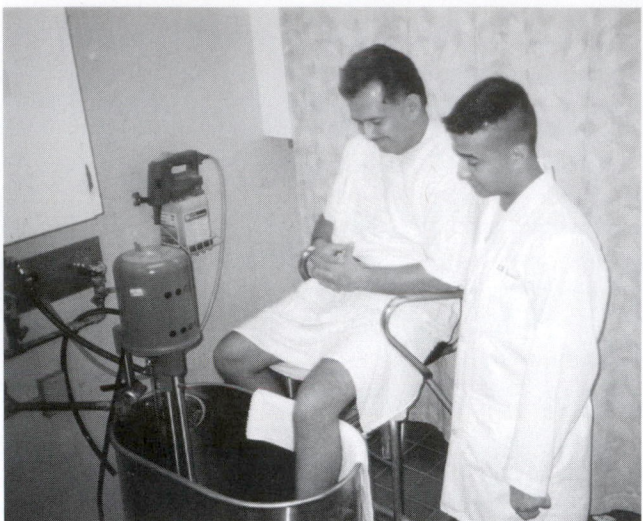

Figure 5-11 Once the determination has been made that whirlpool is appropriate to facilitate wound repair, the patient must be positioned so that there is no undue pressure from the side of the tank on the immersed extremity. The towel cushions the calf and the popliteal space has clearance from the edge of the side of the tank.

Considerations for Hydrotherapy Treatment

In considering hydrotherapy treatment for wound management, the clinician needs to ask the following questions:

- What are the effects of the treatment?
- When do the effects facilitate healing, and when are they detrimental?
- How should the effects be used?
- Are there other treatment options?

Hydrotherapy can be used for debridement, cleansing, hydration, circulatory stimulation, and analgesia. Care should be given to maintain appropriate patient positioning to guard against increased pressure (Fig. 5-11).

Debridement

Debridement is the rapid removal of necrotic and devitalized tissue to allow reepithelialization and granulation. Necrotic and devitalized tissue impedes granulation and prevents or slows migration of epithelial cells across the wound.[25,26] Debridement is indicated for wounds with extensive necrotic tissue. This tissue delays healing and provides potential for bacterial growth and infection.[27] Hydrotherapy can be used to debride, soften, and loosen adherent devitalized tissue in preparation for manual or enzymatic debridement (Fig. 5-12).

Hydrotherapy provides nonselective debridement, with removal of viable tissues along with necrotic devitalized tissue and debris. Nonselective debridement may cause injury to new endothelial and epithelial cells, disrupting the formation of new blood vessels (neovascularization) and the formation of new skin (reepithelialization).

Modality

The provision of hydrotherapy for wound care may be done with different types of modalities, such as whirlpools, pulsatile lavage, and irrigation. With each, the goals will be the same; however, the modalities will provide different benefits versus disadvantages. For example, if a patient is nonam-

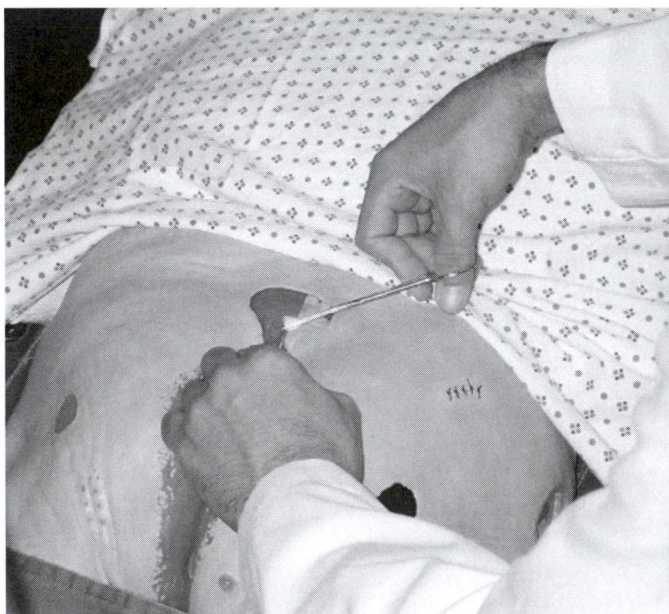

Figure 5-12 This patient has been transported the hydrotherapy area of the department and transferred to a gurney that can be raised and lowered into the Hubbard tank for treatment. As long as the gurney is lowered so that the head is angled above the surface of the water, this position will potentially provide non-specific debridement to the healing areas without undue pressure.

bulatory and has a small wound, pulsatile lavage may be more appropriate than whirlpool treatment.

Cleansing

Cleansing removes dirt, foreign bodies, exudate, or residue from topical agents and bacteria. Excess exudate, bacterial residue, or foreign substances can prolong the normal inflammatory response and delay the proliferative phase of healing.[28] Dirt and foreign bodies provide a medium for promoting bacterial growth and infection. The critical number for bacteria is considered to be 10^5 organisms/gram of tissue[30]; an excess may result in infection. If there is concern of infection, a culture should be obtained.

Removal of residue from topical agents is done to allow topical antibodies or enzymatic preparations, if used, to reach the wound bed. When using cleansing techniques, avoid concentrations of topical agents that might damage new cells.

Hydration

Hydration provides a moist wound bed that will proceed more rapidly through the phases of healing.[25,30] Dehydration (desiccation) of the wound may result in an alteration of electrical potentials of skin (e.g., a decreased lateral voltage gradient) and adversely affect epidermal migration.[31]

Circulatory Stimulation

Increased circulation obtained with hydrotherapy appears to be the result of thermal rather than mechanical effects.[34] Increasing local circulation can facilitate healing by increasing oxygen levels and metabolite removal.

Increasing circulation in an area of venous insufficiency can facilitate circulatory compromise, increase edema, and impede healing. The blood is entering the area and hydrostatic pressure is increased more than the venous system can compensate.

Mechanical effects of hydrotherapy can be potentially damaging to new endothelial and epithelial cells, slowing healing and decreasing resistance to infection.

Analgesia and Sedation

Mechanical stimulation of skin receptors, such as with gentle whirlpool agitation, can assist in decreasing pain. Thermal effects can assist with pain relief by increasing circulation in areas of compromised arterial flow.

Intrinsic and Extrinsic Factors

Effective utilization of hydrotherapy for wound healing must consider intrinsic and extrinsic factors. Information obtained and documented should include status of the patient, condition of tissues other than the wound, and description of the wound.

Patient Status

Important factors in providing treatment include the following:

- Subjective report, especially of pain and sensory changes
- Duration and intensity of symptoms
- Age
- Occupation
- Alcohol and tobacco use
- Systemic conditions
- Medications
  - Previous
  - Current
- Allergy
  - History of the wound
- Mechanism
- Healing progress or lack thereof
- Previous treatment
- Location of wound

Condition of Surrounding Tissues

The area around the wound or even an entire extremity environment is important in optimal wound healing. The area around the wound or extremity tissues should be assessed for

- Color
- Edema
- Temperature
- Areas of pain or sensory changes
- Trophic changes
- Pulses

Attention should be given to areas of swelling, redness, increased temperature, and pain. During the early inflammatory phase, these are not unexpected, but prolongation may indicate potential for delayed healing or infection.

Description of the Wound

Wounds may be classified according to type of closure:

- Primary
- Delayed primary
- Secondary intention
- Grafts or flaps
- Delayed
- Chronic stage I–IV

Open wounds can be classified according to the three-color concept of Marion Laboratory.[32] This concept uses a color description of the wound bed tissue in order of severity: red, yellow, or black. Documentation of the color or colors present and percentage of each directs treatment toward the most severe or predominant color.

In addition to the type of closure and description of wound bed, the clinician needs to document and describe the location of the wound; its size, shape, and margins; and the amount, color, consistency, and odor of any exudate.

Facilitation of Healing

Indications

Indications for hydrotherapy include debridement or preparation for debridement in wounds healing by second intention, stable flaps or grafts, and stage III or IV chronic ulcers with less than 50% necrotic tissue.

Hydrotherapy may also be indicated for cleansing wounds containing excess or malodorous exudate, loose debris or foreign bodies, or localized infection. A venous insufficiency ulcer may benefit from cleansing techniques that avoid dependent positioning and increased tissue temperature. A desiccated wound bed may be moisturized with hydrotherapy techniques. The patient with arterial insufficiency may obtain some pain relief[33] and increased circulation with gentle agitation–warm temperature treatment.

Precautions and Contraindications

Hydrotherapy, especially whirlpool technique, can be overused, providing no benefits or even detrimental effects to healing wounds. Fresh granulation tissue is fragile and may be damaged by too much turbulence too soon.

The clean, primarily closed, clean reepithelializing or granulating (red), or chronic wound with greater than 50% adherent black eschar will usually not benefit from hydrotherapy. A wound with nonlocalized infection or tissues with cellulitis may be further compromised. Whirlpool treatment should not be used with split-thickness skin grafts before 3 to 5 days and full-thickness skin grafts before 7 to 10 days.

Edematous tissues may incur increased venous compromise with hydrotherapy if the extremity is dependently positioned and provided with increased tissue temperature via warm water. Patient tolerance for treatment, including systemic factors and allergy or sensitivity to additives, is an important consideration.

Clinical Use of Hydrotherapy Techniques

Whirlpool may be indicated for debridement or preparation for debridement, cleansing, circulatory stimulation, hydration, or analgesia. Clinical hydrotherapy techniques include whirlpool, irrigation or flushing, rinsing, and soaking. The technique used will depend on the desired effect, condition of the patient, and status of the wound and surrounding tissues.

Irrigation or flushing with sterile water or saline in a syringe or Water Pik[34] may be indicated for removing superficial nonadherent cell debris or topical agents. Cleansing of malodorous wounds, removal of exudate, and hydration may also be obtained with alternatives to whirlpool, such as use of a faucet or hose, or soaking in a basin. The amount of pressure delivered to tissues with irrigation, rinsing, or flushing is manually controlled and therefore is not consistent, and care must be taken to avoid tissue and wound trauma.

Cleansing or debridement with irrigation, flushing, rinsing, or soaking techniques can be considered as an alternative to whirlpool, more tolerable to a debilitated patient, with avoidance of prolonged dependent positioning, and more efficient in use of time and staff. For example, a cleansing technique other than whirlpool is often appropriate for venous insufficiency ulcers to avoid dependent positioning and increased tissue temperature.

Additives

Bactericidal additives most frequently used are povidone-iodine, sodium hypochlorite, and chloramine-T (Chlorazine). These agents, unless properly diluted, can be injurious to fibroblasts.[35] Patients may also have sensitivity or allergy to additives, and the open wound provides entrance for systemic absorption.[36]

The clinician needs to consider the effects of an additive and, if necessary for bacterial control of wound infection, use a concentration that is bactericidal without injuring fibroblasts. Often, use of sterile water or saline for irrigation, flushing, or soaking and avoidance of any whirlpool additive will provide the best wound environment.

Recommended dilutions of povidone-iodine are 1:1000 and of sodium hypochlorite 1:100.[38] Steve and colleagues[37] recommend use of chloramine-T in concentrations of 50 g per 60-gallon tank and 320 g per Hubbard tank.

Temperature

Recommended temperature for hydrotherapy application in wound treatment is in the neutral range of 92° to 96°F (33.5° to 35.58°C)[33] or no greater than 1°C above skin temperature. Temperature will be based on the indications for hydrotherapy, the condition of the patient, and the area to be treated.

Duration and Agitation

Duration of treatment and amount of whirlpool agitation or force of irrigation or rinsing are determined by the indications for treatment. Considerations are the desired effects, state of the wound and surrounding tissues, and patient tolerance.

There is no absolute standard duration, with soaking, irrigation, or rinsing varying from 1 to 5 minutes, debridement from 10 to 20 minutes, and increasing circulation 20 minutes.[38] A venous ulcer may benefit from 5 minutes or less of rinsing or soaking in tepid water.[36]

When using whirlpool agitation, it is important to remember that increased airflow through the turbine results in increased pressure and that there is increased turbulence toward the water surface.[10] Fragile tissues, such as a split-thickness skin graft at 3 to 5 days or a full-thickness skin graft at 7 to 10 days, should be exposed to only minimal agitation and should not be positioned toward the water surface, due to increased turbulance. Treatment duration initially should be limited to 5 minutes.

Positioning

Patient tolerance and comfort and avoidance of circulatory compromise or nerve compression with posturing or restrictive garments must always be considered when positioning a patient for treatment.

Ambient Temperature

A warm environment is important in ensuring patient comfort and avoiding reflex vasoconstriction and compromised wound healing, which can occur with exposure to cool room air.

Theory Behind Effectiveness Whirlpool affects the *inflammation phase* of healing.

- Warm water increases vasodilatation of the superficial vessels.
- Increased blood flow brings oxygen and nutrients to the tissues and removes metabolites.
- Increased blood flow brings antibodies, leukocytes, and systemic antibiotics.
- Fluid shifts into the interstitial spaces, leading to edema.
- Softening and loosening of necrotic tissue aid phagocytosis.
- Cleansing and removal of wound exudate control infection.
- Mechanical effects of whirlpool stimulate granulation tissue formation.
- Sedation and analgesia are induced by the warm water.

Explanation to Patient

Clinicians need to remember the importance of the patient as a member of the health care team. Explanation of the problems, goals, precautions, and treatment plan is a vital component of optimal care. Example of education to patient would include discussion of nutrition and how this relates to wound healing, contraindications, and instructions on dressing wound.

 ## Summary

Hydrotherapy use can vary from burn management, active sprains, wound care, and buoyancy-assisted or -resisted exercise. Although specific treatment protocols may vary by facility, the decision to include hydrotherapy for treatment should be based on knowledge of the potential benefits of water as a therapeutic medium and the treatment goals. Wound treatment should be based on knowledge of the biologic events in wound healing, effects of techniques used, status of the patient and the wound, and other available options.

Other purposes of hydrotherapy are as follows:

- Hydrotherapy can provide phasic stimuli to the skin afferents, continuously reactivating them.
- It can increase hydrostatic pressure, which may increase lymphatic circulation.
- It can provide a mean for grading exercises (for example, moving a limb with or without turbulence).
- It can provide heat or cold to a large part of the body.
- It can help to decrease weight-bearing.
- It can remove debris and necrotic tissue from wounds and decrease the bacterial load.

Discussion Questions

1. The use of whirlpool agitation provides which method of debridement?
2. Why is nonselective debridement possibly detrimental to wound healing?
3. What alternative method to whirlpool might be more appropriate for the treatment of venous insufficiency ulcer?
4. Is whirlpool treatment indicated for a wound described as having 100% red granulation bed? Why?
5. What precautions should be considered with use of additives in whirlpool treatments?
6. What are some safety issues with aquatic pools?
7. What are some contraindications to aquatic therapy?
8. What is more difficult for a patient with weight-bearing precautions in the aquatic pool? Walking in deep water or walking in shallow water? Why?
9. What are some educational issues that would need to be addressed before a patient is discharged from an aquatic environment?

CASE STUDY

Mary is a 72-year-old woman with rheumatoid arthritis affecting mainly her hands, feet, knees, and shoulders. She ambulates with two canes in a flexed posture due to flexion deformities at her hips and knees. This patient loves heat and finds the pool very soothing. She was admitted 3 weeks earlier with an acute flareup and is now in the subacute phase.

- What are the goals of hydrotherapy?

- Describe what would be the best method of entry into the pool and the ideal starting position? What treatment approach would you use?

- Because rheumatoid arthritis is a chronic disease for which your treatment is as much preventative as curative, when would you discontinue treatment and with what recommendations?

References

1. Framroze, A: Aquatic rehabilitation Q & A: Judy A Cirullo PT. Rehab Manag 8:43, 1995.

2. Walsh, M: Hydrotherapy: The use of water as a therapeutic agent. In Michlovitz, SL (ed): Thermal Agents in Rehabilitation. FA Davis, Philadelphia, 1986.

3. Skinner, AT, and Thomson, AM: Duffield's Exercise in Water, ed 3. Bailliere Tindall, London, 1983.

4. Bueche, F: Principles of Physics, ed 4. McGraw-Hill, New York, 1982.

5. Johnson, LB, Stromme, SB, Adamczyk, JW, et al: Comparison of oxygen uptake and heart rate during exercises on land and in water. Phys Ther 57:273, 1977.

6. Tovin, BJ, Wolf, SL, Greenfield, BH, et al: Comparison of the effects of exercise in water and on land on the rehabilitation of patients with intra-articular anterior cruciate ligament reconstructions. Phys Ther 74:712, 1994.

7. Wilmore, J, II: Athletic Training and Physical Fitness. Allyn & Bacon, Boston, 1978.

8. Behlsen, GM, Grigsby, SA, and Winant, DM: Effects of an aquatic fitness program on the muscular strength and endurance of patient with multiple sclerosis. Physiotherapy 64:653, 1984.

9. Hanna, RD, Sheldahl, LM, and Tristani, FE: The effect of enhanced preload with head-out water immersion on exercise response in men with healed myocardial infarction. Am J Cardiol 71:1041, 1993.

10. Hellerbrand, T, Holutz, S, and Eubank, I: Measurement of whirlpool temperature, pressure and turbulence. Arch Phys Med Rehabil 32:17, 1950.

11. Costil, D: Energy requirements during exercise in the water. J Sports Med 11:87, 1971.

12. Bullard, RW, and Rapp, GM: Problems of body heat loss in water immersion. Aerospace Med 41:1269, 1970.

13. Toomey, R, Grief-Schwartz, R, and Piper, MC: Clinical evaluation of the effects of whirlpool on patients with Colles' fractures. Physiother Can 38:280–284, 1986.

14. Clemant, DB, Ammann, W, Taunton, JE, et al: Exercise-induced stress injuries to femur. J Sports Med 14:347, 1993.

15. Katz, VL, McMurray, R, Goodwin, WE, and Cefalo, RC: Nonweightbearing exercise during pregnancy on land and during immersion: A comparative study. Am J Perinatol 7:281, 1990.

16. Routi, RG, Toup, JT, and Berger, RA: The effects of nonswimming water exercises on older adults. J Orthop Sports Phys Ther 19:140, 1994.

17. Cassady, SL, and Nielsen, DH: Cardiorespiratory responses of healthy subjects to calisthenics performed on land versus in water. Phys Ther 72:532, 1992.

18. Fyestone, ED, Fellingham, G, George, J, and Fisher G: Effect of water running and cycling on maximum oxygen consumption and two mile run performance. Am J Sports Med 21:41, 1993.

19. Whann, CM, Chung, JK, Gregory, PC, et al: A new improved flotation device for deep-water exercise. J Burn Care Rehabil 12:62, 1991.

20. Shelbourne, KD, and Wilckens, JH: Current concepts in anterior cruciate ligament rehabilitation. Orthop Rev 11:957, 1990.

21. Boyle, AM: The Bad Ragaz ring method. Physiotherapy 67:265, 1981.

22. Voss, DE, Ionta, MK, and Myers, BJ: Proprioceptive Neuromuscular Facilitation. Harper & Row, Philadelphia, 1985.

23. Cole, A, Eagleston, RE, Moschetti, M, and Sinnett, E: Spine pain: Aquatic rehabilitation strategies. J Back Musculoskel Rehabil 4:273, 1994.

24. Saal, JA: Dynamic muscular stabilization in the non-operative treatment of lumbar pain syndromes. Orthop Rev 19:691, 1990.

25. Hunt, TK, and Van Winkle, W: Wound healing: Normal repair. In Dunphy, JE (ed): Fundamentals of Wound Management in Surgery. Chirugecom, South Plainfield, NJ, 1977, p 40.

26. Feedar, JA: Clinical management of chronic wounds. In McCulloch, JM, Kloth, LC, and Feedar, JA (eds): Wound Healing: Alternatives in Management, ed 2. FA Davis, Philadelphia, 1995, p. 151.

27. Agency for Health Care Policy and Research: Treatment of Pressure Ulcers: Clinical Practice Guideline No.15. ACHPR Publication No. 95.0625. U.S. Department of Health and Human Services, Rockville, MD, 1994, pp 6–7, 47–53.

28. Kloth, LC, and Miller, KH: The inflammatory response to wounding. In McCulloch, JM, Kloth, LC, and Feedar, JA (eds): Wound Healing: Alternatives in Management. FA Davis, Philadelphia, 1990, p 3.

29. Alvarez, OM, Mertz, PM, and Eaglstein, WH: The effect of occlusive dressings on collagen synthesis and re-epithelialization in superficial wounds. J Surg Res 35:142, 1983.

30. Pollack, SV: The wound healing process. Clin Dermatol 2:8, 1984.

31. Kloth, LC: Electrical stimulation in tissue repair. In McCullough, JM, Kloth, LC, and Feedar, JA (eds): Wound Healing: Alternatives in Management, ed 2. FA Davis, Philadelphia, 1995, p 298.

32. Walsh, MT: Relationship of hand edema to upper extremity water temperature during whirlpool treatment on normals.

Master's thesis. College of Allied Health Professions, Philadelphia, 1983.

33. Cazell, JZ: Wound care forum—the new RYB color code. Am J Nursing 1342, 1988.

34. Walsh, MT: Hydrotherapy: The use of water as a therapeutic agent. In Michlovitz, SL (ed): Thermal Agents in Rehabilitation, ed 2. FA Davis, Philadelphia, 1990, p 132.

35. Trelstad, A, et al: Water Piks: Wound cleansing alternative. Plast Surg Nursing 9:117, 198.

36. Linneaweaver, W, et al: Cellular and bacterial toxicities of topical antimicrobials. Plast Reconstruct Surg 75:394, 1985.

37. Aronoff, GR, et al: Increased serum iodide concentration from iodine absorption through wounds treated topically with povidone-iodine. Am J Med Sci 279:173, 1980.

38. Steve, L, Goodhard, P, and Alexander, J. Hydrotherapy burn treatment: Use of chloramine-T against resistant microorganisms. Arch Phys Med Rehabil 60:301, 1970.

39. Borrell, R, et al: Comparison of in vivo temperature produced by hydrotherapy, paraffin wax treatment, and Fluidotherapy. Phys Ther 60:1273, 1986.

40. McCulloch, JM, and Houde, J: Treatment of wounds due to vascular problem. In Kloth, LC, McCulloch, JM, and Feedar, JK (eds): Wound Healing: Alternatives in Management, ed 2. FA Davis, Philadelphia, 1990, p 191.

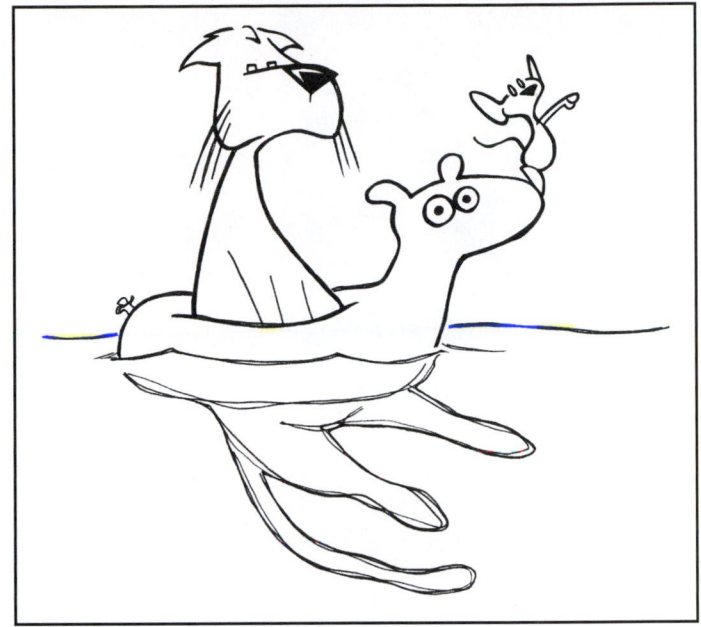

Objectives

- Define the principles of the therapeutic application of traction.
- Describe the theories of cervical and lumbar traction.
- Describe the theories and application of mechanical forms of traction.
- Discuss the clinical uses and safety considerations regarding the use of traction.
- Outline the clinical decision making in the use of traction as a treatment modality.

Key Terms

Angle of pull	Herniation	Manual traction
Distraction	Hypomobility	Mechanical traction
Facet	Impingement	Mobilization
Friction	Intervertebral space	Traction

Burke Gurney, PT, PhD

Soft Tissue Treatment Techniques: Traction

Outline

"Will traction affect my height?"

Traction has long been a mainstay for physical therapists when treating a variety of spinal problems. Many causes of spinal pain, as well as weakness, paresthesia, and pain referred from the spine, have traditionally been treated with traction techniques.

There have been mixed reviews from researchers regarding the physiologic effects of traction.[1] The findings range from claims of profound changes in spinal occlusion[2,3] to studies showing no statistical differences between traction and bedrest.[4] The negative findings have largely been in studies of specific and/or dated methods such as bed traction.

Like some physical therapy treatments, the use of traction has been a subject of ongoing debate amongst physical therapists and physicians. Controversy exists regarding optimal techniques, treatment times, positions, frequency, duration, force of pull, angle of pull, and overall efficacy of traction.

The scrutiny of research has helped drive the evolution of traction over the past several decades. Traction no longer means simply mechanical traction performed by traction machines and can include forms such as polyaxial traction, inversion traction, home traction units, and the assortment of manual traction.

A review of the literature in traction is daunting as there is a seemingly endless variety of treatment techniques and protocols. In attempts to face this problem, several researchers have consolidated the different protocols into useful information,[5-7] such as the general acceptance that supine is preferable to sitting when treating the cervical spine. It also appears that, regarding apparent efficacy, all forms of traction cannot be lumped together. In general, for example, there seems to be a greater body of literature to support the use of cervical traction than the use of lumbar traction.

Some therapists use traction liberally for a number of conditions such as herniated nucleus pulposus and lateral stenosis (a diminution of the intervertebral foramen). Some do not use traction at all. Although controversy remains as to physiologic effects, traction has weathered the test of time as a useful treatment for many spinal problems.[1-3,8-12]

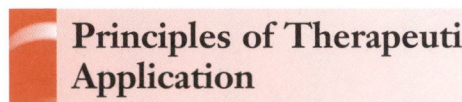

Principles of Therapeutic Application

Terminology and Definitions

Traction

The word traction is defined as a process of drawing apart or pulling. In physical therapy applications, traction refers to any process that results in the separation of bones, usually spinal segments. Two areas of the spine are commonly treated using traction—the lumbar spine (lumbar traction) and the cervical spine (cervical traction). There are many types of traction used in clinics; a partial list of these is given in Table 6-1.

TABLE 6-1 Traction Methods

TYPE OF TRACTION	FEATURES	ADVANTAGES/DISADVANTAGES
Autotraction	Involves the patient using his/her own muscle strength as the distraction source. This can be done in different ways, the use of a three-dimensional autotraction table. Has gained popularity in Europe and is becoming more commonly used in the U.S. In addition, several home lumbar traction units utilize this method.	**Advantage:** Patient can control parameters such as position and amount of force. Some forms can be done at home. **Disadvantages:** Three-dimensional tables are expensive, have been shown to increase intradiskal pressure.
Cervical traction	Traction applied to the cervical spine by applying a force to move the weight superiorly, or mobilization technique used to distract the individual cervical vertebra. This can be done manually, with halters, or through Crutchfield tongs which are inserted directly into the skull.	
Continuous (bed) traction	Traction that is administered for several days to weeks. The traction force is often minimal because of the duration of the treatment. This form of traction has fallen into disuse because of studies indicating that the results are consistent with bedrest alone.	**Advantages:** Can be done at home, inexpensively. **Disadvantages:** Efficacy is questionable.
Elastic traction Gravity-assisted traction	Traction by use of elastic devices such as rubber bands. Utilizes gravity to facilitate localized traction of target issue. This differs from inversion traction in that the body is not suspended in the air.	**Advantages:** Can be done at home, inexpensively. Does not require healthy cardiopulmonary systems as does inversion traction. **Disadvantages:** Traction force is limited by body weight.
Head traction	Traction applied to the head in the presence of injury to the cervical vertebra.	

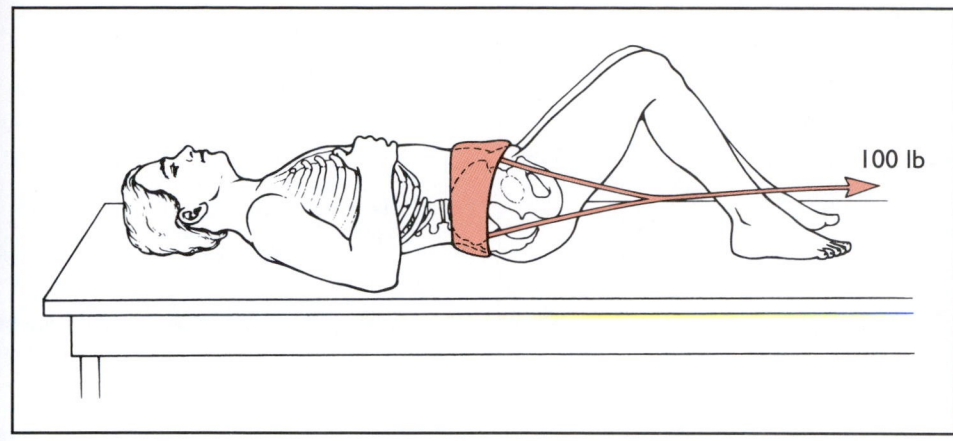

Figure 6-1   Patient is positioned supine with 100 pounds of pull.

Distraction

Perhaps the term distraction should be used instead of traction as it better describes the modality. Distraction is defined as the separation of surfaces of a joint by extension without injury or dislocation of the parts.[13]

Related Physics

A basic understanding of the physical principles of traction is necessary to understand the physiology of traction. Principles to be discussed include definition of force and friction as they pertain to traction.

A force, in the simplest sense, is a push or a pull. In the case of traction, it is generated either by the therapist (manual traction), by a machine (mechanical traction), or by weight (gravitational traction). If a therapist places a 100-pound weight on a cable and attaches it by way of a strap onto a patient, the patient will receive traction force of 100 pounds (Fig. 6-1).

Friction is the resistive force that arises to oppose the motion or attempted motion of an object past another with which it is in contact.[14] Friction results from irregularities of the surfaces of the two bodies. The direction of frictional force is always parallel to the surfaces in contact and in the direction opposing motion (Fig. 6-2).

The maximal frictional force on a body resting on another body is proportional to the normal force pushing the two objects together. For our purposes, the normal force would be the weight of the person on a table. The relationship between the maximal force of friction and the normal force is known as the coefficient of static friction and is designated by μ_s.

Expressed mathematically:

$$r_s = \frac{\text{maximal force of friction}}{\text{normal force (weight of person)}}$$

The coefficient of static friction has no units and is different for any two objects depending on how irregular the surfaces are between the two objects. It has been shown that the coefficient for static friction between a person and a treatment table is about 0.5.

Therefore, by example, if a person lying on a table weighed 160 pounds (normal force), the force of friction between the person and the table would be 80 pounds (Fig. 6-3).

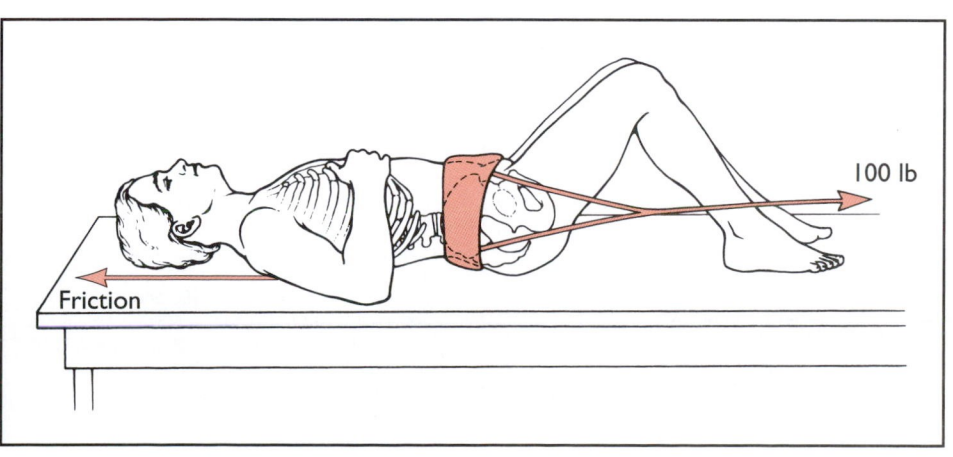

Figure 6-2   Patient is positioned with 100 pounds of traction pull, and the force of friction is depicted.

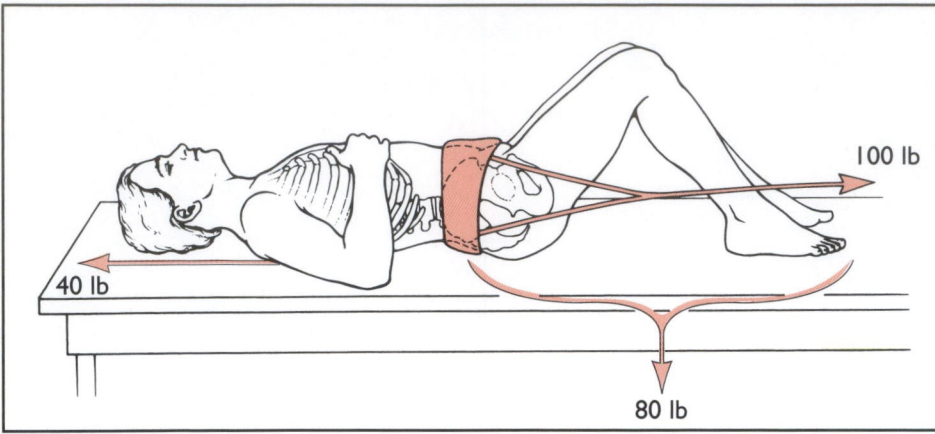

Figure 6–3 Patient is positioned supine with 100 pounds of traction pull, and the force of friction is indicated. The resultant pull is equivalent to 60 pounds once the coefficient of friction is calculated into the formula. The weight of the individual was 160 pounds, and 50% of the weight of the individual (80 pounds) was distributed between the legs and pelvis. The coefficient of friction was 50%. Summary: 160-pound patient (80 pounds below the waist), coefficient of friction = 50% or 40 pounds to move the pelvis and legs. Traction force applied = 100 pounds − 40 pounds for the pelvis and legs = 60 pounds of traction force. With the coefficient of static friction of 0.5, the 160-pound patient would have a frictional force of 80 pounds.

With lumbar traction, a thoracic harness is often used to keep the upper body from sliding along the table. Therefore, only half (the lower half) of the patient's body weight is involved in the traction. In our example, then, the amount of body weight involved would be 80 pounds, and the frictional force would be 40 pounds. In this case, the force of traction would be 60 pounds (Fig. 6-4).

In most clinics, however, this frictional force is eliminated by use of a split traction table that allows half of the table to glide horizontally on rollers independent of the other half of the table (Fig. 6-5). The use of a split traction table in combination with a thoracic harness ensures that very little force is lost to friction; therefore, the pull of traction can be substantially less.[15] This equipment is necessary only with lumbar traction.

With cervical traction, the coefficient of static friction between the head and the table has been calculated to be 0.62.[16] If the weight of the head were 15 pounds, for example, the traction force would have to be 9.3 pounds to overcome friction.

Theory of Application

Brief Historical Perspective

The use of traction may well date back to the time of the Egyptians and is documented at least to the times of Hippocrates (460–376 BC). The original traction table, or *Scamnum Hippocratis* ("the bench of Hippocrates"), was used by Galen (130–200 AD) and others (Fig. 6-6). The Turks have used a traction device for over 500 years, and the Italians used a traction table in the mid-sixteenth century that was based on the Hippocratic model.[17] Traction came into disuse for some time based in part on studies challenging its efficacy.

Traction enjoyed a renaissance starting with an orthopedist named James Cyriax in the 1950s and others who developed new and creative approaches to traction treatment. This spurred new research that verified some physiologic effects such as vertebral separation and reversal of spinal nerve root impingement.[12]

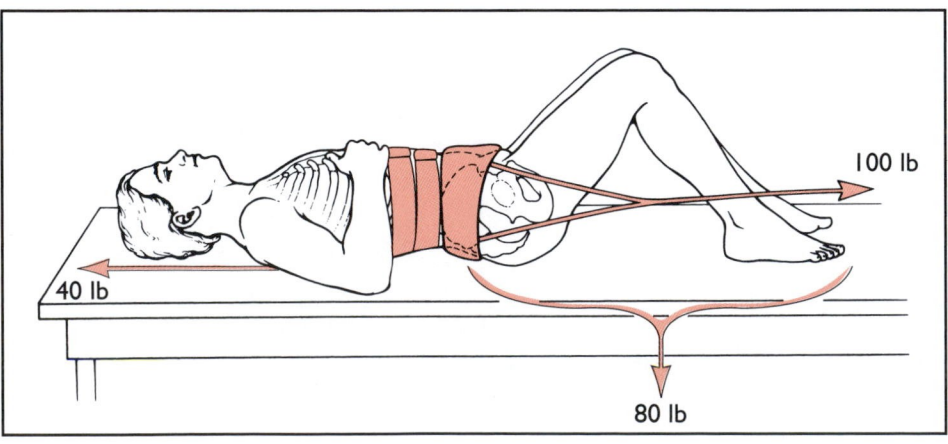

Figure 6–4 Patient is positioned supine with 100 pounds of traction pull, and the force of friction is indicated. The resultant pull is equivalent to 60 pounds once the coefficient of friction is calculated into the formula. The weight of the individual was 160 pounds, and 50% of the weight of the individual (80 pounds) was distributed between the legs and pelvis. The coefficient of friction was 50%. Summary: 160-pound patient (80 pounds below the waist), coefficient of friction = 50% or 40 pounds to move the pelvis and legs. Traction force applied = 100 pounds minus 40 pounds for the pelvis and legs = 60 pounds of traction.

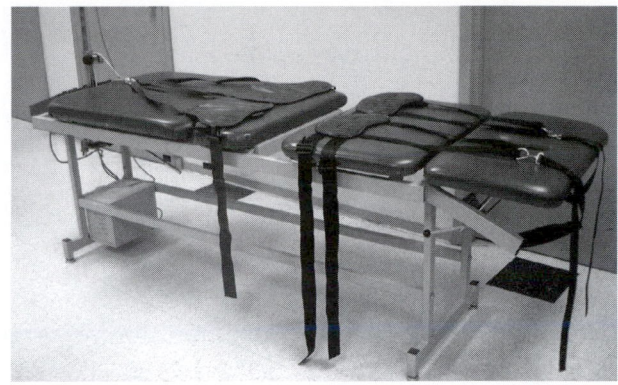

Figure 6-5   Split traction table, which lowers the coefficient of friction to close to zero. Traction force to cause movement or separation is greatly reduced through the use of a split table.

Current Trends and Research

Modern research involving traction has been going on since at least the 1950s and involves studies of the physical and physiologic effects and efficacy of traction and comparisons of different protocols of traction such as optimal patient positioning, intermittent versus continuous pull, angle of pull, and time and frequency of application. Some of the problems that arise when researching traction (and many other modalities) are (1) conclusively defining the population base; (2) objectively measuring variables, that is, pain and dysfunction levels, nerve decompression, etc.; and (3) eliminating or accounting for unwanted, e.g., confounding, variables.[18] It is probable that the future of traction research will be enhanced by better imaging equipment such as magnetic resonance imaging (MRI) and computerized axial tomography (CAT) scans. This will allow researchers to better categorize their diagnostic groups and better assess physiologic changes.

General Treatment Goals for Traction

Traction should be used, as all physical agents, with careful regard to desired physiologic effects[1] and should usually be combined with active components of treatment[19] such as strengthening, stretching, postural/proprioceptive training, and patient education. Goals of traction include reduction of radicular signs and symptoms associated with conditions such as disc protrusion, lateral stenosis, degenerative disc disease, and subluxations (i.e., spondylolisthesis). Other goals of trac-

Before You Begin

You need to ask yourself how much the patient weighs so that you can use an appropriate amount of weight for lumbar traction.

tion include reduction of muscle guarding/spasm via prolonged stretch; reduction of joint pain via neurophysiologic pathways (gating mechanism); and increasing range of motion (ROM) via distraction/mobilization of joint surfaces. Traction has also been used for fracture immobilization. Examples include immobilization of cervical spine fracture via Crutchfield or Burton tongs and immobilization of lower-extremity long bones via skeletal or skin traction, that is, Buck's traction or Russell's traction. Further discussion of traction for fracture immobilization is beyond the scope of this book. The remainder of this chapter will address the issues of lumbar and cervical traction methods.

Cervical Traction

Physiologic Effects and Clinical Uses

Cervical traction is a mainstay in physical therapy treatment for various cervical conditions. As noted earlier, a close review of the literature reveals that clinical efficacy of cervical

Why Do I Need to Know About...

APPLICATION OF WEIGHT

- If distraction of the vertebral bodies is the desired goal, then the amount of weight used must be great enough to overcome friction.
- If the weight used is not sufficient to overcome friction, no therapeutic action will occur.

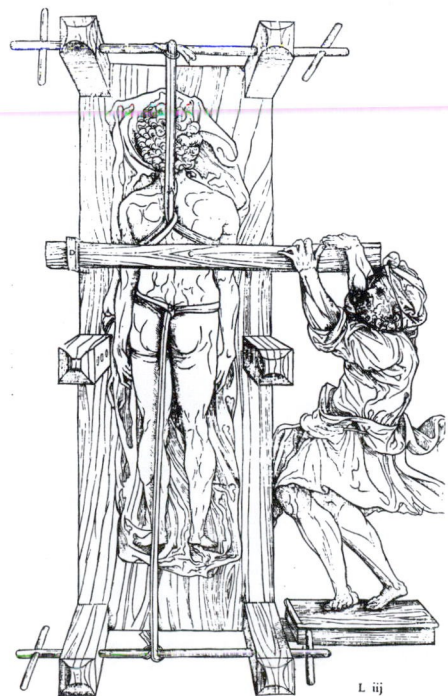

Figure 6-6   Hippocratic method.

traction is less controversial than that of lumbar traction. Results of studies have reported cervical traction alone and in conjunction with other modalities to be beneficial in cases of osteoarthritis,[20] cervical radiculopathy,[21–23] disc herniation,[24–26] and tension headaches.[27,28]

The physiologic effects of cervical traction include increasing cervical vertebral separation,[12,25] reducing cervical electromyographic (EMG) activity,[23] reducing nerve conduction disturbances,[29] increasing H reflex amplitude,[22,30] reducing alpha-motor neuron excitability,[31] increasing blood flow to cervical musculature,[32] and restoring cervical lordosis.[33] In contrast, there are studies that show that cervical traction actually increases EMG activity in cervical musculature,[32] has no effect on cervical muscle EMG activity,[34,35] and decreases the H reflex pathway for the soleus muscle.[36]

Mechanical Techniques

Mechanical traction is the use of free weights and traction machines to create a pulling force. Programmable traction units are primarily used because of their versatility. Traditional halters pull from both the occiput and the mandible (Fig. 6-7). There is evidence that mandibular pull

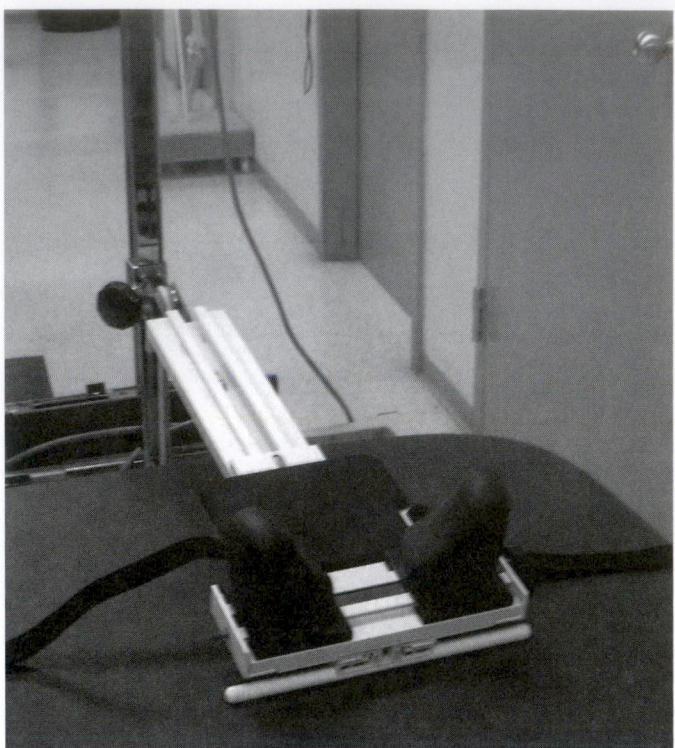

Figure 6-8   A cervical traction appliance that does not apply any pressure to the mandible.

can create and aggravate temporomandibular joint problems.[37] Occipital halters have largely replaced traditional halters (Fig. 6-8). They have no mandibular strap and pull exclusively from the occiput. In addition, some models are capable of pulling the head into side flexion and rotation.

Position

Supine position has been shown to be preferable to sitting for most treatments.[38] There are those that prefer prone as a position of choice in cases of low back pain (LBP) involvement.[39]

Poundage

The head weighs approximately 14 pounds. The poundage used for cervical traction varies according to the source, but it is generally accepted that to produce elongation of the spine, 25 to 30 pounds (11.25 to 13.5 kg) is necessary.[7] Greater amounts produce greater separation only to a point, and excessive traction may produce muscle guarding that can overcome up to 55 pounds of traction force.[12] It appears that the upper cervical spine requires less traction force to cause separation than does the lower cervical spine.[6] Weight approaching 120 pounds was necessary to cause a disc rupture at the C5-6 level.[40] One paper indicates that application of cervical traction can reproduce low back radiculopathy in patients with past episodes,[41] so care should be taken to use the least amount of force that is clinically effective.

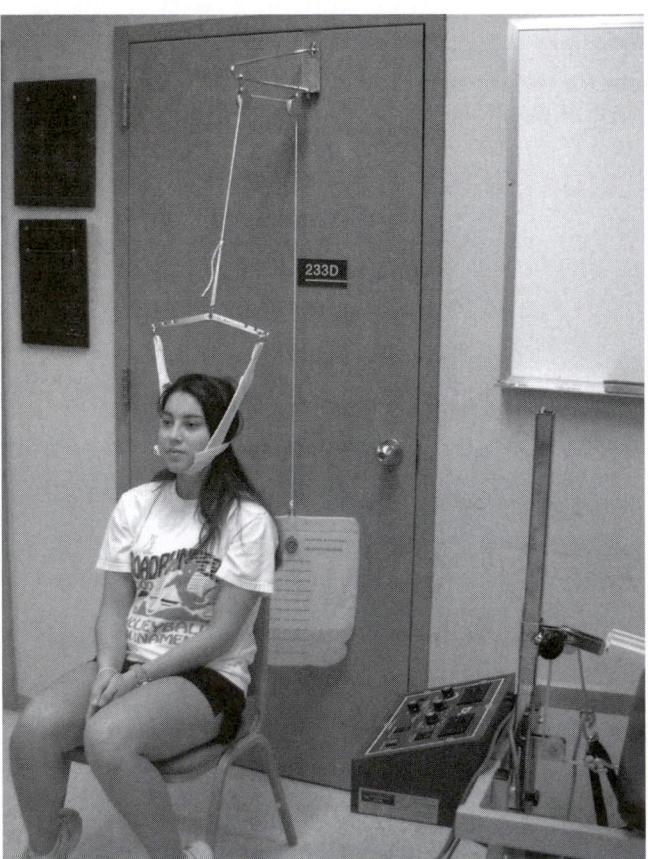

Figure 6-7   Traditional halter that pulls from both the occiput and the mandible.

Angle of Pull

The angle of pull varies according to target tissue. For maximal perpendicular facet separation, the angle would be 0° at the atlanto-occipital (A/O) joint and increasing amounts of extension to C6-7 (Fig. 6-9). Prolonged positioning of the neck in extension should be done with discretion, however, as it causes a reduction in the intervertebral separation posteriorly.[42] Beyond that, the relationship between angle of pull and posterior vertebral separation is unclear. Although one study contends that greater amounts of flexion causes greater separation more distally down the cervical spine,[43] another study showed that traction with a neutral spine position actually causes more posterior separation at C6-7 than the same force of traction performed with 30° of flexion.[42] For increasing the intervertebral space overall, it is generally accepted that about 25° of flexion is optimal.[44] A slightly different angle on the subject was given by the authors of a study that concluded that the maximal force acting on the cervical spine as a whole was obtained with a 35° traction inclination.[16] Too much flexion has been shown to actually decrease intervertebral space because of encroachment of the ligamentum flavum on the intervertebral foramen.[5,45] For some disc problems, a neutral spine is indicated because it causes the ligaments to be lax and the traction can be transmitted more completely to the disc. Three-dimensional or polyaxial traction is becoming more popular because of its ability to maximally gap vertebral segments unilaterally (Fig. 6-10).

Static Versus Intermittent

There is little agreement on one over the other, but intermittent traction seems to be more comfortable for most

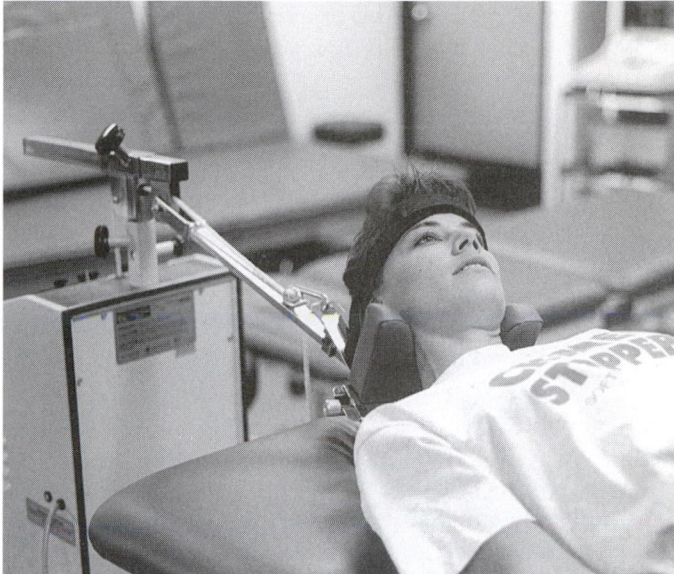

Figure 6-10 Example of cervical three-dimensional or polyaxial traction.

patients. The shorter the time of pull, the more poundage can generally be tolerated. Muscle relaxation and facet joint capsule stretching applications might respond better to low-load, long-duration stretch (static traction). Facet mobilization techniques could best be mimicked by shorter and equal on time and off time (10 seconds/10 seconds), and patients with herniated disc problems to longer on-off times with a ratio of approximately 3:1 (60 seconds/20 seconds), and static pulls.

Facet problems seem to respond better to shorter and equal on time versus off time (10 seconds/10 seconds), and herniated disc problems to longer on-off times with approximately 1:3 ratios (20 seconds/60 seconds), and sustained pulls.

Treatment Time

The optimal amount of time that traction is administered ranges from 2 minutes[46] to 24 hours.[47] One study showed that maximal vertebral separation per pull phase occurs after 7 seconds with intermittent traction.[48] One study found that no significant muscular relaxation was found on EMG after 10 minutes of traction and concluded that if muscle relaxation does occur with traction, the effects are not immediate.[35] In general, therefore, the minimum amount of time that traction should be applied to allow full muscular relaxation is 20 to 25 minutes.[7] Treatment time for cervical degenerative joint disease (DJD) should be approximately 25 minutes; for acute disc protrusion, no more than 8 minutes. Traction for longer than 8 minutes with disc protrusions can cause the disc to imbibe excess fluid and increase intradiscal pressure.[6]

Frequency of Treatment

The number of times per week the patient is treated is dependent on type and severity of the problem and duration

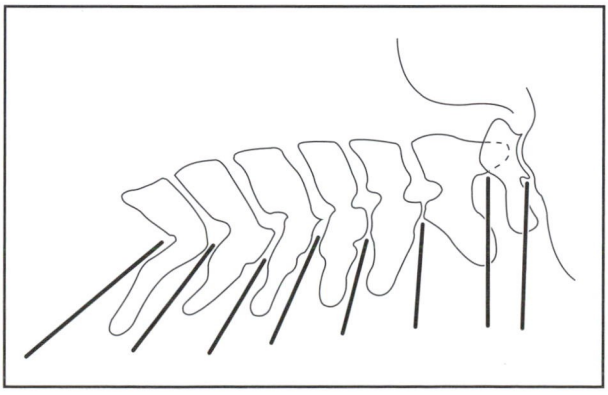

Figure 6-9 Orientation of the facets of the cervical spine.

of relief from traction. The frequency should generally be greater when the problem is more acute, as in the presence of neurologic findings.

Other Equipment for Traction of the Cervical Spine

Autotraction Autotraction of the cervical spine has become more popular recently. The traction force is controlled by the patient through a footboard or other device. This allows constant adjustments to be possible at the patient's discretion and creates an active role of the patient in therapy. The Goodley polyaxial cervical traction unit (E-Z-Em, Westbury, NY) has the advantage of allowing the therapist to administer the line of force through three dimensions. Results using this method have been promising.[8]

Home Units The use of the "over-the-door" variety of home units has endured despite the necessity to perform the traction sitting (see Fig. 6-7). The maximal weight of these units is 20 pounds. When considering the weight of the head at 14 pounds, this means the maximum force on the cervical spine can be only 6 pounds. It has already been established that 25 pounds is necessary to create a significant distraction of the cervical vertebra. In addition, less cervical muscle activity occurs in supine position than in sitting.[35] Despite this, however, there are several studies that have shown symptomatic relief for patients with spondylosis syndromes[49] and whiplash-type injuries[50] as well as improved pain and ROM in patients with cervical disc herniation.[51]

Other home units are available that allow the patient to be treated in supine and can deliver traction forces sufficient to allow vertebral separation (Figs. 6-11 and 6-12). Traction forces in these units can be generated by gravity assistance, pneumatic pressure, and springs.

Although the supine systems tend to be more expensive, in two separate studies, patients seemed to prefer supine pneu-

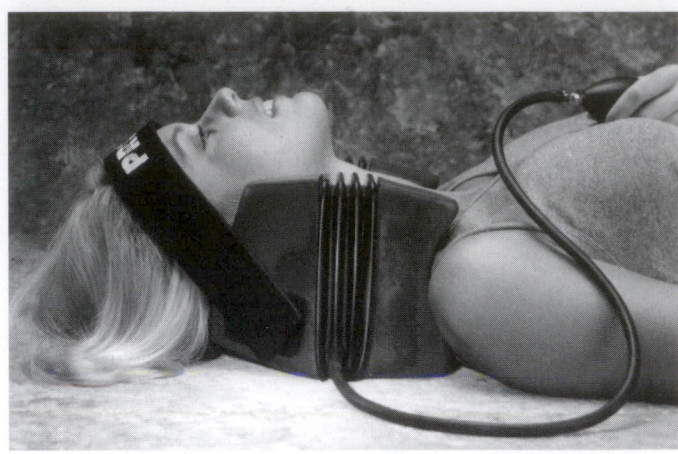

Figure 6-12 Pronex system, another type of home traction unit. (Courtesy of EMPI, St. Paul, MN.)

matic cervical traction units to the conventional over-the-door counterweight systems[52] and had specific preferences within the supine models.[53] It seems that if cost is not an issue, supine systems should be a consideration for home use.

Manual Traction

Cervical manual traction techniques are commonly used by therapists, probably due to ease in application of a three-dimensional force and the ability to continually assess the patient during treatment. It has been shown that experienced physical therapists are able to apply a reliable force of traction force over repeated trials.[54] Manual traction, like mechanical traction, has been shown to decrease the number of alpha motor neurons firing in upper extremity musculature.[31] Techniques ranging from simple occipital distraction (Fig. 6-13) to various segmental locking techniques in unison with three-dimensional distraction to isolate specific vertebral levels are commonly applied. Specific techniques of manual traction are beyond the scope of this text.

Positional Traction

Positional distraction techniques are inviting because the patient can perform them at home with little to no equipment. The general principle is to place the neck in positions that either enhance limited ROM or maximize intervertebral foraminal space to release impinged tissues. The components of motion to maximally open facets would be forward flexion, contralateral side flexion, and ipsilateral rotation, whereas the components of motion necessary to maximally open up the foramen is forward flexion, contralateral side flexion, and contralateral rotation (Fig. 6-14). The forward flexion position of 15° was found to significantly increase the foraminal volume and isthmus area at C5-6. Interestingly, this same study showed that adding 25 pounds of traction in this posi-

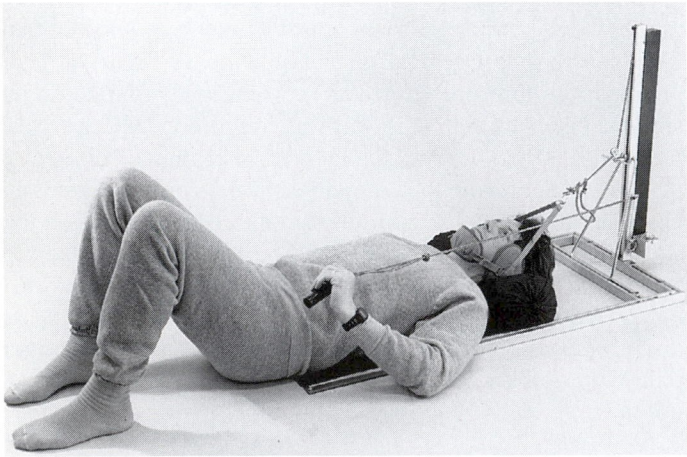

Figure 6-11 Home traction unit. (Courtesy of C-Tract, Granberg International, Richmond, CA.)

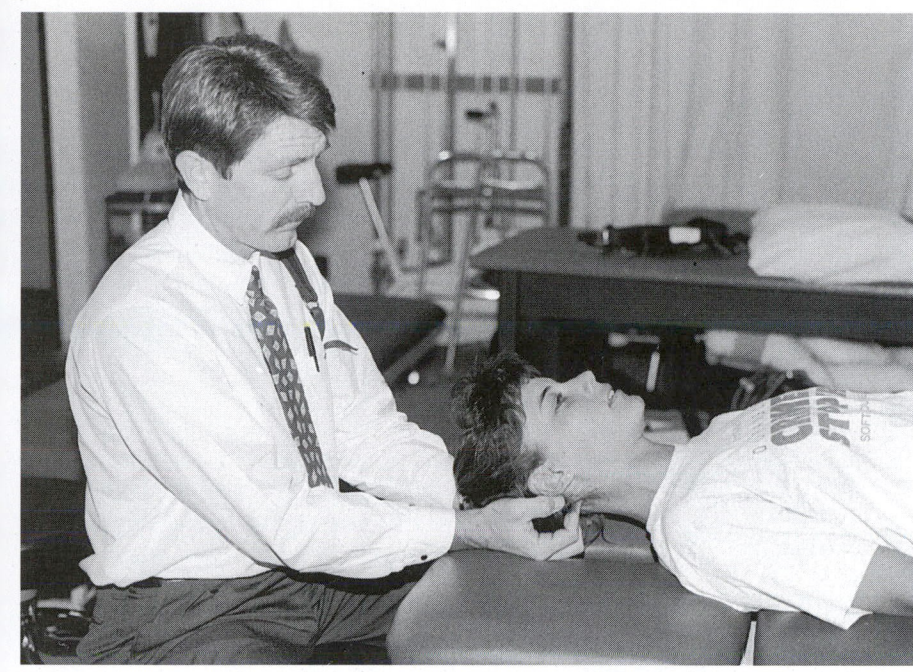

Figure 6-13 Proper positioning of both the patient and the clinician for manual cervical traction. Great care must be taken to ensure an appropriate line of pull.

tion did little to further increase foraminal opening.[55] Placing one side of the spine in maximal facet or foraminal opening places the other side of the spine in a more closed position, and caution should always be taken to avoid prolonged positions that would place the facet joints or foramen in a closed position.

Procedure for Mechanical Cervical Traction

Before starting a mechanical cervical traction treatment, the following should be done:

1. Review the chart, including diagnosis, indications, contraindications, precautions, and plan of care.

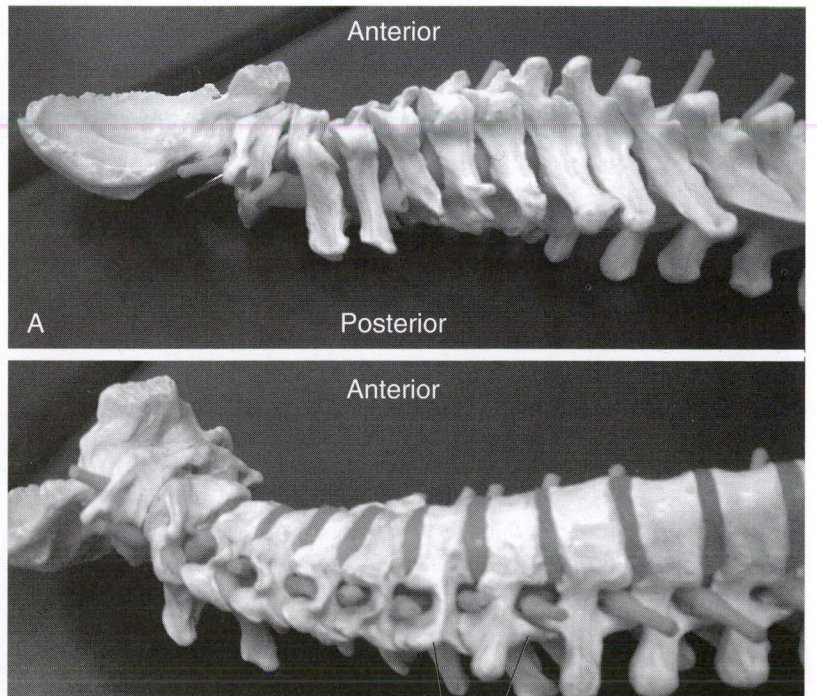

Figure 6-14 Positional distraction of the cervical spine. (A) Position of maximal opening of the cervical facets. (B) Position of maximal opening of the intervertebral foramen.

2. Prepare the table, including halter, pillows, draping sheets, call bell, and timer.

3. Preset treatment time, poundage, time on and off, and duration and angle of pull as per plan of care.

4. Explain fully the effects of traction to the patient, and answer all questions and concerns of the patient.

5. Use a mouthpiece or soft insert between the teeth if no occipital halter is available, to reduce compression forces on the temporomandibular joint (TMJ).

6. Position patient according to desired effect, that is, supine with 258° of cervical flexion in the case of intervertebral foraminal separation. Provide pillows for support and comfort.

7. Adjust the halter according to desired effect. Traditional halters should be positioned so that the patient feels the majority of the pull from the occiput. The posterior (occipital) part of the halter should cradle the occiput at the level of the inferior nuchal line to both mastoid processes. Place a tissue between the anterior (chin) pad and the chin. If properly applied, the anterior pad should cradle the mandible and be snug to patient's tolerance.

8. Attach halter to spreader bar, and remove all slack from the rope.

9. Double check all settings.

10. Turn on the machine, and stay with patient at least through one entire cycle to ensure proper setup.

11. Explain the use of the call bell or safety switch before leaving.

 ## Lumbar Traction

Physiologic Effects and Clinical Uses

The evidence regarding the clinical efficacy of lumbar traction is conflicting, due in part to the wide variety of treatment protocols used and the open range of pathologies for which traction is used.[1] In a recent survey of physical therapists' approach to treatment of LBP, use of lumbar traction was infrequent.[56] Studies have found various forms of lumbar traction be to useful alone and in conjunction with other treatments in cases of disc herniation[2,3,10,57–64] and generalized LBP with and without radicular findings.[65–70] Other research has not been supportive of lumbar traction. In several studies, there was no statistically significant difference between patients treated with lumbar traction compared with controls.[4,71–73] A recent systematic review of randomized controlled trials using lumbar traction concluded that the use of traction in LBP remains inconclusive because of the lack of

methodologic rigor and the limited application of clinical parameters as used in clinical practice.[74]

The physiologic effects of lumbar traction include increase in vertebral separation,[75–80] decrease in intradiscal pressure,[81] reduction of disc protrusion,[2,3,59–61] increase in lateral foraminal opening,[82,83] distraction of the apophyseal joints,[61] temporary reduction of scoliosis,[84] temporary increase in lordosis with extension traction,[85] decrease in lumbar paraspinal EMG activity,[86] and temporary increase in stature.[87] In contrast, there are studies that show no decrease in lumbar paraspinal EMG activity with lumbar traction[88] and no reduction of disc protrusion or altered intradiscal pressure.[89]

Mechanical Techniques

Mechanical traction using a traction machine is the most frequently used method. Free weights have largely been abandoned due to the large amount of weight needed.

Equipment

A programmable traction unit is generally used because of its versatility (Fig. 6-15).

Position

Lumbar traction has traditionally been performed with the patient in supine with knees and hips flexed to varying degrees. It has been demonstrated that, during traction, posterior vertebral separation of the lumbar spine increased as hip flexion increased from 0° to 90°.[75] Colachis and Strohm[80] found that, with traction in 70° of hip flexion, there was an increase in vertebral separation at all lumbar levels.

As with the cervical spine, excessive lumbar flexion can decrease intervertebral foraminal space because of encroachment of the ligamentum flavum on the intervertebral foramen.[5,45]

Current trends include positioning the patient in supine with hips and knees extended and prone, depending on the target tissue and desired effect. Prone has the advantage of accessing the back for modalities to be performed concurrently. It appears that there is no difference in myoelectric activity in back musculature between prone and supine positions.[88]

Poundage

As described under the physics of traction, the poundage necessary to overcome the frictional forces of the lower body (with a thoracic harness, and in the absence of a split traction table) is one-fourth body weight. When using a split traction table, the frictional force is negligible. The protocol for optimal tractional force varies according to source, ranging from 300 pounds[10] to the minimum one-fourth body weight.[5] Maximal tolerance of the T11-12 discs in cadavers was found to be 440 pounds,[40] although estimates for the lumbar spine in living persons are considerably higher than that. One author contends that based on a review of the literature, there

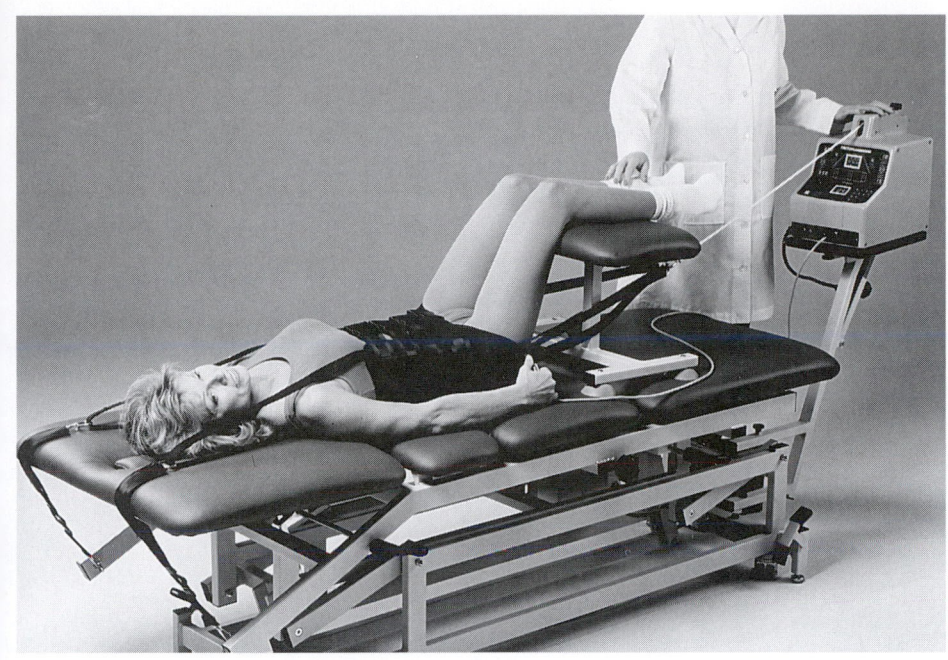

Figure 6-15 Commercial mechanical traction unit. (From Chattanooga Corporation, Chattanooga, TN, with permission.)

is no relationship between dose (poundage) of traction and response and advocates low dosages,[89] others suggest that one of the reasons therapists have poor results with lumbar traction is that they use inadequate traction forces.[5] One study showed that LBP patients showed improvements in pain-free straight leg raise range when 60% and 30% of body weight traction force was used, but none was reported with 10% body weight.[65] Another study showed similar results; most outcome measures of LBP patients improved more with 44% of body weight traction force compared with 19%.[66] As a starting point, then, perhaps Judovich[15] was correct when he proposed that a minimum of one-half body weight be used to have a therapeutic effect.

Angle of Pull

The angle of the traction force on the pelvis can ultimately determine the low back position during traction and can actually be more important than patient position.[44] To maximize separation, the pull of the traction should occur perpendicular to the surfaces acted upon. In the case of the upper lumbar discs, then, the angle of the pull of the rope should be relatively horizontal. In the case of the L5-S1 level, however, there is a normal 30° lumbosacral angle (Fig. 6-16) posterior to the transverse plane. To ensure a pull as close to perpendicular as possible, the patient should either be placed in supine with maximal hip flexion to minimize the shearing angle or, better still, placed in prone with a 30° angle of pull

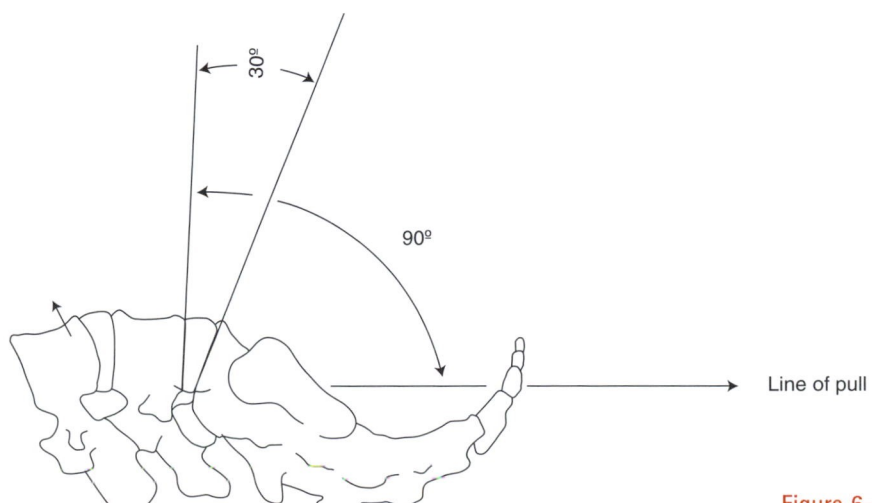

30°

90°

Line of pull

Supine

Figure 6-16 The 30° lumbosacral angle.

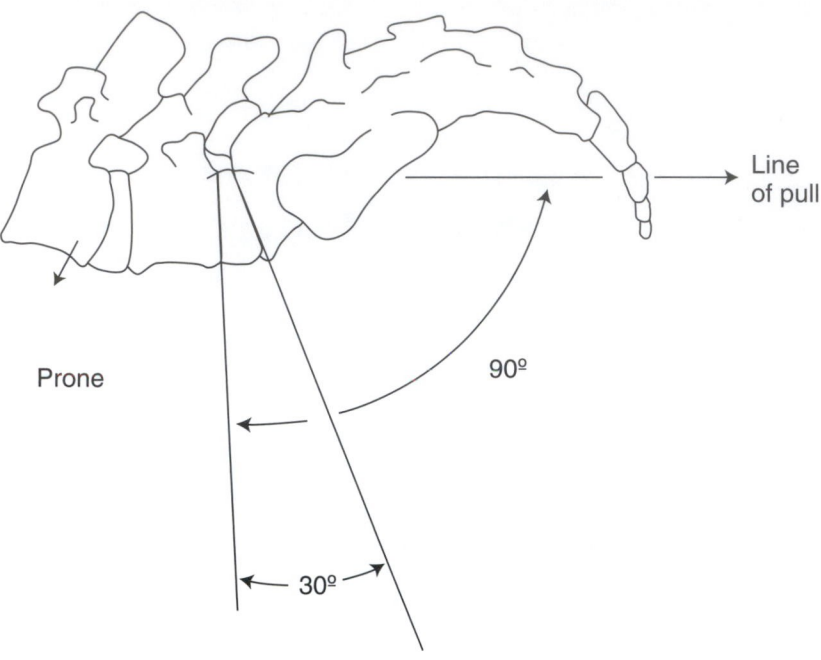

Figure 6-17   Lumbopelvic area in prone, with a 30° angle of pull and its perpendicular orientation to L5-S1.

(Fig. 6-17). Perhaps this is why in several studies traditional angles of pull had minimal effects of joint separation at the L5-S1 level. Colachis and Strohm[80] found that, with supine traction, the least amount of increase in vertebral separation occurred at the L5-S1 interspace. Similarly, Kane et al[82] found that with gravity traction mean intervertebral foraminal separation was significant at all levels except L5-S1.

With the use of modern harnesses, a pull can be generated in the lumbar spine to promote either lordosis or kyphosis depending on the relative placement of the two halves of the harness. Therefore, supine with knees and hips straight with a lordosis pull might be indicated in cases of a disc protrusion, whereas supine with knees and hips bent to 90° with a kyphosis pull might be indicated in the case of lateral stenosis secondary to spondylosis.

Unilateral traction has the advantage of allowing side flexion and rotational forces to occur. This can be of use in cases of lateral disc protrusion or unilateral foraminal stenosis, to name a few. Unilateral traction can be performed by either positioning the patient askew to the line of force or applying the traction pull on one side without the use of a spreader bar (Fig. 6-18).

Static Versus Intermittent

As with cervical traction, the physiologic differences of static versus intermittent traction force are poorly understood,

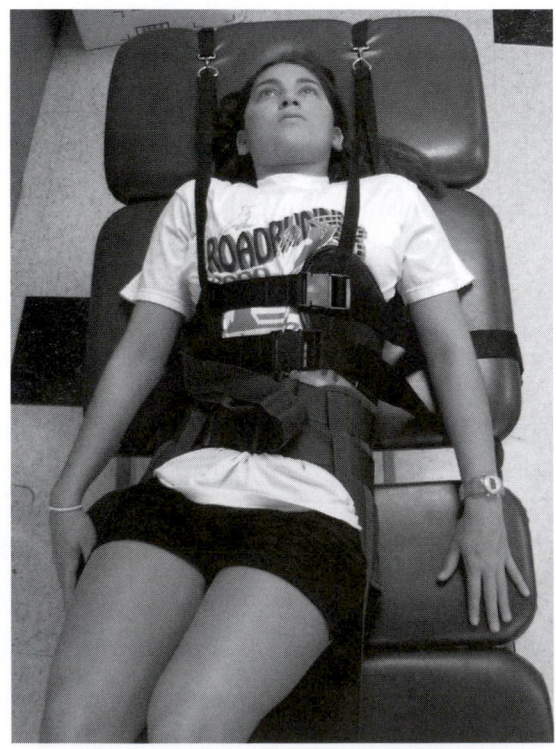

Figure 6-18   Unilateral pull of lumbar traction force.

although intermittent traction allows the therapist to use greater traction forces. One study concludes that there is no significant difference in magnitude of myoelectrical activity between static and intermittent lumbar traction.[88] Muscle relaxation and facet joint capsule stretching applications might respond better to low-load, long-duration stretch (static traction). Facet mobilization techniques could best be mimicked by shorter and equal on time and off time (10 seconds/10 seconds), and herniated disc problems to longer on-off times with approximately 1:3 ratios (20 seconds/60 seconds), and static pulls.

Treatment Time

The length of time for treatment depends on the desired effect and tends to be shorter for disc herniations (8 minutes or less) and longer for spondylosis (about 25 minutes). Traction for longer than 8 minutes with disc protrusions can cause the disc to imbibe excess fluid and increase intradiscal pressure.[6]

Frequency of Treatment

The number of times the patient is treated per week depends on the type of problem and severity. Generally, the more severe the problem, the greater is the frequency.

Other Equipment for Traction of the Lumbar Spine

Autotraction The term autotraction can be used in the broad definition to mean any form of traction where the patient uses his or her own muscle force to generate the traction force, but autotraction is also used to mean a specific type of traction that uses a table that is capable of pivoting on three dimensions. The patient uses his or her own muscle power to create the traction force, so the patient, with the therapist's guidance, can create a varied three-dimensional traction treatment. This latter type of autotraction has gained support in parts of Europe and the United States. There are several studies addressing the clinical efficacy of autotraction. Autotraction was shown to reduce the incidence of surgery in a population of LBP patients compared with controls at 6 months postintervention.[62] In one study, the use of autotraction compared with sustained mechanical traction showed significantly better results,[57] although the methods of this study have been questioned.[90] Another study comparing autotraction with manual traction showed them to be equally successful.[58] These studies sound favorable; however, the use of autotraction has been shown to increase intradiscal pressure, probably due to the patient creating a contraction of his or her abdominal musculature.[91]

Gravity-Assisted Traction Including Inversion Traction

Gravity-assisted traction is the use of body weight as a distractive force, and it is used both in the clinic and as a home treatment. Various devices have evolved, including inversion traction, where the weight of the suspended body, either fully or from the waist down, is used as a tractive force. Both inversion techniques create a lumbar traction force of about 40% of body weight. This method of traction is acceptable only in patients without cardiopulmonary or cardiovascular compromise or hypertension, as it has been shown to raise both systolic and diastolic blood pressure significantly and to increase oxygen uptake.[76,92,93]

Inversion traction has been shown to have effects similar to mechanical traction, including vertebral separation[76,80] and intervertebral foraminal separation.[82] Patients can also be suspended without being inverted in various ways by use of harnesses that allow the lower body to exert a traction pull on the lumbar spine. This type of gravitational traction reduces the possible cardiovascular concerns and has been shown to increase intervertebral space by greater than 3 mm at all levels between L2 to S1.[78] In one study, noninversion gravitational traction was shown to be efficacious for use with LBP patients without true disc herniation but ineffective with those patients with a diagnosis of extruded disc.[67] A more recent study shows this type of traction to be superior to bed rest in pain reduction and objective gains in subjects with radicular pain.[68]

In other studies using noninversion gravitational traction, lumbar lengthening has been measured as well as lordosis reduction.[77]

Home Units

Many of the home units for lumbar traction use the patient's own muscle strength as a traction force and therefore would be considered autotraction. In addition, various other home units use traction force from gravity, hydraulics, spring-loaded, and various other mechanical systems (Fig. 6-19).

Manual Traction

Manual traction techniques can be as simple as providing a simple longitudinal traction force to locking techniques used in unison with three-dimensional pulls to create joint-specific traction in any desired direction.

Positional Traction

Positional traction is used frequently in the lumbar area by therapists because it can be done at home and requires little or no equipment. The forces can be three-dimensional and can be significant, because the weight of the legs can be used as the traction force. The components of motion to maximally open facets would be forward flexion, contralateral side flexion, and ipsilateral rotation, whereas the components of motion necessary to maximally open up the foramen are forward flexion, contralateral side flexion, and contralateral rotation. One study confirmed radiographically that the lumbar neuroforamen was increased by an average of 4 mm with

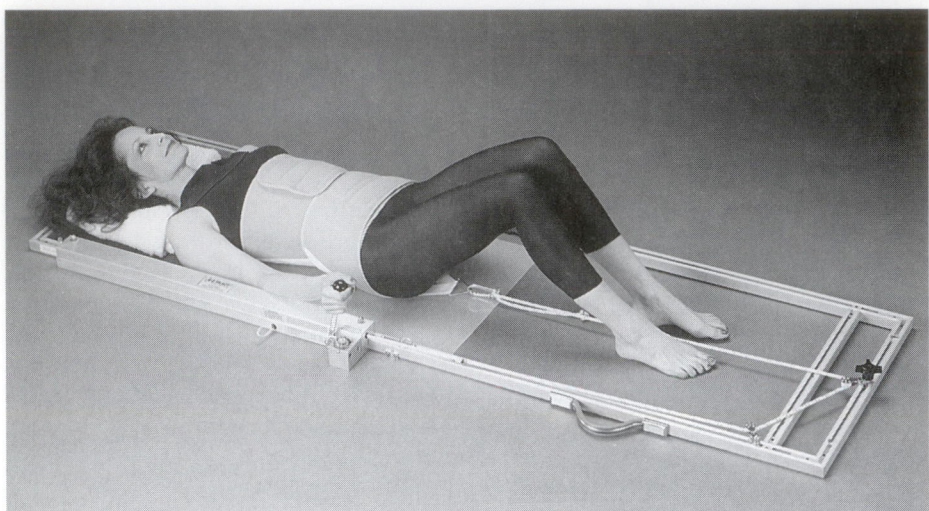

Figure 6-19 An "E-Z track" traction unit. (Courtesy of Granberg International, Richmond, CA.)

positional distraction.[83] As with the cervical spine, the position that either enhances limited ROM or maximizes foraminal size would be encouraged and positions that create a closed-packed position over a prolonged period of time should be avoided.

Procedure for Lumbar Traction

Before initiating lumbar traction, the following should be done:

1. Review the chart, including diagnosis, indications, contraindications, precautions, and plan of care.

2. Prepare the table, including harnesses, pillows, draping sheets, call bell, and timer. Always use a split traction table if available.

3. Preset treatment time, poundage, time on and off, and duration and angle of pull as per plan of care.

4. Explain fully the effects of traction to the patient, and answer all questions and concerns of the patient.

5. Remove clothing from around belt sites, and drape patient appropriately. Position patient according to desired effect, that is, supine with knees and hips flexed to 45°. Provide pillows for support and comfort.

6. Adjust harnesses according to desired effect. Place a folded towel between patient's abdomen and traction harness. Attach traction (pelvic) harness first; the superior part should be in line with the umbilicus. The countertraction (thoracic) harness should then be positioned so that the superior part fits snugly around ribs 8, 9, and 10. If properly applied, the two belts should overlap slightly and be snug to patient's tolerance.

 Before You Begin

Make sure that you ask patients if they need to use a restroom to relieve themselves before securing the traction harnesses.

7. Attach harness to spreader bar, and remove all slack from the rope.

8. Double check all settings.

9. Turn on machine and wait for one complete cycle so that all of the slack is taken up; release catch of split table (during off cycle if using intermittent traction).

10. Explain the use of the call bell or safety switch before leaving.

 ## Clinical Uses and Safety Considerations

Indications and Effects

Herniation of Disc Material

Traction has been a treatment for impingement or irritation of nerves secondary to a variety of causes, including disc material contacting the spinal nerve roots. There is a measurable increase in intervertebral space with traction to both the cervical[11,12,18,25,48] and lumbar[2,10,59,75-80] spine. The debate to date revolves around how much separation occurs with specific distractive forces. There are studies that seem to indicate that the application of traction can reverse spinal obstruction secondary to disc protrusion.[2,3,25,60] It has been proposed that in the presence of increased volume of the disc, intradiscal pressure would be lessened. In other words, the negative pressure that should accompany the increased volume should "suck" the disc material back into the disc.[9,25,60,61,81] This is generally accepted, although one study found that intradiscal pressure either remains the same or actually increases during the application of different forms of traction.[91] In summary, although the precise mechanisms of action are unclear, traction has been found to be effective in treatment of herniated discs.[2,10,11,18,24–26,48,59–64]

Degenerative Joint Disease

With degenerative joint disease (DJD) of the spine, there are at least two clinically significant occurrences: (1) a decrease of intervertebral space with an associated decrease of the intervertebral foraminal space and (2) osteophyte production into the intervertebral space coming from the facet joint and the vertebral body. Collectively, this progression leads to lateral stenosis, which is a reduction of the intervertebral foraminal size. As mentioned, traction has been shown to increase intervertebral space and, with it, the size of the intervertebral foramen. Although the increase in foraminal size seen with traction should return to pretreatment size after the treatment is over, the decrease in pain can last for a prolonged time. Once the nerve is decompressed, perhaps the swelling in the nerve subsides and the existing foraminal size is sufficient to accommodate the smaller-diameter nerve. Traction has been shown to be an effective treatment for impingement of the spinal nerve secondary to spinal stenosis.[5–7,9,10,17,20,82,85]

Muscle Spasm or Guarding

In the presence of spinal pain, be it cervical, thoracic, or lumbar secondary to muscle spasm or guarding, traction can be of use to cause a slow, prolonged stretch of the muscles. Although some sources state that prolonged stretch via traction can cause a reflex inhibition of the muscle,[31,47,86] others disagree.[32,34,35,88] Possible explanations include Golgi tendon organ involvement, a "resetting" of the muscle spindle to a longer length, a stretching of joint receptors or even skin receptors,[94] and relaxation of nociceptive reflexes.

Joint Hypomobility

In studies discussed earlier, it has been shown that traction is capable of vertebral separation in both the cervical and lumbar spines. This separation would have to occur at both the intervertebral bodies and the facet joints. In the presence of generalized decreased spinal ROM, therefore, spinal traction will mobilize the joints by moving the articular surfaces on each other and distract the surfaces and decrease articular pressure.[61] In addition, intermittent traction should have the effect of increasing synovial fluid production and thus nutrifying the cartilage as well as firing mechanoreceptors to "gate" the pain transmission. Treating patients with specific areas of hypomobility would be difficult with generalized traction; however, manual traction and mobilization or three-dimensional traction might be indicated in this case.

Facet Impingement

The facet joints have a capsule that can theoretically become impinged within the joint space.[95] Traction techniques, especially in combination with positions that maximize specific joint separation, will cause a decompression of the facet joints and thus could be of some use in treating impingements.[61] Although standard mechanical traction could be used for this condition, polyaxial autotraction, positional traction, and manual traction would be the preferred methods because of their ability to isolate specific joints.

Contraindications

The following are potential contraindications to the use of traction:

1. Spinal infections (i.e., spinal meningitis, arachnoiditis) that could be spread by the use of traction

2. Rheumatoid arthritis (RA) or other acute inflammatory disorders affecting the joints. Ligaments, such as the transverse ligament of the atlantoaxial joint, are particularly vulnerable with RA.

3. Osteoporosis—traction may exceed the tolerance of the structurally compromised bone.

4. Spinal cancers—traction may increase the chance of metastasis of cancer cells.

5. Spinal cord pressure—in the presence of impingement directly on the spinal cord secondary to a central disc herniation or spinal tumor, traction has not been shown to be effective and may aggravate the condition.

Precautions

The following are precautions to the use of traction:

1. Joint hypermobility—in the presence of hypermobile joints, traction could aggravate the condition.

2. Acute inflammation—in almost all cases, traction could aggravate the condition.

3. Claustrophobia or other anxiety associated with traction—if the patient is not relaxed, muscle guarding can overcome strong traction forces.

4. Cardiac or respiratory insufficiency, both with inversion traction and mechanical lumbar traction[96]

5. Pregnancy—due to constriction of the abdomen, as well as joint laxity secondary to endogenous production of relaxin

6. Patients whose symptoms increase with traction—for example, with cervical traction, preexisting lumbar radiculopathy that was aggravated by traction

7. With cervical traction, TMJ dysfunction when using a chin strap

8. With cervical traction, there is a small risk of internal jugular vein thrombosis.[97]

9. Patients with blood pressure issues, as decreases in both systolic and diastolic blood pressure were seen in patients undergoing cervical traction[98]

Patient Education

As with all treatments, the patient should be as completely informed as possible regarding the effects and goals of traction treatment. Patient compliance markedly increases when patients understand the treatment they are to receive. The use of a spinal model with spinal nerves and drawings of the physical effects are useful tools for traction education. For example, the therapist, upon explaining the effects of cervical traction to treat lateral stenosis, might use a finger to represent a nerve and form an "O" with the finger and thumb of the other hand to represent the foramen, then pass the "nerve" through the "foramen," demonstrating the normal relationship. Inflammation of the nerve might be represented by using two fingers side by side. Radiculopathy can be represented by making the "O" too small for the nerve. Next, the therapist might show on a spinal model how distraction can increase the size of the foramen to allow the nerve unimpeded passage. If you prescribe positional distraction for your patient, the effect of positional distraction on the diameter of the foramen can be represented by making the "O" larger to depict the position used for positional distraction.

Patient Perspective

Remember that your patient may not understand what you are going to do with him or her. He or she might even have images of "the rack" in his or her mind when you mention the word traction. Be calm and provide patient education in terms that are easily understood. Some patients may not realize how claustrophobic they are until after they have been set up with mechanical traction. For this reason it is critical to check on the patient within the first 5 minutes and also to provide access to a call system should it be necessary.

PATIENTS' FREQUENTLY ASKED QUESTIONS

- Will I be taller after traction?
- Why are the straps so tight?
- Can I read while I have traction for my neck?
- What do I do if I need to use the restroom while I am receiving traction?
- Why did the pain that went down in my leg go up into my back after traction? My back didn't hurt before.

If the patient is to be given a home traction device or technique to perform, the therapist should demonstrate the use of it and have the patient demonstrate the use to the therapist. Have the patient bring the device in the next treatment (or use a similar model available in the clinic) and demonstrate the proper use again. These "pop quizzes" will give the therapist valuable information regarding compliance and will alert one to improper use of the modality. Improper use of traction units and improper positional traction positioning can aggravate many conditions.

 ## Clinical Decision Making

During the patient's treatments, certain questions can help prevent problems from arising. The following is an example of some of the questions to ask patients that could yield valuable information.

Questions to rule out contraindications and precautions include the following:

1. Is your pain in both legs (arms)? Contraindication—spinal tumor or central spinal cord impingement

2. Are you having problems going to the bathroom? Contraindication—spinal cord tumor or central spinal cord impingement

3. Have you had any swelling or pain in other joints for no reason (without a traumatic event)? Contraindication—rheumatoid or other systemic inflammatory disorders

4. Tell me about any bones that you have broken. Contraindication—osteoporosis

5. Have you had a fever or sweating and unusual tiredness as of late? Contraindication—spinal infection

6. Is your pain worse at night, any changes in your appetite, sleep patterns, etc.? Contraindication—spinal tumor

7. When did you last injure your back or neck? Precaution—acute inflammation, avoid excessive forces in traction

8. Does all movement hurt your back or neck or specific movements and do you experience any excessive popping, clicking, or other noises with movement? Precaution—hypermobility, avoid excessive forces in traction

9. Do you get short of breath easily? Precaution—respiratory insufficiency, avoid inversion traction

10. Do you have high blood pressure? Precaution—cardiac insufficiency, avoid inversion traction

11. Do you have popping or clicking in your jaw, jaw pain, or frequent headaches? Precaution—TMJ dysfunction

12. Have you ever received traction before, and if so, did it aggravate your condition? Contraindication/precaution—all of the above

Patient Positioning and Draping Considerations

Patient positioning is especially important when dealing with problems for which traction is indicated.

Although there remains controversy about extension versus flexion when treating spine patients, patient comfort is paramount. As mentioned earlier, if the patient is in an uncomfortable position and is in spasm, the strength of the spinal muscles will overcome any desired physiologic effects of traction. Because patient position greatly affects intradiscal pressure,[38] it is of particular importance for patients with disc herniations.

Lumbar Spine

Prone positions tend to increase lumbar extension (lordosis) of the spine with a relative anterior wedging of the disc, decreased intervertebral foraminal space, and increased weight-bearing forces on the facets (closed-packed position). Prone positioning might be indicated with disc bulges without total dissociation of the nuclear material. It would be contraindicated with severe osteoarthritis with lateral stenosis.

The supine position without leg support can also create lumbar extension (lordosis), which has the same effects as above. Supine with knees and hips flexed creates flexion of the lumbar spine and produces a relative posterior wedging of the disc, increased intervertebral foraminal space, and decreased weight-bearing forces on the facets. Excessive lumbar flexion has actually been shown to decrease intervertebral space, probably because of the movement of the ligamentum flavum into the foraminal space.

Cervical Traction

When performing cervical traction, positioning is usually performed either sitting or supine. As mentioned earlier, there is less muscle activity in the paraspinals when supine compared with sitting, and therefore this appears to be the position of choice if the patient can tolerate it. Prone positioning creates an extension bias and should be avoided unless the therapist can create a neutral spine with supports. The supine position maintains an approximately neutral cervical spine in patients with normal thoracic kyphosis. Patients with excessive kyphosis or a dowager's hump are apt to experience a position of excessive cervical lordosis when supine without at least one pillow for support. A position of slight hip and knee flexion during cervical traction prevents lumbar lordosis in persons with tight hip flexors and can relax the patient to ensure greater efficacy.

Patient draping should be consistent with room temperature and patient modesty and expose only the skin necessary to perform techniques effectively.

Summary

Traction has endured as a treatment technique for hundreds of years because of its ease of application and versatility. Although traction is not a panacea, it can be an effective treatment technique for a variety of spinal disorders and can be used with a modicum of equipment both in the clinic and in the home setting. Although there is a plethora of research that substantiates the efficacy of certain traction methods, there is also a body of literature to refute the physiologic effects and clinical efficacy of traction, most notably lumbar traction. Either way, more research needs to be done to validate (or invalidate) specific methods of traction treatment in all of its applications.

Discussion Questions

1. Why would position make a difference in the treatment outcome when using either cervical or lumbar traction?
2. Of what significance is the presence of a lordosis in the lumbar spine if lumbar traction is used?
3. How does knowledge of the coefficient of friction influence your decision regarding the amount of traction required to cause distraction of the joint surfaces?
4. How would you explain the purpose of cervical traction to a patient who was referred for treatment with a diagnosis of a cervical strain with radiating pain and paresthesia in the right upper extremity following an automobile accident?
5. Describe the differences between the use of an occipital pull harness and a typical head halter for cervical traction.

CASE STUDY 1

Ms. Jones is a 68-year-old left-handed woman who complains of neck pain, predominantly on the left. She has no specific underlying cause but seems to remember falling about 8 years ago and experiencing some pain in her neck for a week or so later. She has pain with extension and side flexion to the left. She reports that her left arm often feels heavy and clumsy but denies sensory changes. She says, "It's not as bad in the morning and gets worse as the day goes on"; she has problems looking overhead and doing her sewing. Your examination reveals she has limitations with extension, side flexion left, and rotation to the right. She has somewhat diminished reflexes on the left triceps compared with the right and has a 4/5 wrist extension on left when compared to right. She has decreased right side glide to the right in slight extension of C6 on C7 and has tenderness over her left C6-7 facet with deep pressure. Her radiograph shows some degenerative changes at this level with some spurring of the facet joint encroaching on her lateral foramen. She also exhibits some tightness in her upper trapezius, anterior scalenes, and levator scapula on both sides. The category she falls under using *The Guide to Physical Therapist Practice* is impaired joint mobility, motor function, muscle performance range of motion, and reflex integrity associated with spinal disorders with the interventions to include intermittent mechanical traction. You elect to start with supine traction with 25° of flexion 15 seconds on, 5 seconds off with 20 pounds of traction for 15 minutes on the first treatment to assess efficacy.

Patient education includes using a stepstool to ensure the work space is at eye level or below; self-ranging of the neck with emphasis on flexion and side flexion right, stretching of the upper trapezius, scalenus, and levator scapula; and instruction in use of a home cervical traction unit. She has been instructed to use an over-the-door unit in sitting, while facing the door with 15 pounds of force for 20 minutes in the morning. In addition, she has been given information on the anatomy of the cervical spine including the lateral foramen, and she has been shown how the nerve in her lower neck is being pinched due to the bony changes in her spine and how to maximally open up the lateral foramen using the position of forward flexion, side bending right, and rotation right (see **Fig. 6–14**). She was instructed in the use of pillows and positioning to facilitate this position.

CASE STUDY 2

Mr. Jones is a 27-year-old carpenter with a history of low back pain that started with an episode about 3 months earlier, where he was reaching across a sawhorse to lift some wood off a shelf. He felt immediate pain in the right side of his low back. He went to the emergency department, where they took a radiograph, which was negative, and gave him some nonsteroidal anti-inflammatory drugs and muscle relaxants. He stated the pain kept getting worse and he started developing pain shooting into the posterior leg to the back of the knee. He went to see his primary care physician, who ordered a magnetic resonance image, which was also negative for disc herniation. The physician sent him to the therapist, who found that the patient had a negative straight leg raise test on the right, pain and limitations with forward bending, pain-free extension, painful rotation and side bend left. The patient also complained of some discomfort with posterior-anterior glides at L4-5, which did reproduce his pain in the low back and leg. Joint plays revealed a hypomobility in facet opening at L4-L5 and L5-S1 on the right. Segmental passive range of motion revealed a failure of the L4-5 facet to open on the right. There was no evidence of changes in sensation, reflexes, or strength in the lower extremity.

The category the patient falls under using the *Guide to Physical Therapist Practice* is "Impaired joint mobility, motor function, muscle performance, range of motion and reflex integrity associated with spinal disorders" with the interventions to include static mechanical traction. The therapist elects to perform mechanical traction in supine starting with one-half body weight to cause a therapeutic effect of joint separation. He sets the patient in 90° of flexion of the hips and knees to ensure posterior pelvic tilt and reduction of lumbar lordosis and the angle of pull at 20° above horizontal to maximize facet separation. The therapist elects to do static traction to promote a reduction in muscle guarding and to induce a possible elongation of scar tissue that may have formed at the facet joint capsule.

Patient education for this patient would include an understanding that positional traction in left side lying with a pillow under his left hip, knees to chest, and left rotation can maximize the separation of his facet joints on the right. He is told to maintain this position for at least 30 minutes at least once a day.

References

1. Pellecchia, GL: Lumbar traction: a review of the literature. J Orthop Sports Phys Ther 20:262–267, 1994.
2. Mathews, J: Dynamic discography: a study of lumbar traction. Ann Phys Med 9:275, 1968.
3. Gupta, R, and Ramarao, S: Epidurography in reduction of lumbar disc prolapse by traction. Arch Phys Med Rehabil 59:322, 1978.
4. Pal, B, et al: A controlled trial of continuous lumbar traction in the treatment of back pain and sciatica. Br J Rheumatol 25:181, 1986.
5. Saunders, H: Lumbar traction. J Orthop Sports Phys Ther 1:36, 1979.
6. Saunders, H: The use of spinal traction in the treatment of neck and back conditions. Clin Orthop Rel Res 179:31, 1983.
7. Harris, P: Cervical traction: review of literature and treatment guidelines. Physical Therapy 57:910, 1977.
8. Walker, G: Goodley polyaxial cervical traction: a new approach to a traditional treatment. Physical Therapy 66:1255, 1986.
9. Larsson, U, et al: Auto-traction for treatment of lumbago-sciatica. Acta Orthop Scand 51:791, 1980.
10. Cyriax, J: The treatment of lumbar disk lesions. Br Med J 2:1434, 1950.
11. Judovich, B: Herniated cervical disc. Am J Surg 84:649, 1952.
12. Bard, G, and Jones, M: Cineradiographic recording of traction of the cervical spine. Arch Phys Med Rehabil August:403, 1964.
13. Taber's Cyclopedic Medical Dictionary, ed 17. FA Davis, Philadelphia, 1993.
14. Hewitt, P: Conceptual Physics, ed 6. HarperCollins, New York, 1989.
15. Judovich, BD: Lumbar traction therapy—elimination of physical factors that prevent lumbar stretch. JAMA 159:549, 1955.
16. Pio, A, et al: The statics of cervical traction. J Spinal Disord 7:337–342, 1994.
17. Natchev, E: A Manual of Auto-traction Treatment for Low Back Pain. Folksam, Stockholm, Sweden, 1984.
18. Goldie, I, and Reichmann, S: The biomechanical influence of traction on the cervical spine. Scand J Rehabil Med 9:31, 1977.
19. Tan, JC, and Nordin, M: Role of physical therapy in the treatment of cervical disk disease. Orthop Clin North Am 23:425–449, 1992.
20. Gilworth, G: Cervical traction with active rotation. Physiotherapy 77:782–784, 1991.
21. Moetti, P, and Marchette, G: Clinical outcomes from mechanical intermittent cervical traction for the treatment of cervical radiculopathy: a case series <corrected>. J Orthop Sports Phys Ther 31:207–213, 2001.
22. Abdulwahab, SS: The effect of reading and traction on patients with cervical radiculopathy based on electrodiagnostic testing. J Neuromusculoskeletal System 7:91–96, 1999.
23. Lee, MY, Wong, MK, Tang, FT, Chang, WH, and Shiou, WK: Design and assessment of an adaptive intermittent cervical traction modality with EMG biofeedback. J Biomech Eng Trans ASME 118:597–600, 1996.
24. Constantoyannis, C, et al: Intermittent cervical traction for cervical radiculopathy caused by large-volume herniated disks. J Manipulative Physiol Ther 25:188–192, 2002.
25. Chung, TS, et al: Reducibility of cervical disk herniation: evaluation at MR imaging during cervical traction with a nonmagnetic traction device. Radiology 225:895–900, 2002.
26. Saal, JS, et al: Nonoperative management of herniated cervical intervertebral disc with radiculopathy. Spine 21:1877–1883, 1996.
27. Fitz-Ritson, D: Therapeutic traction: a review of neurological principles and clinical applications. J Manipulative Physiol Ther 71:39–49, 1984.
28. Stone, RG, and Wharton, RB: Simultaneous multiple-modality therapy for tension headaches and neck pain. Biomed Instrum Technol 31:259–262, 1997.
29. Hattori, M, Shirai, Y, and Aoki, T: Research on the effectiveness of intermittent cervical traction therapy, using short-latency somatosensory evoked potentials. J Orthop Sci 7:208–216, 2002.
30. Haraoka, K, and Nagata, A: Modulation of the flexor carpi radialis H reflex induced by cervical traction. J Phys Ther Sci 10:41–45, 1998.
31. Brandman, L, Rochester, L, and Vujnovich, A: Manual cervical traction reduces alph-motoneuron excitability in normal subjects. Electromyogr Clin Neurophysiol 40:259–266, 2000.
32. Nanno, M: Effects of intermittent cervical traction on muscle pain. Flowmetric and electromyographic studies of the cervical paraspinal muscles.
33. Harrison, DE, et al: A new 3-point bending traction method of restoring cervical lordosis and cervical manipulation: a nonrandomized clinical controlled trial. Arch Phys Med Rehabil 83:447–453, 2002.
34. Jette, DU: Effect of cervical traction on EMG activity of upper trapezius. Phys Ther 65:730, 1985.
35. Murphy, MJ: Effects of cervical traction on muscle activity. J Orthop Sports Phys Ther 13:220–225, 1991.
36. Hiraoka, K, and Nagata, A: The effects of cervical traction on the soleus H reflex amplitude in man. Jpn J Phys Fitness Sports Med 47:287–294, 1998.
37. Shore, A, et al: Cervical traction and temporomandibular joint dysfunction: report of case. J Am Dent Assoc 68:4, 1964.
38. Deets, D, et al: Cervical traction: a comparison of sitting and supine positions. Physical Therapy 57:255, 1977.
39. Sood, N: Prone cervical traction. Clin Manag 7:37, 1987.
40. DeSeze, S, and Levernieux, J: Les traction vertebrales. Semin Hip Paris 27:2075, 1951.
41. LaBan, M, et al: Intermittent cervical traction: a progenitor of lumbar radicular pain. Arch Phys Med Rehabil 73:295, 1992.
42. Wong, AM, et al: The traction angle and cervical intervertebral separation. Spine 17:136–138, 1992.
43. Hseuh, TC, et al: Evaluation of the effects of pulling angle and force on intermittent cervical traction with the Saunder's Halter. J Formos Med Assoc 90:1234–1239, 1991.
44. Saunders, H: Evaluation, Treatment, and Prevention of Musculoskeletal Disorders, ed 3. WB Saunders, Philadelphia, 1993.
45. Maslow, G, and Rothman, R: The facet joints, another look. Bull NY Acad Med 51:1294, 1975.
46. Frazer, H: The use of traction in backache. Med J Aust 2:694, 1954.
47. Crue, BL, and Todd, EM: The importance of flexion in cervical halter traction. Bull Los Angeles Neurol Soc 30:95, 1965.

48. Colachis, SC, and Strom, BR: Cervical traction: relationship of traction time to varied tractive force with constant angle of pull. Arch Phys Med Rehabil 46:815, 1965.

49. Swezey, RL, et al: Efficacy of home cervical traction therapy. Am J Phys Med Rehabil 78:30–32, 1999.

50. Olson, VL: Whiplash-associated chronic headache treated with home cervical traction. Physical Therapy 77:417–424, 1997.

51. Baker, P, and Marcoux, BC: The effectiveness of home cervical traction on relief of neck pain and impaired cervical range of motion. Phys Ther Case Rep 2:145–151, 1999.

52. Waylonis, GW, et al: Home cervical traction: evaluation of alternative equipment. Arch Phys Med Rehabil 63:388–391, 1982.

53. Venditti, PP, et al: Cervical traction device study: a basic evaluation of home-use supine cervical traction devices. J Neuromuscoskeletal System 3:82–91, 1995.

54. Sailors, ME, et al: Force reproduction in submaximal manual cervical traction applied by experienced physical therapists. J Manual Manipulative Ther 5:27–32, 1997.

55. Humphreys, SC, et al: Flexion and traction effect on C5-C6 foraminal space. Arch Phys Med Rehabil 79:1105–1109, 1998.

56. Li, LC, and Bombardier, C: Physical therapy management of low back pain: an exploratory survey of therapist approaches. Physical Therapy 81:1018–1028, 2001.

57. Tesio, L, and Merlo, A: Autotraction versus passive traction: an open controlled study in lumbar disc herniation. Arch Phys Med Rehabil 74:871, 1992.

58. Ljunggren, A, et al: Autotraction versus manual traction in patients with prolapsed lumbar intervertebral discs. Scand J Rehabil Med 16:117, 1984.

59. Mathews, W, et al: Manipulation and traction for lumbago sciatica: physiotherapeutic techniques used in two controlled trials. Physiother Pract 4:201, 1988.

60. Onel, D, et al: Computed tomographic investigation of the effect of traction on lumbar disk herniations. Spine 14:82, 1989.

61. Goldish, G: Lumbar traction. In Tollison, CD, and Kriegel, M (eds): Interdisciplinary Rehabilitation of Low Back Pain. Williams & Wilkins, Baltimore, 1989.

62. Tesio, L, et al: Natchev's auto-traction for lumbago-sciatica: effectiveness in lumbar disc herniation. Arch Phys Med Rehabil 70:831–834, 1989.

63. Weinert, AM, and Rizzo, TD: Nonoperative management of multilevel lumbar disk herniations in an adolescent athlete. Mayo Clin Proc 67:137–141, 1992.

64. Guvenol, K, et al: A comparison of inverted spinal traction and conventional traction in the treatment of lumbar disc herniations. Physiother Theory Pract 16:151–160, 2000.

65. Meszaros, TF, et al: Effect of 10%, 30% and 60% body weight traction on the straight leg raise test of symptomatic patients with low back pain. JOSPT 30:595–601, 2000.

66. van der Heijden, GJM, et al: Efficacy of lumbar traction: a randomized clinical trial. Physiotherapy 81:29–35, 1995.

67. Oudenhoven, RC: Gravitational lumbar traction. Arch Phys Med Rehabil 59:510–512, 1978.

68. Moret, NC, et al: Design and feasibility of a randomized clinical trial to evaluate the effect of vertical traction in patients with a lumbar radicular syndrome. Manual Ther 3:203–211, 1998.

69. Werners, R, et al: Randomized trial comparing interferential therapy with motorized lumbar traction and massage in the management of low back pain in a primary care setting. Spine 24:1579–1584, 1999.

70. Corkery, M: The use of lumbar harness traction to treat a patient with lumbar radicular pain: a case report. J Manual Manipulative Ther 9:191–197, 2001.

71. Beurskens, AJ, et al: Efficacy of traction for nonspecific low-back pain. 12-week and 6-month results from a randomized clinical trial. Spine 22:2756–2762, 1997.

72. Beurskens, AJ, et al: Efficacy of traction for nonspecific low-back pain: a randomized clinical trial. Lancet 346:1596–1600, 1995.

73. Borman, P, et al: The efficacy of lumbar traction in the management of patients with low back pain. Rheumotol Int 23:82–86, 2003.

74. Harte, AA, et al: The efficacy of traction for back pain: a systematic review of randomized trials. Arch Phys Med Rehabil 84:1542–1553, 2003.

75. Reilly, JP, et al: Effect of pelvic-femoral position on vertebral separation produced by lumbar traction. Physical Therapy 59:282–286, 1979.

76. Gianakopoulos, G, et al: Inversion devices: their role in producing lumbar distraction. Arch Phys Med Rehabil 66:100–102, 1985.

77. Janke, AW, et al: The biomechanics of gravity-dependent traction on the lumbar spine. Spine 22:253–260, 1997.

78. Tekeoglu, I, et al: Distraction of lumbar vertebrae in gravitational traction. Spine 23:1061–1063, 1998.

79. Twomey, LT: Sustained lumbar traction, an experimental study of long spine segments. Spine 10:146–149, 1985.

80. Colachis, SC, and Strohm, BR: Effects of intermittent traction on separation of lumbar vertebrae. Arch Phys Med Rehabil 50:251–258, 1969.

81. Ramos, G, and Martin, W: Effects of vertebral axial decompression on intradiscal pressure. J Neurosurg 81:350–353, 1994.

82. Kane, MD, et al: Effect of gravity-facilitated traction on intervertebral dimensions of the lumbar spine. JOSPT 6:281–288, 1985.

83. Creighton, DS: Positional distraction, a radiological confirmation. J Manual Manipulative Ther 1:83–86, 1993.

84. Hales, J, et al: Treatment of adult lumbar scoliosis with axial spinal unloading using the LTX3000 Lumbar Rehabilitation System. Spine 27:E71–E79, 2002.

85. Harrison, DE, et al. Changes in sagittal lumbar configuration with a new method of extension traction: nonrandomized clinical controlled trial. Arch Phys Med Rehabil 83:1585–1591, 2002.

86. Falkenberg, J, et al: Surface EMG activity of the back musculature during axial spinal unloading using an LTX 3000 Lumbar Rehabilitation System. Electromyogr Clin Neurophysiol 41:419–427, 2001.

87. Bridger, RS, et al: Effect of lumbar traction on stature. Spine 15:522–524, 1990.

88. Letchuman, R, and Deusinger, RH: Comparison of sacrospinalis myoelectric activity and pain levels in patients undergoing static and intermittent lumbar traction. Spine 18:L1361–L1365 1993.

89. Krause, M, et al: Lumbar spine traction: evaluation of effects

and recommended application for treatment. Manipulative Ther 5:72–81, 2000.

90. Trudel, G: Autotraction. Arch Phys Med Rehabil 75:234–235, 1994.
91. Andersson, G, et al: Intervertebral disc pressures during traction. Scand J Rehabil Med 9:88, 1983.
92. Ballantyne, B, et al: The effects of inversion traction on spinal column configuration, heart rate, blood pressure, and perceived discomfort. J Orthop Sports Phys Ther 7:254, 1986.
93. LeMarr, J, et al: Cardiorespiratory responses to inversion. Phys Sport Med 11:51, 1983.
94. Katavich, L: Neural mechanisms underlying manual cervical traction. J Manual Manipulative Ther 7:20–25, 1999.
95. Paris, S: The spine: etiology and treatment of dysfunction including joint manipulation. Course notes, 1979.
96. Quain, BM, and Tecklin, JS: Lumbar traction: Its effect on respiration. Physical Therapy 65:1343–1346, 1985.
97. Simmers, TA, et al: Internal jugular vein thrombosis after cervical traction. J Internal Med 241:333–335, 1997.
98. Balogun, JA, et al: Cardiovascular responses of healthy subjects during cervical traction. Physiother Canada 42:16–22, 1990.

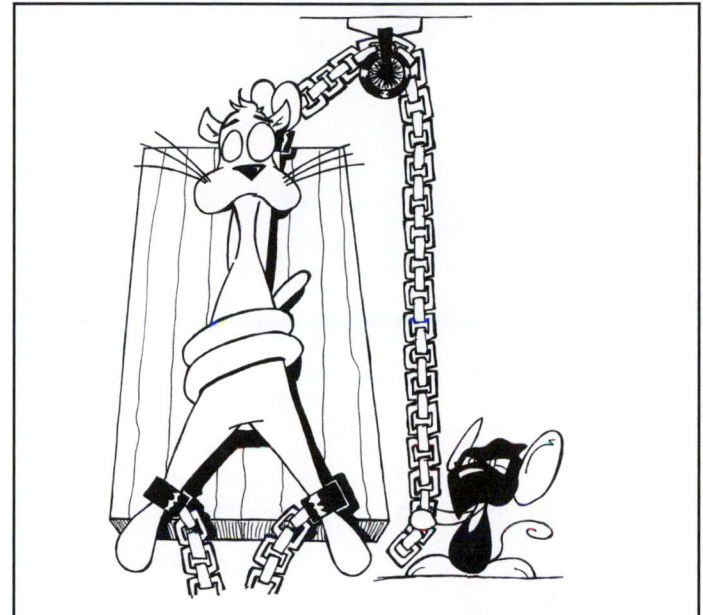

Objectives

- Discuss the pathophysiology of edema and identify different types of edema.
- Discuss the specific interventions to address edema.
- Discuss the factors that determine the appropriate intervention for edema reduction.
- Discuss the clinical decision-making process for determining the effectiveness of the chosen intervention for edema reduction.

Key Terms

Lymphatic system
Lymph transport
Interstitial space
Musculoskeletal pump

Low versus high
    protein edema
Primary lymphedema

Secondary lymphedema
"RICE"
Risk reduction

Joy C. Cohn, PT CLT-LANA

Soft Tissue Management Techniques: Edema Management

Outline

Pathophysiology of Edema	Examination of Patient
Types of Edema	Goals and Expected Outcomes
Management of Edema	Summary
Interventions for Edema	Patient Education

"I thought I could put my cancer behind me, but now this swelling is a daily reminder."

Edema is an abnormal accumulation of fluid in the interstitial space. This is a seemingly simple definition, but it in fact reflects a very complex interaction between physiologic and anatomic facts. Edema can present as an acute event in a localized area of the body as is commonly seen, for example, after a sports injury. Or an individual may experience a more sustained effect and less-localized swelling of a limb, for example, as a consequence of treatment for cancer. The intervention required can be very different in these two instances. As is true in all areas of practicing physical therapy, a precise understanding of the mechanisms giving rise to the edema is critical to determining the appropriate intervention.

Pathophysiology of Edema

Fluid travels through the body in three major pathways—the circulatory system, the lymphatic system, and in the interstitial spaces between the cells. The circulatory system has a "pump"—the heart—that pushes the fluid through an extensive network of vessels divided into an arterial and a venous side. These sides are divided by the capillary bed in the interstitial spaces where fluid and nutrients leave the capillary bed on the arterial side and fluid and byproducts of metabolism are reabsorbed on the venous side. In the normal state, 90% of the fluid that filters out of the capillary bed on the arterial side is reabsorbed on the venous side.[1] The 10% of the remaining fluid and all proteins and other debris are removed by the lymphatic vessels that lie in intimate contact with the capillaries in the interstitial space. The removal of proteins along with the excess fluid cannot be emphasized too strongly because *"this removal of proteins from the interstitial spaces is an essential function without which we would die within about 24 hours."* [2] Fluid and proteins in the interstitial space are held primarily in a "gel matrix" that serves several purposes: it acts as a spacer between the cells, it prevents excessive movement of the fluid into the lower body when we stand, and it prevents the rapid spread of bacteria through the tissues.[2]

The lymphatic system is analogous to a "sewer system" and is not often thought of unless the "water backs up into the street" and edema becomes clinically symptomatic. It serves three important functions in the body: regulation of fluid balance through transport of fluid and proteins, defense against infection/cancer as a part of the immune system, and transport of digested fat from the gut. It is a system with a one-way flow from the periphery to its termination at the jugular angles just above the heart where the lymph fluid is returned to the circulatory system. The vessels of the lymphatic system gradually progress from fragile, very superficial capillaries to deeper "collectors" that lie in parallel to the deep veins in returning fluid to the circulatory system. The absorbing lymphatic capillaries are vessels with walls of endothelial cells in a single layer. They are anchored into the tissues by fine filaments. Fluid enters these vessels through gaps between the cells that are opened by the anchoring filaments in response to changes in local tissue pressure from movement or an increase in the hydrostatic pressure in the tissue space. These gaps are larger than those in the blood capillaries and also allow proteins and debris to be absorbed. The deeper lymphatic vessels have valves like the veins that prevent backflow. They also have intrinsic muscle in their walls and pulsate in response to being stretched or from stimulation from the autonomic nervous system to help propel fluid toward the heart. Lymph transport relies on several extrinsic mechanisms because there is no intrinsic pump (the heart) as in the circulatory system. These include the musculoskeletal pump, respiratory pressure changes, the intrinsic pulsation of the deep lymphatic vessels, close proximity to the pulsating arteries, and gravity. All of these mechanisms should be kept in mind when treating an individual with edema.

The lymphatic system normally transports approximately 2 to 2.5 liters of fluid per day and 80 to 200 g of protein back to the circulatory system.[3] The fluid is filtered through nodes that are responsible for the removal of foreign substances and are the site of lymphocyte activity to fight infection. It has the capacity to increase its flow up to 10 times the normal volume of fluid carried as the hydrostatic pressure increases,[1] but not for the long term.

Types of Edema

Edema becomes apparent when the interstitial fluid has reached a level at least 30% above normal.[2] Due to the capacity of the lymphatic system to increase its flow rate by 10-fold and because the gel matrix is able to absorb 30% to 50% more fluid than in the normal state before free fluid accumulates, if edema is apparent, it represents, at least in the short term, a failure of the normal compensatory mechanisms in the tissues.

Localized acute edema usually occurs due to tissue injury, in response to trauma of a mechanical, infectious, or toxic nature. This causes inflammation that is characterized by localized redness, warmth, swelling, and pain. The patient may be unable to move comfortably or weight bear on the affected limb. The edema in this case is caused by a substantial increase in the capillary permeability allowing large quantities of fluid and protein to escape the capillaries and flood the interstitial space. Actual bleeding with hematoma formation is also possible. The capillary permeability is changed by actual trauma to the vessels, the inflammatory response to an injury, and the secondary release of chemicals that stimulate the healing response but also increase capillary permeability.[4] The edema fluid has a relatively low protein content in this type of situation. An acute edema usually occurs in conjunction with a normal venous and lymphatic system. This type of edema usually resolves in a limited timeframe (weeks to months), although more extensive injuries may progress to a more chronic form. The therapist's intervention focuses on enhancing the normal physiological mechanisms to resolve the edema via venous and lymphatic return. Examples of this type of edema would include a sports injury to soft tissue or a joint, a wound in the skin, a localized infection, or a reaction to an insect or snake bite (Table 7-1).

Acute edema of a widely affected area of the body is usually due to metabolic disease states such as malnutrition or liver, kidney, or heart disease. Congestive heart failure (CHF)

TABLE 7-1 Types of Edema

TYPE	SIGNS AND SYMPTOMS
Acute	Rapid onset after known injury
	Redness
	Warmth
	Painful to palpation or movement
	Localized
Venous	Slowly progressive
	Moderate warmth
	Dusky color or brownish staining of skin
	Achy pain as day progresses
	Normal contours of leg are lost
Lymphatic	Slowly progressive
	Mild warmth
	Color changes rare
	Usually painless
	Sensation of fullness or heaviness in limb
	Soft and pitting or hard
	Asymmetrical in comparison of limbs
Systemic edema (heart, kidney, and liver disease)	Abdominal swelling (ascites)
	Generalized, varying edema
	Generally pitting
	Bilateral, symmetrical edema
Toxic	Acute
	Localized
	Itchy or painful
	Redness
	Nonpitting

is a good example. In this instance, there is increased capillary pressure due to a venous obstruction from pooling of blood in the veins as the heart fails to adequately pump.[2, p 306] CHF causes a soft, symmetrical swelling in the legs. The causes of cardiac failure are complicated, and the treatment of this type of edema requires the skilled care of a physician and is beyond the scope of this chapter.

Chronic or progressive (slow or rapidly accumulating) edemas can be more accurately described as lymphedemas. This type is due to venous and/or lymphatic obstruction. The edema fluid in this instance has high protein content due to the slow accumulation of proteins in the absence of adequate clearance by the lymphatics. The lymphatic return is limited because of obstruction or failure due to overload in compensating for a lack of adequate venous return. It must be remembered that the lymphatics are the only mechanism to remove protein from the tissues. This type of edema can often be painless and only mildly warm in relation to the contralateral limb. Other symptoms common to this type of swelling include heaviness, warmth, aching, stiffness, tight/shiny skin, loss of skin folds, and inability to wear clothing or jewelry on the affected limb. Lymphedema can be divided into two varieties. Primary lymphedema is a congenital lack of adequate lymphatic drainage. The lymphatic vessels are usually either malformed or reduced in number. There are several presentations (Box 7-1). Secondary lymphedema is due to an acquired injury to the venous or lymphatic system. There are many known causes. Lymphedema is frequently associated with fibrotic skin changes. The fibrosis is due to increased fibroblast activity in response to the high level of proteins in the tissues. The therapist's intervention in this case is aimed at enhancing the remaining venous and lymphatic return to reduce the lymphedema volume, modifying chronic changes in the soft tissue, and teaching strategies to reduce the reaccumulation of fluid.

Management of Edema

Interventions for Edema

Acute localized edema due to a traumatic injury is best treated immediately after injury to minimize the extent of bleeding and edema fluid accumulation. This is important to minimize the proteins that accumulate in the tissues. The protein-rich fluid, or exudate, can determine the extent of the inflammatory reaction that occurs, and the greater the inflammatory reaction, the greater is the risk of a chronic, fibrotic change in the tissues.

RICE therapy has been the intervention of choice since the 1950s in the first 24 to 72 hours after injury.[4] RICE stands for Rest, Ice, Compression, and Elevation of the affected body part. Rest, for the most part, is important to limit the blood flow to the area during the time period that there is excessive capillary permeability and increased pain with movement. This time period for rest, however, is very brief.

The application of ice or cold to the tissues causes a number of important physiological effects: decreases in the local tissue temperature, inflammation, metabolic rate, circulation through vasoconstriction, and pain with treatments lasting more than 2 to 3 minutes in duration. Continuous application of ice is generally limited to time periods of 10 to 20 minutes because extended applications of cold can cause a reflex vasodilation or tissue damage.[4] The application of cold can take many forms: ice massage, a chemical or gel ice pack, an iced towel, an ice bath, or whirlpool. An ice bath or whirlpool is not the treatment of choice in many situations because it does not allow elevation of the body part and is less practical in many settings. Contraindications to the use of cold include intolerance to cold (ask patient of previous experiences), history of Raynaud's phenomenon, ischemic tissue (frostbite injury likely without adequate blood flow), and decreased sensation. Use with caution in a patient with a recent open wound/incision or active bleeding.

Elevation of the body part alone can decrease the edema in an ankle.[6] Elevation allows gravity to assist both the veins and the lymphatic vessels to carry excess fluid and proteins away from the area of injury. Elevation also decreases the hydrostatic pressure in the tissues.[7] Elevation of the body part above the level of the heart is commonly recommended if practical. Elevation has not been shown to help except in the early stages of swelling.[7] The contraindication to elevation is an ischemic limb, because this increase in hydrostatic pressure in the limb will further reduce arterial flow to the limb.

BOX 7-1 Types of Lymphedema [5]

Primary Lymphedema

- Milroy's disease — Presents at birth
- Lymphedema praecox — Presents at adolescence
- Lymphedema tarda — Presents after age 30

Secondary Lymphedema

Lymphatics damaged by:

- Trauma
- Surgery
- Infection
- Obstruction by tumor
- Radiation therapy
- Obstruction by parasite
- Paralysis of a limb
- Chronic venous insufficiency

Compression increases the hydrostatic pressure in the tissues, decreasing ultrafiltration out of the damaged capillaries and increasing the absorption of fluid by the veins and fluid and proteins by the lymphatic vessels.[9] Compression can be accomplished by intermittent compression devices, compression bandaging, compression garments, or a combination compression/cold device. Intermittent compression devices are most commonly air-inflated sleeves that fit over the limb. The sleeves can have only one chamber or various numbers of multiple chambers that fill sequentially.[8] The parameters that can commonly be controlled by the therapist include inflation pressure, on-time/off-time cycle, and total treatment time. Inflation pressures are usually set between 30 and 100 mm Hg. There is a potentially significant problem associated with setting the pressure above the patient's diastolic pressure, as this could occlude the arterial blood supply. Therefore, most manufacturers recommend staying below this level. Recommended pressures are in the range of 30 to 60 mm Hg for the upper extremity and 40 to 80 mm Hg in the lower extremity. Many authors recommend staying at or below 30 to 40 mm Hg pressure in all instances due to inaccurate control of the actual pressures created by the devices[8] or because of the potential damage to the delicate, superficial lymphatics.[9] One author reports complete closure of lymphatic vessels at pressures of 75 mm Hg.[10]

There is no published research regarding the on-time/off-time cycle. In many devices this is not even adjustable. The range of settings could be from 30 seconds on/30 seconds off up to 4 to 5 minutes on/1 to 5 minutes off. Some of these ratios seem to relate more to the time necessary to fill all chambers sequentially than to any actual physiological reason. Patient comfort could probably be used as a deciding factor. The total treatment time recommended also varies widely.[7] Times can range from 30 minutes up to 6 to 8 hours repeated over 2 to 3 days.[11] In practical terms, treatment times range from 30 minutes up to 1 hour. Circumferential measurements should be taken before and after a session of intermittent compression to evaluate the response. The choice of a single-chamber pump as opposed to pumps with multiple chambers is also not clear. There is a theoretical advantage in a pump with multiple chambers that fill sequentially as they ascend the limb. This would then be pushing edema fluid along through the limb. This advantage has not been proved.[12,13] It has been recommended that a trial of different pumps be completed before long-term use at home.[7] The contraindications for use of an intermittent pump include CHF, active infection, unstable fractures, recent thrombophlebitis, and pulmonary emboli.

Compression can also be applied with bandaging or garments. The intent of static external compression is to decrease ultrafiltration by increasing hydrostatic pressure, to decrease the present edema by improving the musculoskeletal pump, and to soften fibrotic tissue.

TABLE 7-2 **Compression Bandages**	
Short stretch	<70% stretch
Medium stretch	70% to 140% stretch
Long stretch	<140% stretch

Types: short, Comprilan (BSN Medical, Charlotte, NC), Rosidal (BSN Medical, Charlotte, NC); medium, Coban; long, Ace bandages.

Compression bandaging is available in three varieties: short stretch, medium stretch, and long stretch (Table 7-2). Short stretch bandages provide a low pressure at rest and a high pressure when the limb is working (Fig. 7-1). Long stretch bandages provide a high pressure at rest due to the increased elasticity but a lower pressure when the limb is working because of the "give" inherent to the bandage. Short stretch bandages are preferable to reduce edema because they provide a better pumping effect in combination with the muscles when the patient moves (Fig. 7-2). Long stretch bandages are inexpensive and frequently adequate for acute, localized swellings. A long stretch bandage should always be removed at night and replaced by elevation of the limb to avoid arterial occlusion. Arterial occlusion is possible at night due to decreased limb perfusion with elevation, decreased perfusion without assistance from the musculoskeletal pump, and the danger of rolling or shifting of the bandage, which can produce a tourniquet effect. An Unna boot is a type of very short stretch bandage that can be applied to the leg. It is a zinc oxide–impregnated gauze bandage that keeps the skin moist while creating a "soft cast" on the limb, thereby improving the musculoskeletal pump and preventing additional fluid accumulation. It is frequently used in managing the

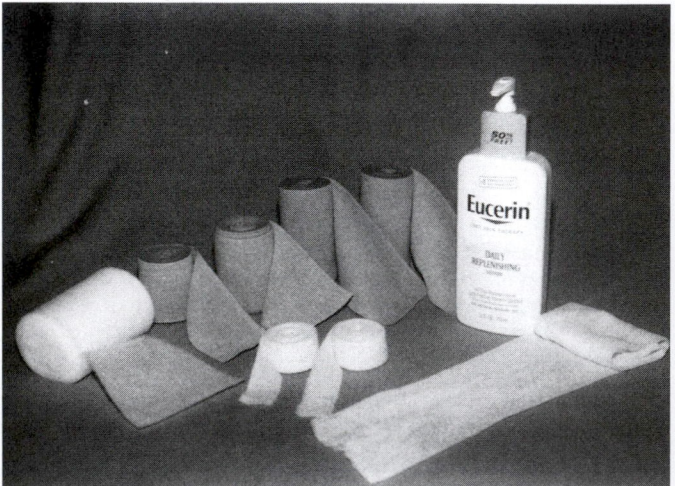

Figure 7-1 Short stretch bandages of varying widths are used to conform to a limb and apply a low resting pressure and high working pressure. Padding materials and soft elastic gauze are included to protect bony prominences and to add pressure to fingers or toes.

edema associated with a venous wound and can be left in place for up to 1 week. Another bandaging scheme to manage edema with wounds is to combine short and medium stretch bandages in layers used in the same way as Unna boots. All bandaging should include adequate padding of bony areas by felt, foam, or soft cotton to prevent excessive pressure and skin breakdown. Contraindications to the use of bandaging include active infection, recent thrombophlebitis or pulmonary embolus without adequate anticoagulation, and CHF. Precautions for bandaging include arterial disease, diabetes mellitus, decreased sensation, and metastatic disease.

Compressive garments are similar in action to bandaging and are used to maintain a limb size and to prevent reaccumulation of fluid during the day when a limb is dependent. They are a compromise compared with short stretch or inelastic supports, which allow greater freedom of movement and comfort. Compression garments cannot be expected to reduce a chronic edema.[7,15] They are more appropriately fitted to a limb once the edema volume has reduced and reached a plateau. A randomized, controlled study of compression bandaging followed by compression garments versus compression garments alone demonstrated that the combination therapy led to double the reduction achieved by compression garments alone.[16] A compression garment is manufactured to place the most pressure at the wrist or ankle and then progressively less through the remainder of the limb[17] (Fig. 7-2). This is described as a gradient pressure on the limb. Compression garments are available as off-the-shelf sizes and as custom made. The off-the-shelf garments **must** fit correctly at the wrist or ankle as this is the location where the maximum compression is applied. A custom-made garment is much more expensive but essential if a limb is disproportionate, such as a small ankle with a very large calf, or irregular in size. There are many other factors that should be considered when choosing a garment for a patient (Box 7-2). The compression class chosen varies by the limb and degree of edema. For treatment of a lymphedema, generally an arm sleeve/glove is prescribed in a compression class I or II and a

BOX 7-2	Factors to Consider in Choosing a Compression Garment[18]

- Coverage
- Compression class
- Appearance
- Custom made versus off the shelf
- Material or fabric
- Construction
- Suspension
- Skin condition/sensitivity/wounds
- Ability of patient to don/doff
- Cost and source of payment

leg garment in compression class II or III. (Table 7-3). After an acute injury such as an ankle fracture, many patients can benefit from a compression class I knee-high garment to control the swelling in the rehabilitation phase after immobilization. The contraindications for compression garments are acute thrombophlebitis/infection, cardiac edema, malignant lymphedema (relative), arterial disease (relative), and acute vascular blockages.[17, p 56,18] Garments should be used with caution in patients with active cancer, decreased sensation, or arterial compromise.

Exercise enhances venous and lymphatic flow.[4, 5, 19] Exercise in combination with compression of any kind further enhances the musculoskeletal pump.[20] This can include isometric exercises during intermittent compression pumping, walking with a compressive bandage on the lower leg, simple arm exercises while wearing a compression bandage or compressive sleeve, or specific exercise programs designed for

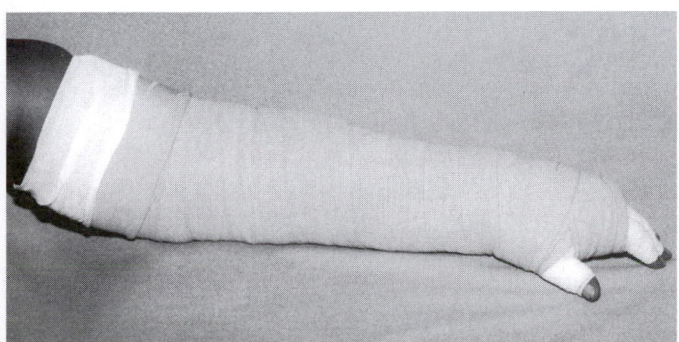

Figure 7–2 A completed compression bandage for an upper extremity from the fingers to the axilla.

TABLE 7-3	Compression Classes for Medical-Grade Garments [1,17]	
Class I	20 to 30 mm Hg	Minor varicose veins, minor varicosities of pregnancy, mild lymphedema of the arm
Class II	30 to 40 mm Hg	Significant varicose veins with edema, post-traumatic swelling, postphlebitis swelling, significant varicosities of pregnancy, lymphedema of the arm
Class III	40 to 50 mm Hg	Chronic venous insufficiency, status post venous ulcers, lymphedema of the arm or leg
Class IV	50 to 60 mm Hg	Lymphedema

patients with lymphedema.[5] Exercise programs for lymphedema management usually are performed in a specific sequence where more central regions are exercised before the more distal portions of the limb. This allows more central "reservoirs" to be emptied before edematous areas are exercised.[5] Elevating the limb while performing exercise enhances edema reduction. Aerobic exercises are often prescribed for patients with edema. An athlete with an acute injury may wish to maintain his or her level of fitness while recovering. An individual with a chronic lymphedema may be deconditioned due to a decreased level of activity. Aerobic exercise is accompanied by an increased heart rate and respiratory rate. Lymph flow is enhanced by both the pressure differential in the thorax that occurs with breathing and increased pulsation of the arteries.[21]

Aquatic exercise is particularly beneficial for individuals with leg swelling of nonmetabolic origin and with a stable cardiovascular system. Water exerts a gradient compression on a body when immersed, with the most distal portions of the limb under greatest pressure. For example, an individual with a 32-inch inseam standing in groin-deep water has a pressure of 60 mm Hg exerted on the foot/ankle.[5] Combined with the musculoskeletal pump activity with exercise, an individual with acute edema could experience a notable difference in swelling after an aquatic therapy session. The edema reduction is often considered a side benefit to the ease of movement achieved because of the reduction in weight-bearing and active assistance for joint motion from buoyancy. Excessive warmth, however, can have a deleterious effect due to an increase in local blood flow. Increased blood flow adds to the hydrostatic pressure in the tissues and can cause increased ultrafiltration into the interstitial space, leading to more edema volume.

Electrical stimulation can be used to achieve rhythmic contraction of muscles in an area of localized edema, thereby enhancing the musculoskeletal pump. Electrical stimulation below the threshold to elicit muscle contraction can also be used to repel proteins. Proteins and plasma in the interstitial space have a negative polarity, and when treated with negative polarity, they are repelled, causing a movement from the local area of edema. As the water is attracted to the proteins, it is also shifted from the area (see Chapter 10). This treatment is most easily used for hand edema.[22]

Examination of Patient

In the American Physical Therapy Association's *Guide to Physical Therapist Practice*,[23] the practice pattern 6H–Impaired Circulation and Anthropomorphic Dimensions Associated with Lymphatic System Disorders addresses all of the pertinent data that should be included in a thorough examination. Certain aspects of the initial examination warrant particular attention once general demographic, social, employment, habits, and living environments have been considered.

1. Timing of symptoms of edema: When did the swelling begin? Is there an event that precipitated the edema? Has the swelling improved, worsened, or remained unchanged? Is the edema worse as the day goes on? Is the edema gone first thing in the morning?

2. Medical/surgical history: Includes history of cancer treatment, other medical conditions, all surgical procedures, and history of previous injury

3. Pain: Intensity, quality, and what causes an increase or a decrease

4. Has the patient self-treated or received any treatment up until now and with what response?

5. Medications/tests: Has the patient taken any over-the-counter or prescribed medications? Has the patient had any medical tests, and what were the results?

6. What functional limitations does the patient report?

The results of this part of the examination can help to classify a generalized limb edema as lymphedema and allow determination of whether it is a primary or secondary lymphedema. Lymphedema is described by stages, which describe the amount of progression (Box 7-3).

Tests and measures to document the particular impairments of the patient are chosen based on the initial interview of the patient, but in the presence of edema, they should always include the following:

1. Musculoskeletal survey including range of motion, strength, stability of joints, and posture

2. Neurological status including sensation and signs of neural tension

3. Skin integrity including color, breaks or irritations in the skin, presence of scars, tattoos demarcating an area of previous radiation therapy, and temperature

4. Edema including circumferential measurements or volumetric measurements, pitting or nonpitting, and extent of edema

5. Cardiovascular/circulatory status including blood pressure, pulses, heart rate, rubor with dependency, and venous filling time

---

BOX 7-3   Stages of Lymphedema [14]

Stage I	Reversible: edema reverses with elevation, pitting edema with pressure
Stage II	Irreversible: edema remains with elevation. Increased fibroblast activity due to proteins causes fibrosis in the tissues. Minimal pitting to pressure
Stage III	Elephantiasis: extensive tissue hardening, papillomas (wart-like growths), and huge limb size

6. Wounds, if any, should be described by size, depth, presence of drainage, odor, appearance of the depth of the wound, and appearance of the immediate skin area

7. Functional status and activity level including whether the patient has difficulty with clothing or shoes, reaching overhead, ambulation, or transfers

Anthropomorphic characteristics of the limb or area of the edema can be documented by circumferential measurements or volumetric measurements. A simple body diagram is also very useful. Measurements should ideally always be taken at the same time of day and by the same person. Circumferential measurements are taken with a nonstretch tape measure of a material that can be easily cleaned with alcohol between uses. The tape must have a lead at the beginning meaning that the zero mark must be easily discerned and not hidden or missing. All measurements must be taken at reproducible landmarks that should be documented or at regular intervals. Casley-Smith and Casley-Smith[5] describe taking measurements at 4- or 10-cm intervals with no loss in accuracy or reproducibility. This has become a commonly used method in lymphedema management because it is inexpensive, it can be accomplished in any location, and it is convenient. This method is sensitive to varying degrees of change in a limb. These measurements can used to obtain a calculated volume by a "truncated cones" method.[5] The measurements can be used to calculate a rough estimate of the difference in "volume" between two limbs by summing all of the measurements of each limb and comparing the sum for the affected to the unaffected side. A percentage difference can also be calculated. This very simple method allows the therapist to learn how the limb changes over time in comparison with the opposite limb with little error compared with more rigorous mathematical determinations of volume.[5] The comparisons can be expressed as a percentage difference.

A volume measurement can also be obtained by use of a volumeter that follows the principle of water displacement (Fig. 7-3). This method is excellent when assessing the edema in a hand or foot/ankle injury because of the irregular surfaces. This method requires a volumeter designed for the hand or foot filled preferably with tepid or lukewarm water. The patient immerses the body part to a standard depth, and the water displaced is collected as it runs out of a spout (Fig. 7-4A). The volume of fluid displaced is measured[22] (Fig. 7-4B). This method is less convenient, not easily transportable, and more expensive as the clinic must own a volumeter. Additionally, it provides only one measure of change in the body part and is not sensitive to varying amounts of change in different parts of the limb. However, this "total volume" can be used to make direct comparisons over time to assess overall response to treatment. Either method (water displacement or calculated volume) is acceptable as they have been shown (for the upper extremity at least) to have concurrent validity though they are not interchangeable.[24,25]

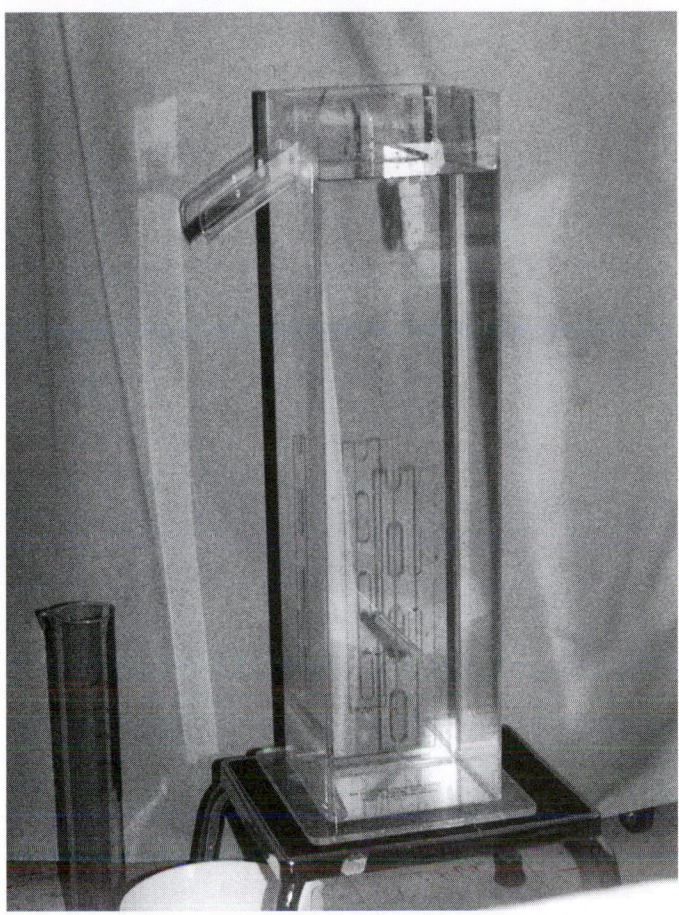

Figure 7-3 A volumeter is generally constructed of Plexiglas with a spout. It is filled with water until a small amount runs out of the spout and stops.

Measurement of and comparison to the contralateral limb gives information as to a "normal" value for the individual being treated.

The quality of the edema is important to note. An acute edema with a large sudden increase in fluid in the tissue space will "pit" when the skin is pressed with a finger. This occurs because, with pressure, the fluid flows through the gel matrix away from the area of pressure and then returns to the original location in 5 to 30 seconds. A scale used commonly by physicians rates pitting edema on a 1-to-4 scale (Box 7-4). With longstanding edema or inflammation, the gel matrix becomes fibrotic due to macrophage activity and will be firm and no longer "pit" with pressure.

Palpation of the skin also serves to provide information as to thickening in the skin and soft tissue. Attempting to lift a skin fold in comparison to the corresponding contralateral area of the body can give a sense of the skin turgor. This is particularly helpful if assessing areas like the trunk for edema. Stemmer's sign[28] is a diagnostic tool of the physical examination. If a skin fold cannot be lifted off of the dorsum of the hand or foot, it is considered to be a positive Stemmer's sign

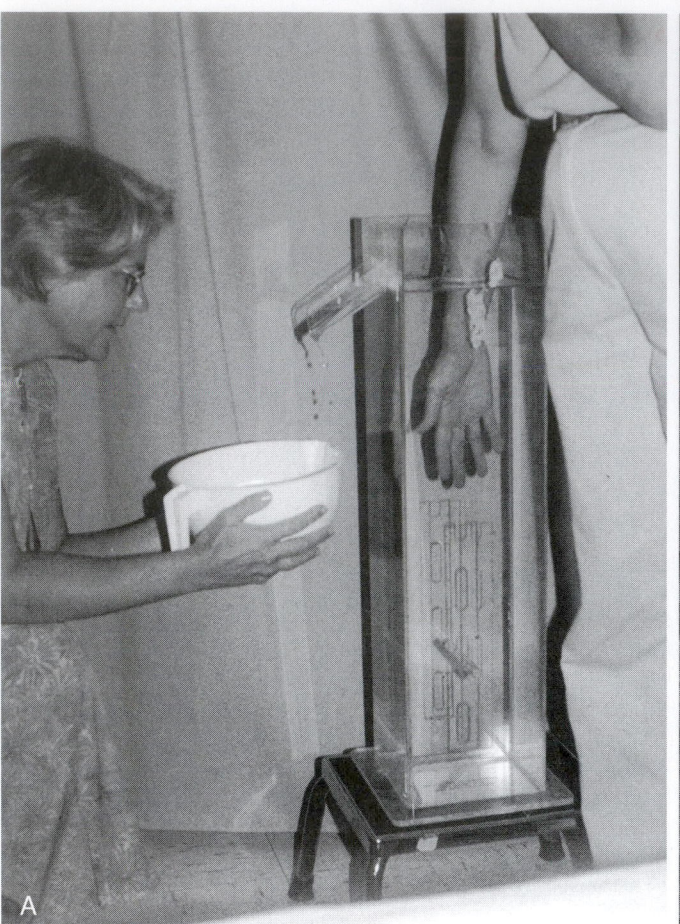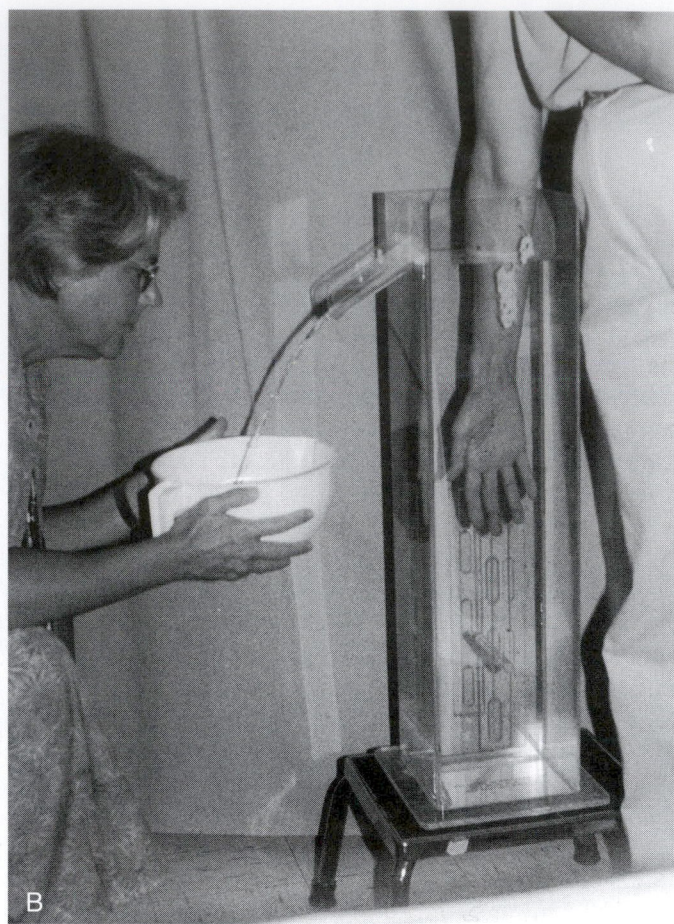

Figure 7-4   The patient inserts the limb slowly (*A*), and the water displaced by the limb is collected and measured (*B*).

for lymphedema. However, if negative, it does not eliminate lymphedema as a diagnosis.

Goals and Expected Outcomes

The American Physical Therapy Association's *Guide to Physical Therapist Practice* Pattern 6H covers the wide range of possible goals to be set in addressing the impairments, functional limitations, and disabilities identified during the initial examination. Goals and outcomes specific to reduction of edema could include the following:

1. Increased range of motion
2. Decreased pain
3. Decreased edema, lymphedema, or effusion
4. Improved skin integrity
5. Normal tissue temperature
6. Independent management of symptoms achieved by patient/caregiver
7. Risk of recurrence reduced through patient education
8. Adequate edema control achieved with appropriate device if indicated
9. Patient/caregiver able to correctly don/doff and care for devices

In the treatment of a stage 2 lymphedema, the literature demonstrates that complete resolution of the swelling is rarely achieved due to the chronic tissue changes that accompany a lymphedema in this stage. An outcome with an edema volume reduction of 50% or better is expected. This reduction, if maintained by consistent self-management, can be expected to continue to improve but more slowly over time.[5]

BOX 7-4   Pitting Edema [26,27]

1+ = Edema that is barely detectable

2+ = A slight indentation is visible when the skin is depressed.

3+ = A deeper fingerprint resolves in 5 to 30 seconds.

4+ = The limb is swollen to 1.5 to 2 times its normal size.

Summary

Patient Education

In any instance where edema is treated, it is essential to educate the patient as to self-care measures to achieve timely reduction in the edema. Providing the patient with an "owner's manual" description of how swelling occurs and what can be done to reduce it gives the patient a sense of control and usually results in better adherence to the suggested treatments. Take-home instructions written in plain English greatly enhance understanding and follow-through. Family members or caregivers are always encouraged to attend a treatment session to learn how to assist the patient with his or her edema management.

Lymphedema is not a well-understood condition among physicians. Lymphedema as a consequence of treatment for cancer is well understood by most surgeons and oncologists, who usually refer their patients promptly for treatment; however, not all patients receive or comprehend timely information in risk-reduction measures after treatment for cancer. Individuals with congenital forms of lymphedema often see many physicians before receiving an accurate diagnosis. Information accessible to the general public regarding lymphedema was even harder to obtain, until recently. The advent of the widespread use of the World Wide Web has made it easier to obtain information. Many patients come for their first visit with a large file of printouts from their Internet searches. It is extremely important to help patients understand that they must be careful to consider the source of any information obtained from the Internet. Two excellent sources of information about lymphedema are the Lymphoedema Association of Australia and the National Lymphedema Network (Box 7-5). In recent years, there have been several excellent texts published on lymphedema and treatment as well.

Of special concern to people at risk for lymphedema is how to "prevent" it from developing. There is no research to date that demonstrates that lymphedema can be prevented. There are several known factors that do increase the risk of lymphedema in women who have been treated for breast cancer[29]: radiation therapy of the axilla, an axillary node dissection, and obesity. Despite a lack of research in this area, a number of lists of "do's and don'ts" have been developed as guidelines based on an understanding of normal physiology and the pathophysiology of lymphedema.[30] The most well known of these lists are the "18 Steps to Prevention" published by the National Lymphedema Network for people at risk for upper extremity or lower extremity lymphedema. In practice, these lists are frequently very upsetting to patients, because they seem overwhelming. In our practice, we have developed a somewhat condensed version for breast cancer patients that we believe puts more emphasis on understanding the "why" of risk reduction.[31]

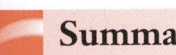

Patient Perspective

PATIENTS' FREQUENTLY ASKED QUESTIONS
1. What is the cause of the swelling?
2. How do I reduce the swelling effectively?
3. How do I keep the swelling from returning?

Recommended Books for Lymphedema

Modern Treatment for Lymphedema, ed 5, by Judith R. Casley-Smith and J. R. Casley-Smith, Lymphoedema Association of Australia, Adelaide, Australia, 1997.

Textbook of Lymphology for Physicians and Lymphedema Therapists, by M. Foldi, E. Foldi, and S. Kubik, Urban and Fischer, Munich, Germany, 2003.

A Primer on Lymphedema, by Deborah G. Kelly, Prentice Hall, Upper Saddle River, NJ, 2002.

Lymphedema: Diagnosis and Therapy, ed 3, by H. Weissleder and C. Schuchhardt, Viavital Verlag GmbH, Koln, Germany, 2001.

Lymphedema: A Breast Cancer Patient's Guide to Prevention and Healing, by Jeannie Burt and Gwen White, Hunter House, Alameda, CA, 1999.

Researching the Literature

An essential reference for understanding and treating lymphedema is Textbook of Lymphology for Physicians and Lymphedema Therapists, by M. Foldi, et al. This book can be ordered through The National Lymphedema Network at www.lymphnet.org

Discussion Questions

1. Your patient has come to physical therapy today and is in the waiting area. You observe that the patient is sitting with his legs, outstretched and crossed, supported by his ankles on the chair in front of him. He was scheduled to see you for treatment of an acute ankle sprain/strain with pronounced edema. He had also previously reported knee and back pain. During this patient's last visit, you had instructed him in the proper use of axillary crutches with weight bearing as tolerated (WBAT), and you had also instructed him to keep his leg elevated.
   A. What patient education needs to be revisited and why?

BOX 7-5   Internet Resources for Lymphedema Information

Lymphoedema Association of Australia	www.lymphoedema.org.au
National Lymphedema Network	www.lymphnet.org
American Cancer Society	www.cancer.org
Oncolink–University of Pennsylvania Cancer Center Site	www.oncolink.upenn.edu

B. What do you expect to find when you reassess edema for this patient and why?

C. How could you prevent this in the future?

2. You observe a patient who has been scheduled for physical therapy for lymphedema following a mastectomy; she is wearing spandex clothing.

A. Is this something that is of concern to you as a clinician? Why or why not?

CASE STUDY 1

Acute Ankle Sprain

Patient Description The patient is a 40-year-old accountant who sustained an acute inversion injury of the right ankle playing basketball with friends 2 days ago. He was been sent to your clinic after a fracture has been ruled out by an x-ray examination in the emergency department. He was treated immediately with ice and elevation, which he continued at home. He presents with significant nonpitting edema and ecchymoses in the region of the lateral malleolus and lateral foot. The ankle is painful to palpation over the anterior talofibular ligament. A figure-of-eight girth measurement is 2.8 cm larger than on the opposite ankle. His active ankle dorsiflexion and plantarflexion are limited and painful, and he is unable to bear weight on that extremity without crutches.

Diagnosis Acute ankle sprain (inversion)

Plan of Care Intermittent compression

Compressive bandaging/compressive ankle support

Active range of motion exercises

Progressive weight-bearing as tolerated

Balance/proprioceptive training

Return to work and leisure specific activities

Intervention After completion of the initial examination, the patient was positioned with the right lower leg elevated. A length of stockinette was applied from the toes to the knee, and a three-chamber sequential compression boot was slipped on over the extremity. The limb was treated for 30 minutes at a pressure setting of 30 to 40 mm Hg adjusted to the patient's pain tolerance. The patient was encouraged to gently pump the foot inside the boot and to use the calf muscle during the off time of the pump cycle. Posttreatment figure-of-eight measurements were taken. The patient was compressively bandaged with low stretch bandage with a posterior kidney-shaped malleolar pad behind the lateral malleolus. An alternative method for compression would be a thermoplastic ankle stirrup brace with a built-in air bladder for compression. The stirrup brace is preferable if the patient can tolerate weight-bearing because it combines compression with protective medial lateral

stability. The patient is given written take-home instructions, including the following:

1. Ambulate as tolerated (with appropriate assistive device if needed).

2. Elevate and continue to ice for 20 minutes at a time.

3. Perform gentle ankle pumps four or five times per day.

4. Wear bandage/ankle support full time when not in bed.

The patient attended six additional sessions over the next 2 weeks, with gradual resolution of the edema/inflammation and decreased pain with AROM/weight-bearing. Intermittent compression was discontinued after two additional sessions, and strengthening exercises were gradually added and progressed. Functional skills to improve balance and proprioception were added as tolerated, and the patient was to be weaned from his ankle support as tolerated when AROM and strength returned to normal.

CASE STUDY 2

Postmastectomy Lymphedema

Patient Description The patient is a 56-year-old woman who was treated for breast cancer 4 years earlier with a right lumpectomy/axillary node dissection, followed by chemotherapy for six cycles and radiation therapy to the right breast/chest wall and axilla. The patient saw her oncologist last week with a complaint of 2 weeks of swelling in her right hand and difficulty buttoning the cuff of her blouse. The patient states that the swelling is better but not gone when she arises and that it is worse as the day goes on, with an achy discomfort in the forearm by the end of the working day as a secretary. The patient is right-handed. Highlights of her examination were as follows. After disrobing to the waist, the patient was examined. It was observed that the patient had a dropped right shoulder with moderate protraction of the right scapula. Her active range of motion (ROM) was limited to 0 to 150 degrees of right shoulder flexion, 0 to 160 degrees of shoulder abduction, and 0 to 70 degrees of shoulder external rotation. All other ROM measurements were within normal limits. The patient reported "pulling" in the right breast and axilla with all extremes of ROM. Strength was graded as either 4- or 4/5 in all muscle groups of both upper quadrants. Inspection of the skin revealed a healed but puckered and relatively immobile lumpectomy incision in the upper lateral quadrant of the right breast and swelling of the posterior axillary region compared with the left. Tattoos delineating the radiation field were sought and noted.

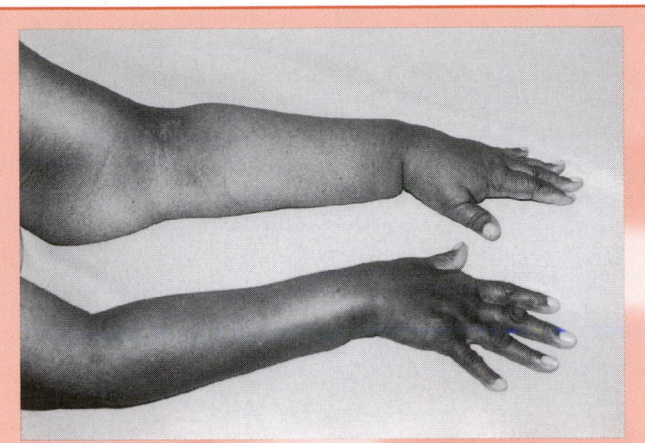

Clinical presentation of a woman with a postmastectomy lymphedema of the left upper extremity. This represents a stage 2 secondary lymphedema caused by damage to the lymphatic drainage of the left arm due to removal of lymph nodes in the left axilla and subsequent radiation therapy.

Circumferential measurements of both arms were taken using the most distal wrist crease as the 0 mark and measuring every 4 cm distal (to the metacarpal joints) and proximal (to the axilla). Each finger was individually measured just distal to the metacarpophalangeal joint. The patient had a 10% difference (right larger than left).

Diagnosis Early stage II lymphedema of the right upper extremity and trunk secondary to breast cancer/lumpectomy

Plan of Care Education re: diagnosis and pathophysiology

Education re: reduction of risk and skin care

Postural and flexibility exercises

Diaphragmatic breathing exercises

Lymph drainage massage

Compressive bandaging of the right upper extremity

Instruction in a home exercise program for increased lymphatic flow

Scar modification

Fitting of compression garment at end of treatment

Intervention After completing the initial examination, the patient was provided with written educational material on lymphedema and its treatment, and the plan of care was discussed. The patient was instructed in gentle postural and flexibility exercises to address the limited ROM and postural faults seen. The patient was scheduled to be seen two or three times

a week over the next 3 weeks. At the next session later that week, the patient was instructed in how to moisturize the skin with a low pH lotion and then apply a lightweight compression bandage (see photograph) to be worn full time and removed for showering. The patient was also instructed in a simple exercise program of diaphragmatic breathing and gentle massage of adjacent regional lymph nodes combined with movement of the limb. The goal of exercise was to enhance the musculoskeletal pump through movement combined with compressive support from bandaging. The patient was encouraged to supplement her exercise with a 15- to 20-minute walk at a moderate pace to enhance the effect of the respiratory pressure change on lymphatic flow. At the next session, the patient's arm was remeasured, and a reduction to 6% larger than the left arm was seen. Manual lymphatic massage and gentle mobilization of the lumpectomy scar were initiated, the arm was bandaged again, and the exercise program was reviewed. The ROM of the right shoulder had improved by 10 degrees in flexion, abduction, and external rotation. A small, high-density foam pad was cut, and after it was covered with stockinette, it was tucked into the patient's bra on the lateral chest wall to provide a gentle compression to the posterior axilla. The patient was encouraged to very gently mobilize the lumpectomy scar after showering every day. At subsequent visits, her exercise program was advanced to include strengthening exercises with 2- to 3-pound free weights. After five sessions, measurement demonstrated a reduction of the lymphedema to the right arm being only 2% larger than the left with minimal swelling over the dorsum of the hand. As the patient is right-handed, a small differential in size was expected due to increased muscular development of a dominant limb. The patient was fitted with a compression sleeve of 20 to 30 mm Hg from the wrist to the axilla and a gauntlet of the same compression to place pressure on the dorsum of the hand. She was instructed in donning/doffing of the sleeve and care of the garments. She was instructed to wear the garment daily. She was to remove it at night and replace with compression bandaging. All of these instructions were given in written form. The patient was scheduled for a follow-up visit in 1 week and instructed to call immediately if any unusual swelling was experienced. In 1 week's time, the patient returned with full active range of motion of the right arm, improved posture, and a stable limb size and demonstrated she was independent in all aspects of self-management. She was instructed to replace her compression garments every 4 to 6 months.

CASE STUDY 3

Edema following Patellar Surgery

Patient Description   The patient is a 72-year-old retired male schoolteacher who fell 6 weeks ago and had a comminuted fracture of the left patella. He was treated by surgical repair and an immobilizer for 4 weeks. He began physical therapy 2 weeks ago to regain range of motion (ROM) and strength and was progressing well. When he started therapy, he had minimal nonpitting edema at the ankle. As he used the immobilizer less and was on his feet more, he began to notice increased swelling at the end of the day. This afternoon, he demonstrates +2 pitting edema to the mid calf without pain. The other leg is not swollen. He states that there was no swelling when he got up this morning. Despite a low level of suspicion for a deep vein thrombosis, the patient was referred back to his surgeon because of the change in his status.

Diagnosis   Mild venous insufficiency

Plan of Care   Fitting of knee-high compression garment

Instruction in donning, care, wearing, and replacement schedule

Intervention   After the patient had a negative Doppler ultrasound study, he was referred back to continue his physical therapy. He was scheduled for an early morning appointment when his edema was minimal and measured and fit with a 20 to 30 mm Hg knee-high garment. Due to limited knee ROM, he was unable to reach his foot to don his garment independently, so his wife was instructed in don/doff skills. He was instructed to remove the garment at night. He was encouraged to wear his garment daily for at least 1 to 2 months and then to have his need for continued compression therapy reassessed. He continued the rehabilitation of his patellar fracture without further edema.

References

1. Foldi, M, Foldi, E, and Kubik, S: Textbook of Lymphology for Physicians and Lymphedema Therapists. Urban & Fischer, Munich, Germany, 2003, p 208.
2. Guyton, AC, and Hall, JE: Textbook of Medical Physiology, ed 9. WB Saunders, Philadelphia, 1996.
3. Weissleder, H, and Schuchhardt, C: Lymphedema: Diagnosis and Therapy, ed 3. Viavital Verlag, Koln, Germany, 2002, p 26.
4. Leadbetter, WB, Buckwalter, JA, and Gordon, SL: Sports-Induced Inflammation. American Academy of Orthopaedic Surgeons, Park Ridge, IL, 1990, p 12.
5. Casley-Smith, JR, and Casley-Smith, JR: Modern Treatment for Lymphoedema, ed 5. The Lymphoedema Association of Australia, Adelaide, Australia, 1997, p 55.
6. Sims, D: Effects of positioning on ankle edema. J Orthop Sports Ther. 8:30–33, 1986.
7. Brennan, MJ, DePompolo, RW, and Garden, FH: Focused Review: Postmastectomy Lymphedema. Arch Phys Med Rehabil 77:S74–S80. 1996.
8. Segers, P, Belgrado, JP, LeDuc, A, LeDuc, O, and Verdonck, P: Excessive pressure in multichambered cuffs used for sequential compression therapy. Phys Ther 82:1000–1008, 2002.
9. Foldi, E: Editorial: Massage and damage to lymphatics. Lymphology 28:1–3, 1995.
10. Miller, GE, and Seale, J: Lymphatic clearance during compressive loading. Lymphology 14:161–166, 1981.
11. Pappas, CJ and O'Donnell TF: Long term results of compression treatment for lymphedema. J Vasc Surg 16:555–564, 1992.
12. Klein, MJ, Alexander, MA, Wright, JM, Ward, LC, and Jones, LC: Treatment of adult lower extremity lymphedema with the Wright Linear Pump: Statistical analysis of a clinical trial. Arch Phys Med Rehabil 69:202–206, 1988.
13. Zanolla, R, Monzeglio, C, Balzarini, A, and Martino, G. Evaluation of the results of three different methods of post mastectomy lymphedema treatment. J Surg Oncol 26:210–213, 1984.
14. Foldi M, and Foldi, E: Lymphoedema (translation from German: Das Lymphodem, ed 5.) Lymphoedema Association of Victoria Inc, Victoria, Australia, 1993, pp 48–49.
15. Kloth, LC, McCullouch, JM, and Feedar, JA: Wound Healing: Alternatives in Management. FA Davis, Philadelphia,1990, p 191.
16. Badger, CMA, Peacock, JL, and Mortimer, PS: A randomized, controlled, parallel-group clinical trial comparing multilayer bandaging followed by hosiery versus hosiery alone in the treatment of patients with lymphedema of the limb. Cancer 88:2832–2837, 2000.
17. Hohlbaum, GG: The Medical Compression Stocking. Schattauer, Stuttgart, 1989, p 34.
18. Cohn, JC, and Lowry, AL: It's all in the stocking. Rehab Management June/July:36–40, 2002.
19. Mortimer, PS. Managing lymphedema. Clin Exp Derm 20:98–106, 1995.
20. LeDuc, O, Peters, A, and Bourgeois, P: Bandages: Scintigraphic demonstration of its efficacy on colloidal protein resorption during muscle activity. Progr Lymphol XII:421–423, 1990.
21. Wittlinger, H, and Wittlinger, G: Textbook of Dr. Vodder's Manual Lymph Drainage, ed 6. Karl F. Haug Verlag, Heidelberg, Germany, 1998, p 53.
22. Villeco, J, Mackin, EJ, and Hunter, JM: Edema: Therapist's Management in Rehabilitation of the Hand and Upper Extremity, ed 5. Mosby, St Louis, 2002, p 192.
23. Guide to Physical Therapy Practice. Phys Ther 77:577–593, 1997.
24. Karges, JR, Mark, BE, Stikeleather, SJ, and Worrell, TW: Concurrent validity of upper extremity volume estimates: Comparison of calculated volume derived from girth measurements and water displacement volume. Phys Ther 83:134–145, 2003.
25. Megens, AM, Harris, SR, Kim-Sing, C, and McKenzie, DC:

Measurement of upper extremity volume in women after axillary dissection for breast cancer. Arch Phys Med Rehabil 82:1639–1644, 2001.

26. Guyton, AC: Textbook of Medical Physiology, ed 7. WB Saunders, Philadelphia, 1986, p 367.

27. Kelly, DG: A Primer on Lymphedema. Prentice Hall, Upper Saddle River, NJ, 2002, p 37.

28. Weissleder, H, and Schuchhardt, C: Lymphedema: Diagnosis and Therapy, ed 3. Viavital Verlag, Koln, Germany, 2002, p 34.

29. Rockson, SG: Precipitating factors in lymphedema: Myths and realities. Cancer 83:S2814-S2816, 1998.

30. Ridner, SH: Breast cancer lymphedema: Pathophysiology and risk reduction guidelines. Oncol Nursing Forum 29:1285–1293, 2002.

31. Cohn, JC: Lymphedema: Understanding and decreasing your risks. Living Beyond Breast Cancer Newsletter Fall 2000. Available at:www.lbbc.org/docs/nlfall00.pdf.

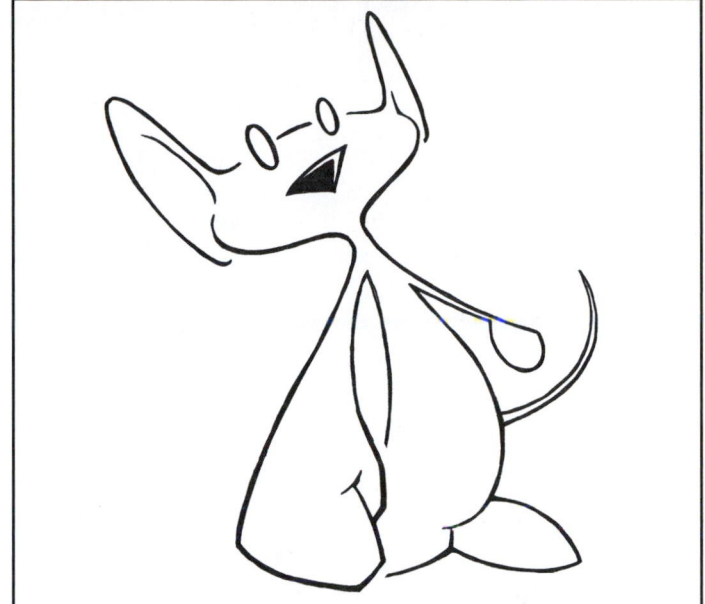

Electrical Stimulation

Objectives

- Introduce the basic concepts, terminology, and physiology of electrical stimulation.
- Guide selection of optimal current parameters for effective and safe delivery of electrical stimulation.
- Understand adjustment of treatment parameters to meet the needs and responses of individual patients.
- Present clinical decision-making considerations regarding application of electrical stimulation.

Key Terms

Accommodation	Current	Impedance	Resistance
Alternating current	Decay time	Ohm's law	Rise time
	Direct current	Pulse duration	Voltage
Amplitude	Duty cycle	Pulse trains	Waveform
Capacitance	Frequency	Pulsed current	Modulation

Cheryl A. Gillespie, PT, DPT, MA

Foundations of Electrical Stimulation

Outline

> *"Every beat of the heart, every twitch of a muscle, every stage of secretion of a gland is associated in some way with electrical changes."*[1]

This chapter will use the standardized electrotherapeutic terminology defined by the American Physical Therapy Association section on Clinical Electrophysiology.[2] Use of standardized terminology is essential for consistent communication of the parameters of treatment in research and practice.

Application of Electrical Stimulation

The history of electricity and electrotherapeutics is well documented by numerous authors.[3–7] Two fields have emerged from this early research and use of electricity. Electrotherapy applies electricity to treat disease and dysfunction. Electroneuromyography (ENMG) is used to diagnosis disease by interpreting the response of nerves and muscles to electrical stimulation. ENMG combines the diagnostic procedures of nerve conduction studies (NCV) and electromyography (EMG). A flourishing area of electrical stimulation is the field of biomedical technology. Manufacturers are developing more highly technical and versatile stimulator units. Small portable stimulators have augmented electrical stimulation for home use, initially for pain management and now for many conditions requiring neuromuscular stimulation. The development and improvement of neural prostheses for implantation are expanding to multiple patient populations.

Therapeutic Goals

The goals and applications of electrical stimulation, popularly communicated by acronyms, are identified in APTA's *Guide to Physical Therapist Practice*.[8] Electrical muscle stimulation (EMS) is stimulating denervated muscle to maintain muscle viability. Electrical stimulation for tissue repair (ESTR) uses electrical stimulation for edema reduction, enhancement of circulation, and wound management. Neuromuscular electrical stimulation (NMES) is stimulation of innervated muscle to restore muscle function and includes muscle strengthening, spasm and spasticity reduction, atrophy prevention, enhancement of range of motion, and muscle reeducation. Functional electrical stimulation (FES) activates muscles with electrical stimulation to perform functional activities. NMES and FES are often used interchangeably but really represent two different applications of electrical stimulation. NMES can be used to evaluate the patient for long-term management with electrical stimulation which usually incorporates the use of a neural implant.[9] FES uses neural implants to improve function and includes such devices as cardiac pacemakers,[10] electrophrenic respirators,[11]

dorsal column stimulators,[11–13] and visual and auditory implants.[11] Neural implants are also used to manage urinary and anal incontinence[11,14,15] and substitute for orthotics.[11] Trancutaneous electrical nerve stimulation (TENS) has become synonymous with stimulation for pain management. This application of electrical stimulation is usually associated with a group of small battery-powered electrical stimulators called TENS units that were developed specifically to achieve this goal. Because TENS is the application of electrical stimulation across the skin, all stimulators are really TENS units and can be used for pain management providing they have appropriate current parameters. The commercial TENS units have the advantage of portability.

Characteristics of Electricity

Electricity is most often described by its *strength* (charge), *rate of flow* (current), *driving force* (voltage), and *opposition* (resistance/impedance). Table 8-1 presents a review of these terms.

The relationship between current, voltage, and resistance is defined by Ohm's law and is illustrated in Figure 8-1. Current flow is directly proportional to voltage. An increase in voltage when resistance remains constant will increase current. Current flow is inversely proportional to resistance. An increase in resistance when voltage is constant will decrease current. The magnitude of current therefore increases when voltage increases or resistance decreases. High resistance requires high voltages to produce necessary current flow in the tissues below.[16]

Excitable tissues and nonexcitable biological tissues possess an inherent resistance. The opposition to current flow in the body is more accurately described by the term impedance rather than resistance. The body's opposition essentially results from the combination of resistive and capacitive reactance properties of tissue. *Capacitance* is the ability to store charge in an electric field and oppose change in current flow. Nerve and muscle membranes are examples of capacitors.

TABLE 8-1 Terminology of Electricity

ELECTRICITY	WATER
Electron	Water drop
Coulomb	Gallon of water
Current	Water flow
Voltage	Water pressure
	Low voltage: in old house
	High voltage: Water Pik
Resistance (impedance)	Water pipe: Narrow pipe
	Hair clog

$$Current = \frac{Voltage}{Resistance}$$

$$\frac{Voltage}{Resistance} = Current$$

$$\frac{Voltage}{Resistance} = Current$$

Figure 8-1 The relationships in Ohm's law.

The body tissues also function as resistors and model a parallel or series arrangement. When resistors are in series, there is only one pathway for electricity to flow and that is through each resistor in turn. When resistors are in parallel, the current has a choice of pathways and will always flow through the path of least resistance. Skin and adipose tissue function as resistors in series, whereas muscle, blood, tendon, and bone act like resistors in parallel.[17] Electric current therefore takes the path of least resistance once skin and subcutaneous tissues have been penetrated.

Tissue impedance varies throughout the body and conductivity depends on the water content of tissue. High water content decreases impedance and improves conductance. Healthy skin contains a thin layer of water containing salt, yet it offers one of the highest impedances (1000+ V)[18] to current flow because the outer layer of the epidermis contains little fluid. The amount of moisture in the deeper layers is determined by age and the number of sweat glands. Skin resistance is also inversely proportional to its temperature.[19] Heat increases moisture and surface salt content, which promotes conductivity. Bone, fat, tendons, and fascia are also poor conductors with low water contents of 20% to 30%.[20] The intracellular components of nerve and muscle have high water contents of 70% to 75%,[20] but their membranes have a high capacitive reactance that opposes charge movement.

Impedance can dramatically influence the ability to electrically generate an adequate response in underlying muscle. A greater intensity of current would be necessary to obtain a motor response in an area covered by adipose tissue (such as the gluteus maximus muscle) compared with an area with little fat (such as the anterior tibialis muscle). Increasing the current intensity to a level sufficient to drive current through the adipose to the nerve may make the sensation of the stimulation unbearable for the patient. This may rule out stimulation as a treatment option, or limit its effectiveness. Minimizing impedance is important for all applications of electrical stimulation because this allows current intensity to be reduced and increase patient comfort. Cleaning the skin surface with alcohol prior to electrode application will remove dirt and body oils and will decrease impedance; removing excess body hair beneath electrodes will also reduce

impedance, as will warming the region to be stimulated or warming the electrode gel.

Impedance changes in the presence of injury and disease. It increases with edema, ischemia, atherosclerosis, scarring, and denervation and decreases in open wounds and abrasions.[19]

Characteristics of Current Flow

Current will flow under two conditions: (1) there is a source of energy creating a difference in electrical potential and (2) there is a conducting pathway between the two potentials. In therapeutic electrical stimulation, a charge transfer occurs between the electrical generator and the biologic tissue at the electrode interface.[21] Electron flow converts to ionic flow in the body.[22] Sodium chloride (NaCl) ions are examples of charge carriers in the body.

Ionic flow occurs because of the elementary law underlying electrophysics. This law states *like charges repel, unlike charges attract*.[1] Positive ions (cations) are repelled from the positive electrode and migrate toward the negative electrode (cathode), whereas the negative ions (anions) migrate toward the positive electrode (anode). Because at rest the nerve is positively charged on the outside and negative on the inside, nerves will become hyperpolarized (less excitable) under the anode and more excitable under the cathode. This is demonstrated in Figure 8-2. Although both the anode and cathode are necessary to form a complete circuit, the cathode is often referred to as the active electrode because nerve activation (excitation) takes place more easily under this electrode.

Chemical reactions occur at the interface between the electrode and tissue during the transfer of charge.[23] The positive sodium ions (Na^+) migrate to the negative pole and combine with water, forming the base sodium hydroxide (NaOH). This chemical reaction increases the alkalinity of the area and promotes liquefaction of proteins and the softening of tissues.[17] The negative chloride ions (Cl^-) migrate to the positive pole and combine with water, forming hydrochloric acid (HCl). This chemical reaction increases the acidity of the area, thus promoting coagulation of proteins and the hardening of tissues.[17] Circulation is enhanced as the body attempts to neutralize the changes in the pH.[16] The magnitude of the chemical reaction depends on how long the current flows and how much current flows per square centimeter of surface area. Large charge accumulations occur when the current is too strong and can potentially cause tissue damage such as burns. Small charge accumulations are advantageous to certain electrical stimulation treatments such as wound and fracture healing. Figure 8-3 illustrates current flow and the chemical reactions occurring with electrical stimulation.

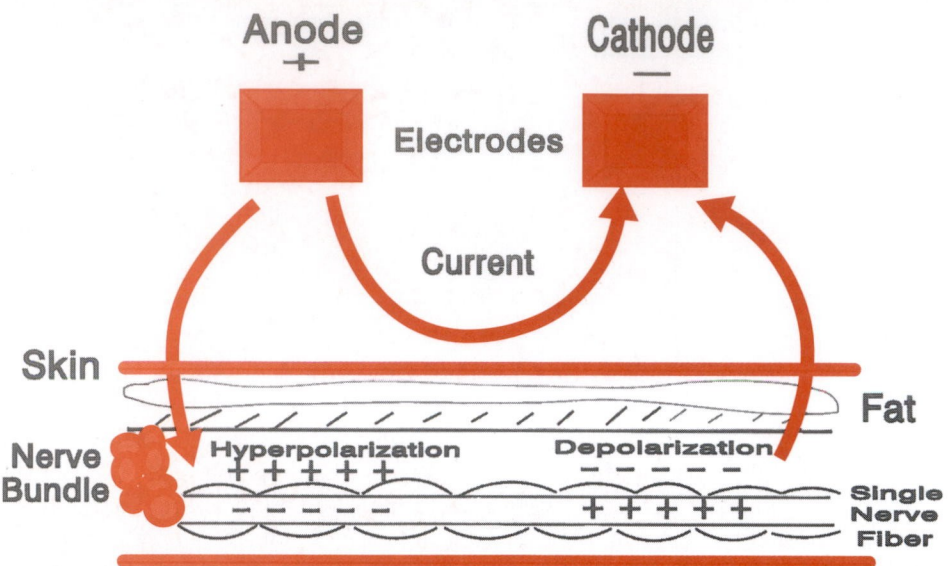

Figure 8-2 The flow of current from surface electrodes to an underlying motor nerve is shown. Hyperpolarization takes place under the anode because positive ions are driven away from this electrode into surrounding tissues. Depolarization, which can lead to an action potential, takes place under the cathode.

Stimulator Outputs

The output of any commercial electrical stimulation machine can be classified as constant-current or constant-voltage. Stimulation units have a safety feature that sets an upper and lower range limit to resistance. This prevents excessive current or voltage output increases when there are large changes in resistance (clinical manifestation of Ohm's law). The selection of a *constant-current* or a *constant-voltage* output for treatment depends on the type of commercial units available in the clinic, and sometimes this is not a choice. If both types of outputs are available, the choice then depends on clinician preference or the therapeutic goal.

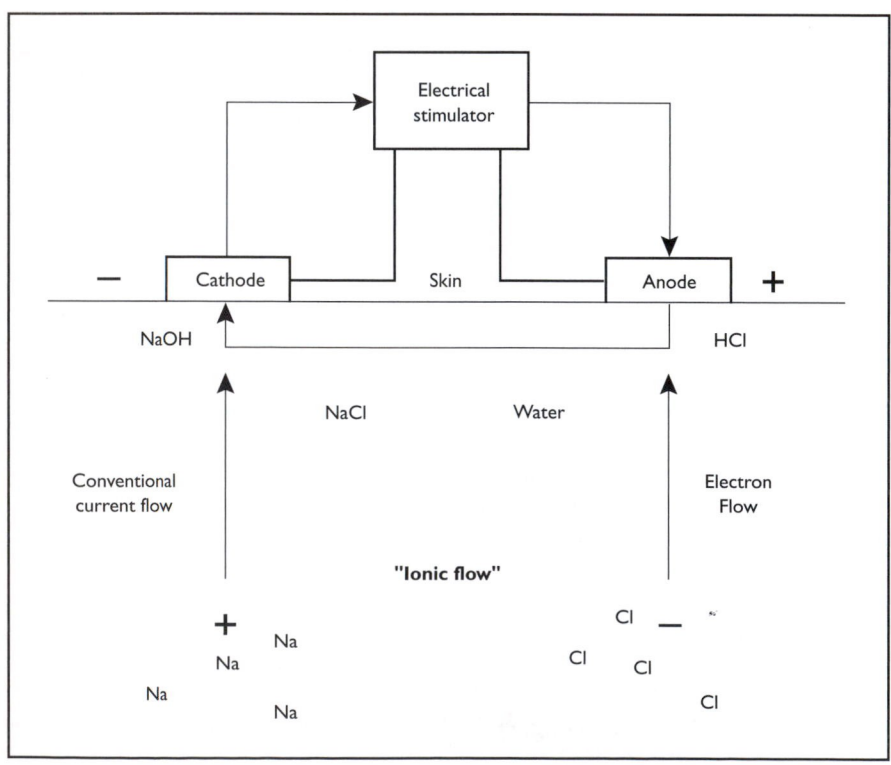

Figure 8-3 Concepts of current and ionic flow with application of electrical stimulation.

There are advantages and disadvantages to both types of output.

Constant-Current Stimulators

A *constant-current* stimulator produces a current that does not vary and is independent of resistance. This generator maintains the same current output regardless of changes in resistance. The voltage output increases or decreases to maintain a constant current flow. The mechanism is similar to cruise control in a car. The car speed (current) is preset and the accelerator (voltage) maintains this constant speed even when the car is going up and down hills (resistance).

The advantage of stimulation with constant current output is consistency of the physiologic response. The quality of the muscle contraction, for example, remains the same throughout the treatment when current level is constant as long as treatment parameters are such that muscle fatigue is avoided or at least minimized.

The disadvantage of this output is the effect on the tissue when resistance changes. Impedance increases as electrode size decreases. Electrode size is decreased with loss of electrode contact or electrode drying. This changes conductivity and increases impedance. The voltage increases to maintain the same level of current flow, which is now focused in a smaller area. The result can be pain with potential for tissue damage.

Clinicians can easily determine on themselves if a machine has a constant-current or constant-voltage output by slowly peeling the electrode away from the skin surface. The machine is a constant-current stimulator if the current sharpens and starts to bite. The machine's output is constant voltage if the current lessens when the electrode is peeled away from the skin.

Constant-Voltage Stimulators

A *constant-voltage* machine produces voltage that does not vary. The current output increases or decreases depending on changes in resistance. This mechanism is similar to conditions of normal driving. The car will decrease speed (current) as it negotiates a steep hill (resistance) or increase speed going down the hill if the same amount of pressure is maintained on the accelerator (voltage).

A constant-voltage stimulator has the advantage of decreased current levels with increased resistance preventing discomfort or damage.

The disadvantage of this output is that the quality of the response, such as muscle contraction, will change with resistance. Current will also increase when initial skin impedance is overcome and resistance decreases. Constant voltage can be a problem if there are large decreases in resistance. The current could increase to levels causing injury to tissue.

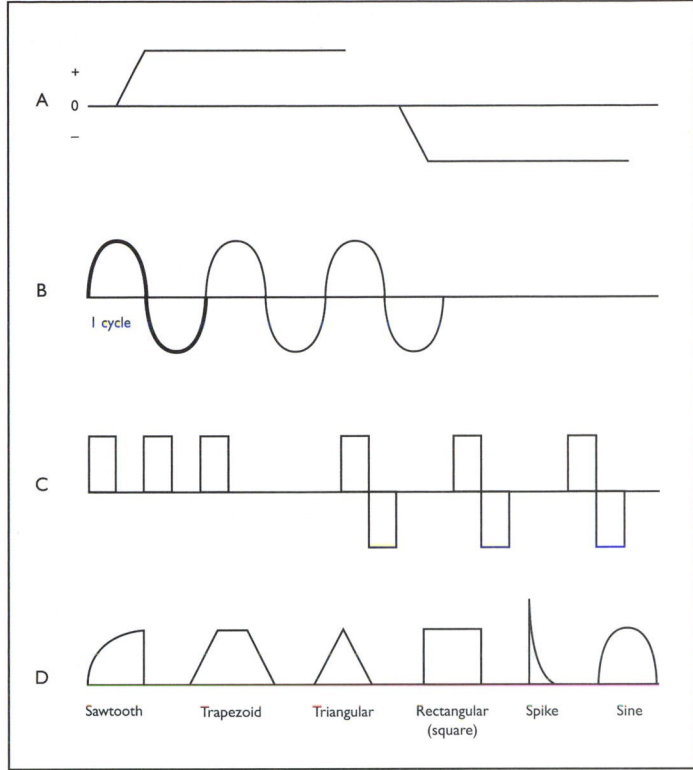

Figure 8-4   Types of current. (*A*) Direct current. (*B*) Alternating current. (*C*) Pulsatile current. (*D*) Common waveform shapes for pulsed current.

Current Classification

Although electrical stimulation treatments are often referred to and documented by the type of commercially named current used, the clinician must be aware of the actual classification of current being produced by the unit. This knowledge is much more important for determining the most appropriate current effective for intervention. All therapeutic electrical stimulation units use one of three generic forms of current: (1) direct current (DC), (2) alternating current (AC), or (3) pulsatile (pulsed) current (Fig. 8-4).

Commercial generators are often named by the manufacturer and include high-volt pulsed current (HVPC), interferential (IFC), Russian stimulator, variable muscle stimulator (VMS), transcutaneous electrical nerve stimulator (TENS), and microelectrical nerve stimulator (MENS) units.

Direct Current

DC (galvanic current) is a continuous unidirectional flow of charged particles with a duration of at least 1 second. One electrode is always the anode (positive) and one electrode is always the cathode (negative) for the period of stimulation. One electrode always receives current from the machine and current is returned to the machine by the other electrode. The polarity of a given electrode is determined by a polarity switch selection on the electrical stimulation unit. Because one electrode is always positive and one is always negative, there is an accumulation of charge, as previously discussed. This accumulation of charge is called a chemical or polarity effect. DC has a strong chemical effect on the tissues.

DC can be delivered continuously to promote absorption of medication through the skin (iontophoresis) or it can be interrupted to stimulate denervated muscle (EMS). DC is the only current form capable of these two treatment protocols.

Alternating Current

AC is an uninterrupted bidirectional flow of charged particles changing direction at least once a second. AC can also be delivered in an interrupted form, sometimes referred to as bursts. Each electrode becomes positive for one phase of the cycle and then negative as the current reverses. Since the electrodes are continuously changing their polarity, charges do not build up in the tissues.

AC is no longer directly used to stimulate tissue. Several commercial stimulators, including Interferential and Russian, use AC as their base or carrier current, which is then modified and delivered to the patient in the form of beats or bursts, respectively.

Pulsatile Current

Pulsed or pulsatile current can take on the directionality characteristics of AC or DC current. It is defined as the unidirectional (like DC) or bidirectional (like AC) flow of charged particles periodically ceasing for less than 1 second (milliseconds or microseconds) before the next electrical event. This small interruption in current, or charge movement, between successive pulses differentiates pulsatile current from AC and DC current forms. Pulsatile current is comprised of individual pulses of short duration delivered in a continuous series called a *pulse train*. This pulse train can be delivered continuously or interrupted as in the AC and DC current forms. Each individual pulse is comprised of one or more phases.

Pulsatile current has a negligible chemical effect in the tissues and the amount of effect depends on whether the pulse is unidirectional like DC or bidirectional like AC. A cathodal or anodal effect will occur under each electrode when the pulse is unidirectional. When the pulse is bidirectional, one phase of the pulse has anodal characteristics and one phase of the pulse has cathodal characteristics so the polarity effect is neutralized.

Current Characteristics

Pulsatile current is the most commonly generated and clinically used current form, and therefore will be the emphasis of discussion for the rest of this chapter.

TABLE 8-2	**Characteristics Describing Pulsatile Current**
SINGLE PULSE	**PULSE TRAIN**
Waveform	Interpulse interval
Amplitude	Frequency
Rise time/decay time	Duty cycle
Intrapulse interval	On-Off time
Duration	Ramp time
Charge	Total current

Manipulating the characteristics of both the single pulse and the pulse train are important for customizing treatment protocols. Table 8-2 lists the characteristics of the single pulse and the pulse train.

Describing a Single Pulse

The pulse is described by time-, amplitude-, and time/amplitude(dependent characteristics.[2]

Waveform

Waveform is a visual representation of the pulse. It is a spatial drawing depicting the shape of the pulse, reflecting amplitude and duration.

Pulses are classified by the number of phases they have: *monophasic*, *biphasic*, and *polyphasic*. Figure 8-5 summarizes the three waveforms.

An additional description is often added to the waveform (see Fig. 8-4), such as square wave or spiked pulse. The body does not distinguish between a square or trapezoid shape, but it does respond to the amplitude and time characteristics of the waveform shape.

Waveforms are diagrammatic only and rarely reflect what is actually going into the patient. Two factors influence the shape of the waveform and account for the difference between the illustrative waveform and the real. The first is the capacitive reactance property of tissue already discussed.[23] A load applied to a current, such as the resistance encountered in the body's tissues, will change the configuration of the waveform. The actual waveform that is delivered when a load (resistance) is applied can be visualized on an oscilloscope. The second factor that determines the actual shape of

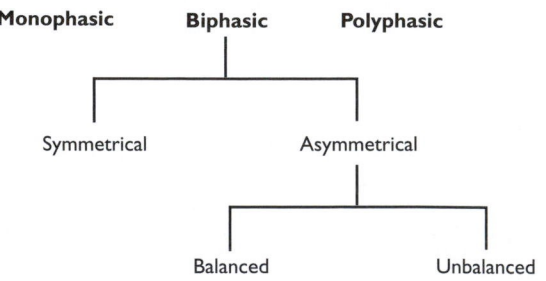

Figure 8-5   Classification of waveforms.

the waveform is whether the equipment has constant-current or constant-voltage output.

Monophasic Waveform A monophasic pulse has one phase. This pulse is unidirectional from the baseline carrying a positive or negative charge; therefore like DC, one electrode is always positive and one is always negative. The polarity or chemical effects are not of the same magnitude as DC because pulsatile current flows for a shorter time period. The tissues are able to neutralize slightly between each pulse. The monophasic pulse is depicted in Figure 8-6.

There is often confusion differentiating between interrupted DC and pulsed monophasic current. These are two different current forms and cannot be referred to interchangeably. Interrupted DC is used for treatment of denervated muscle (EMS). Pulsatile current is unable to do this protocol because of the small interruption in current between each pulse. It is not strong enough. The continuous train of pulses is also not comparable to continuous DC for the same reason and therefore incapable of performing iontophoresis.

The high-voltage commercial units deliver a monophasic pulse.

Biphasic Waveform A biphasic pulse is bidirectional with two phases. One phase deviates from the baseline in a positive direction and the other phase deviates in a negative direction; therefore like AC, the electrodes continuously change their polarity.

Biphasic pulses can be subdivided into two types: (1) symmetrical biphasic and (2) asymmetrical biphasic. The phases of the *symmetrical biphasic pulse* are identical (see Fig. 8-6). The chemicals formed in one phase are neutralized by the reversal of current in the second phase. The charges of the two phases cancel each other out and there is a zero net charge (ZNC) across the baseline. No accumulation of positive or negative charge occurs. The Variable Muscle Stimulator (VMS unit) and some battery-powered neuromuscular units produce this waveform.

A pulse is *asymmetrical biphasic* when the two phases are not identical. The asymmetrical biphasic pulse can be subdivided into (1) balanced and (2) unbalanced. When the charge of one phase is electrically equal to the charge of the other phase, the waveform is an asymmetrical *balanced* biphasic (see Fig. 8-6). The equal charges cancel each other out and a ZNC still exists across the baseline. A pulse is an asymmetrical *unbalanced* biphasic when the electrical charge of one phase is

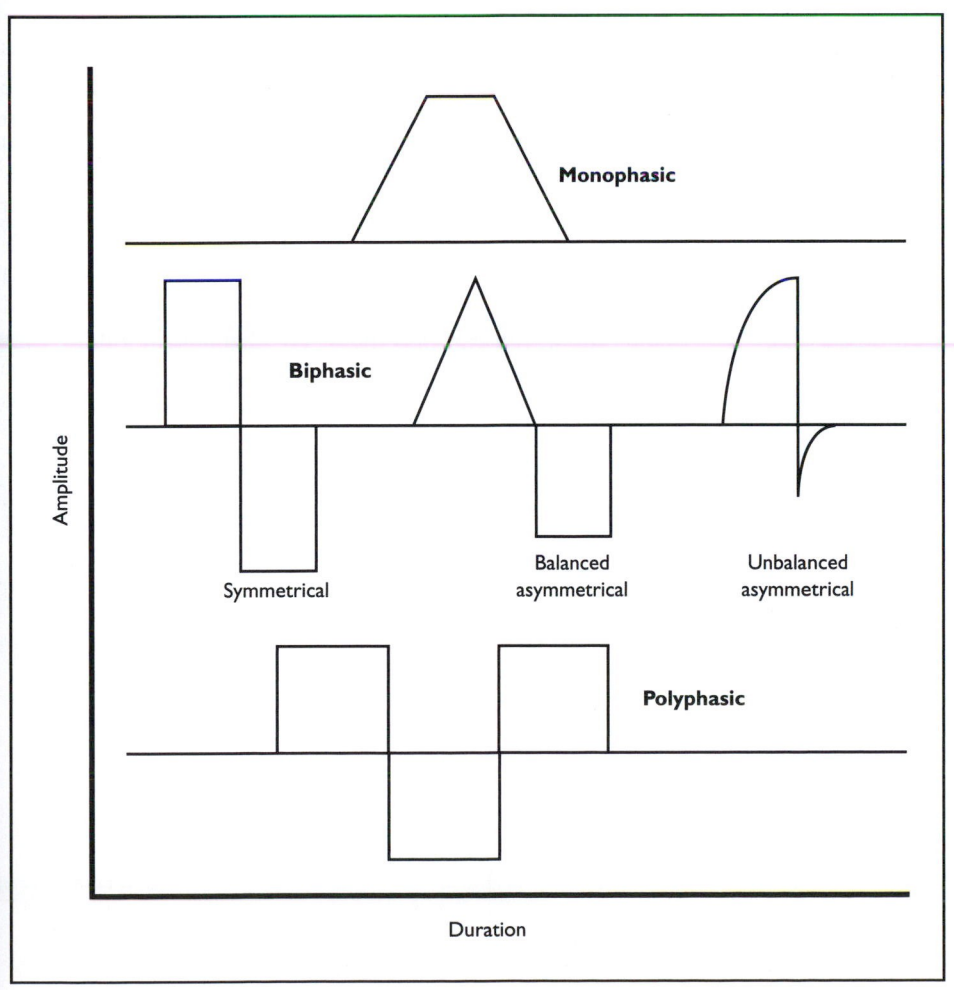

Figure 8-6 Visualization of the various pulsatile waveforms.

greater than the electrical charge of the other phase (see Fig. 8-6). The asymmetrical unbalanced biphasic pulse produces a net charge across the baseline with some residual charge in the tissues. This pulse is similar to the monophasic pulse in that there is accumulation of charge, but the electrochemical reactions are much less because the pulse is biphasic.

Most commercial TENS units and some battery-powered neuromuscular units produce asymmetrical biphasic waveforms.

Polyphasic Waveform   Polyphasic means the pulse is composed of three or more phases (see Fig. 8-6). All polyphasic pulses are bursts. A burst is a finite series of pulses grouped together and delivered to the body as a single charge. A single pulse can be compared with the pull of a trigger on a gun. A single bullet is released. A burst is like the pull of a trigger on a machine gun. Many bullets are released at once. This is illustrated in Figure 8-7. The burst is perceived by the body as a single pulse. It behaves physiologically as a single pulse and has no physiologic advantage over the single pulse.[16] The term burst is also synonymous with the terms packet, beat, and envelope. Although all polyphasic pulses are bursts, not all bursts are polyphasic. A burst can also be a group of monophasic or biphasic pulses delivered as a single charge.

The modified or burst AC produced by the commercial Interferential and Russian stimulators are examples of what may be referred to as a polyphasic pulse.

Phase Versus Pulse   The physiologic effect of current on tissue is determined by the phase not the pulse parameters. The monophasic pulse has only one phase. The phase characteristics therefore describe the whole pulse.

The biphasic pulse has two individual phases. The terms phase and pulse are not the same. The description of one phase is sufficient in the symmetrical biphasic pulse since the phases are equal. The characteristic of each phase needs

to be identified in the asymmetrical biphasic pulse, especially the unbalanced where the charges are not equal.

Waveform Comfort   Many studies have investigated the comfort levels of different waveforms during electrical stimulation.[9,24-28] The symmetrical biphasic waveform is cited as preferred more often. In a comparison between symmetrical biphasic, asymmetrical balanced biphasic, monophasic, and polyphasic waveforms, the biphasic waveforms were most preferred.[9] Between the two biphasics, symmetrical biphasic was preferred with stimulation of large muscles while there was no preference between the two in small muscle stimulation.[9] One conclusion drawn from many of the studies is that there is a variety in preference in a small subgroup of patients. Therefore if one waveform is not tolerated, another should be tried before abandoning electrical stimulation as an intervention. Preference also varies in different muscle groups within the same person.

Waveform Selection   All waveforms are basically effective for activating peripheral nerves, but one consideration on selection should be the waveforms' ability to activate nerves with minimum electrical charge. The symmetrical biphasic waveform meets that qualification and without the potential skin reactions that may occur with the monophasic waveform.[29] Some treatment protocols may dictate the waveform selection. The requirement of specific electrochemical effects in treatment, as in wound healing, precludes the use of the biphasic waveforms. Monophasic waveforms would be the appropriate choice. It was also found that while symmetrical biphasic is preferred on large and small muscles, when used with stimulation of small muscles, it is not discrete in its recruitment and there is overflow.[9] Therefore, asymmetrical balanced biphasic may be a better choice with small muscles. Monophasic and symmetrical biphasic waveforms were found to generate muscle contractions with greater torque than polyphasic waveforms and they were also less fatiguing.[30]

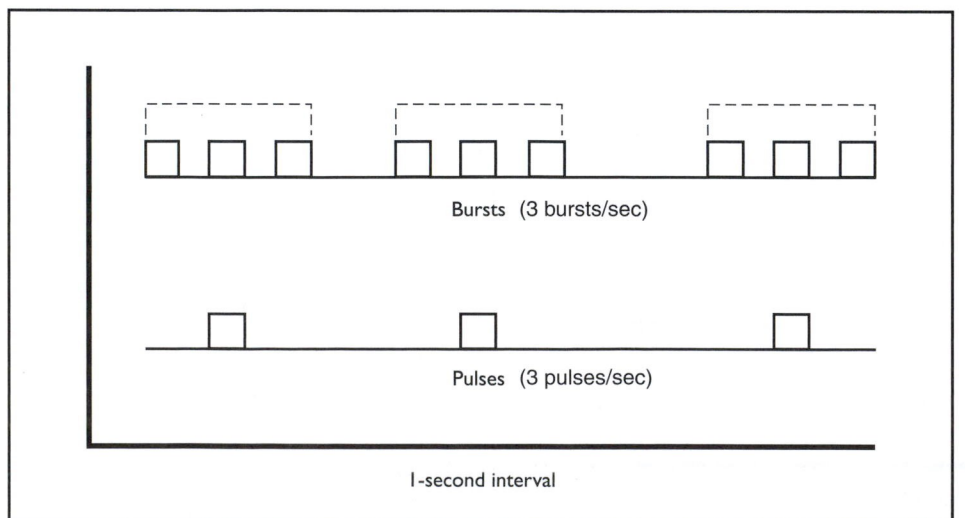

Bursts   (3 bursts/sec)

Pulses   (3 pulses/sec)

1-second interval

Figure 8-7   The burst and single pulse. Example of three bursts and three pulses delivered in a 1-second time interval. Each burst comprises three monophasic pulses in this illustration.

Before You Begin

Remember that the selected waveform of the stimulus will impact:

- Patient comfort
- Fatigue
- Chemical or polarity effects

Amplitude

Peak amplitude (*peak current, peak voltage*) is the maximum current or voltage delivered in one phase of a pulse. It is the magnitude or intensity of the stimulus and it is one factor determining strength of stimulation. It is also one of three criteria necessary for depolarization: *the stimulus must be strong enough.* Peak amplitude describes the maximum amplitude of the monophasic pulse but refers only to the maximum amplitude of one phase of the biphasic pulse.

Peak-to-peak amplitude denotes the maximum current or voltage amplitude over the two phases of biphasic pulses. Peak-to-peak amplitude does not indicate the strength of the pulse because it does not reflect the difference in electrical charge between the positive and negative phases. The peak amplitude of each phase must be compared to determine differences in electrical strength between phases. RMS (root-mean-square) voltage or current describes the average strength of the biphasic pulse. It takes into consideration the opposite charges of the phases. Peak amplitude and peak-to-peak amplitude are shown in Figure 8-8.

Peak amplitude is measured in current (milliamperes or microamperes) or voltage (volts) depending on the electrical stimulation unit. The amplitude is read on either a milliammeter or a voltmeter. The amplitude control on stimulator units is labeled intensity.

Current and voltage are directly related as defined by Ohm's law. A machine with a high-voltage output is capable of producing a high peak current.[16] Most commercial units are low-voltage (0 to 100 V), except for the high-voltage units, which have a maximum output of 500 V.

Peak amplitude is associated with depth of current penetration.[17] Higher peak amplitudes penetrate deeper into tissue. The electrical conductivity of the tissues under the electrode determine how deep this penetration will be. A high-voltage output generating a high peak amplitude will have no more penetration than a low-voltage output if the tissues as adipose and bone are not good electrical conductors.

Electrical stimulation produces three excitatory responses: sensory, motor, and pain.[31] Peak amplitude influences the response of tissue to electrical stimulation. Low peak amplitudes may fail to excite tissue, whereas high peak amplitudes may cause pain and not produce the intended response. The level of current necessary to excite a nerve fiber is inversely proportional to the fiber's diameter.[17] The larger-diameter nerve offers less resistance because of its greater cross-sectional area. The larger sensory fibers are recruited before small pain fibers in "ideal" conditions. The anatomic location of the nerve fiber to the electrode is a factor with electrical stimulation.[22] Sensory fibers will generally fire first with the sensation of tingling, prickling, or pins and needles. Sensory fibers are smaller and have a higher threshold than motor fibers but are usually more superficial and closer to the electrode. Selective discrimination of each excitatory response occurs as amplitude or intensity is increased slowly over time recruiting first sensory, then motor, and finally pain. When amplitude is increased rapidly, all nerve fibers meet threshold simultaneously and the immediate response is pain, usually described as a sharp burning.

Four clinical levels of stimulation are possible with electrical stimulation: subsensory, sensory, motor, and noxious (Table 8-3). The choice of stimulus level depends primarily on the protocol (e.g., ESTR versus NMES). A training period

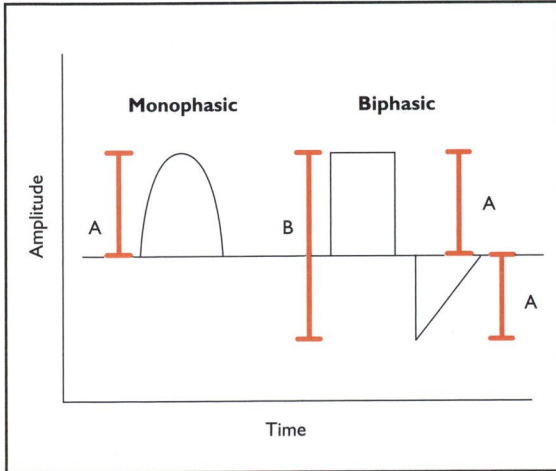

Figure 8-8 Characteristics describing the single pulse. (*A*) Peak amplitude. (*B*) Peak-to-peak amplitude.

TABLE 8-3	Clinical Levels of Stimulation
Subsensory:	No nerve fiber activation
	No sensory awareness
Sensory:	Nonnoxious paresthesias
	Tingling, prickling, or pins and needles
	Cutaneous *A-beta* nerve fiber activation
Motor:	Strong paresthesias
	Muscle contraction
	A-alpha nerve fiber activation
Noxious:	Strong, uncomfortable paresthesias
	Strong muscle contraction
	Sharp or burning pain sensation
	A-delta and *C-fiber* activation

may be necessary for the patient to achieve the target stimulus strength necessary for treatment.

Rise Time and Decay Time

Rise time is the time it takes for the amplitude of the pulse to increase from zero to peak amplitude. The rate of rise directly affects the ability to excite nervous tissue,[17] and it is the second criterion necessary for depolarization: *the stimulus must be fast enough*. Nerve membranes accommodate to slow introductions of current over time (slow rise time) with an automatic rise in threshold. The membrane has time to adjust to the voltage change, and a greater stimulus is then needed to cause depolarization. Increasing amplitude can compensate for waveforms with slow rates of rise. Denervated muscle does not exhibit accommodation and can be selectively excited by current forms with slow rates of rise.[17]

Decay time is the time it takes for the peak amplitude to decrease back down to zero and defines the terminal end of the phase. Rise and decay times are fixed by the pulse shape. Figure 8-9 depicts these parameters.

Intrapulse Interval

The intrapulse interval (*interphase interval*) defines the time period between the end of one phase and the beginning

of the second phase of one pulse when peak amplitude drops to the baseline (Fig. 8-10). It is measured in microseconds and usually fixed by the manufacturer. The monophasic pulse does not have an intrapulse interval.

It has been reported that when the anodal (positive) phase immediately follows the cathodal (negative) phase, the excitation caused by the stimulating cathode phase is depressed and may reverse.[32] Greater peak amplitude is then required for excitation. The introduction of an intrapulse interval abolishes this effect of the anodal phase and decreases the amount of amplitude needed to evoke excitation.[32] There is some discrepancy in the literature concerning the length of the intrapulse interval needed to abolish the anodal effect.[26,32]

Duration

Phase duration is the time period extending from the beginning to the end of one *phase* of a pulse. Pulse duration is the time interval between the beginning and end of all the phases of the *pulse*, including the intrapulse interval. Phase duration is the third criterion for depolarization: *the stimulus must be long enough*. The terms phase and pulse duration are synonymous in the monophasic pulse. The pulse duration of a biphasic pulse includes the *duration of phase 1 + intrapulse interval + duration of phase 2*. Phase and pulse durations are measured in microseconds and are illustrated in Figure 8-11.

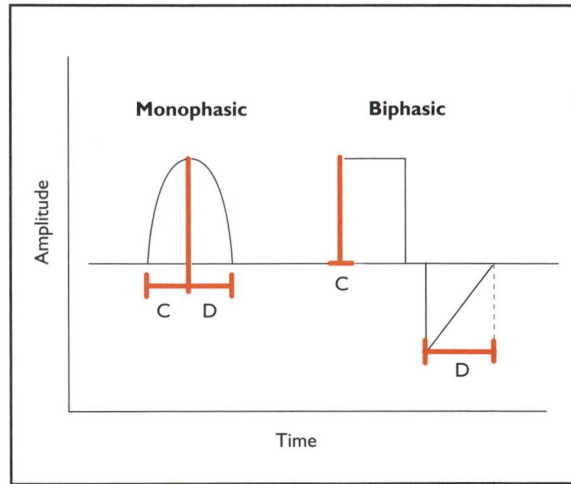

Figure 8-9 Characteristics describing the single pulse. (*C*) Rise time. (*D*) Decay time.

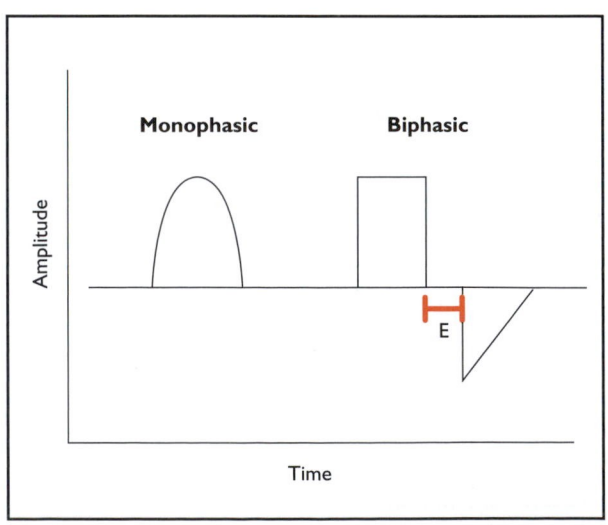

Figure 8-10 Characteristics describing the single pulse. (*E*) Intrapulse interval.

The strength (*amplitude*) and time (*duration*) of current determine tissue excitability. This is the law of excitation.[3] The strength-duration curve (SDC) demonstrates the inverse relationship between these two variables. As phase duration increases, less peak amplitude is required to achieve the desired physiologic response (Fig. 8-12). There is a minimum stimulus duration below which no amplitude of stimulus can cause excitation and a minimum amplitude below which no duration can cause excitation.[17] Nerve and muscle membranes function as capacitors. The membranes are capable of absorbing a certain amount of charge before reaching threshold. The minimum duration necessary to excite muscle is longer than that of a nerve because muscle membranes have greater capacitance than nerve membranes.[17]

Phase duration, like peak amplitude, is associated with discrimination between the excitatory responses. Each excitable tissue has its own SDC. Discrimination, therefore selectivity, is greatest between the different nerve fibers at the shortest durations. The ability to discriminate between the different fibers decreases as phase durations increase,[17] as shown in Figure 8-13. Shorter durations excite the large sensory afferents, whereas the longer durations are necessary to excite the

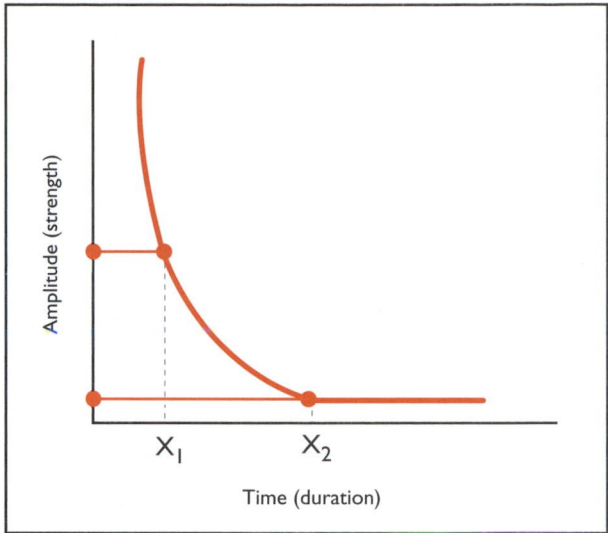

Figure 8-12 Relationship between peak amplitude and phase duration as defined by the strength-duration curve (SDC). Note the different amplitude requirements at durations (X_1) and (X_2). Less current amplitude is required to achieve threshold as phase duration increases.

smaller A delta and C fibers.[22,33,34] Stimulus durations between 20 and 200 microseconds are effective for discrimination.[16] Discrimination ability is lost at phase durations exceeding 1000 microseconds (1 millisecond).[35]

Phase duration affects comfort of stimulation. Comfort decreases as phase duration increases. No optimal phase duration has been defined for surface electrodes. Several studies have indicated that 50 to 1000 microseconds may be within an optimal range with 300 microseconds being the most comfortable duration compared 50- and 1000-microsecond durations.[9,24,26]

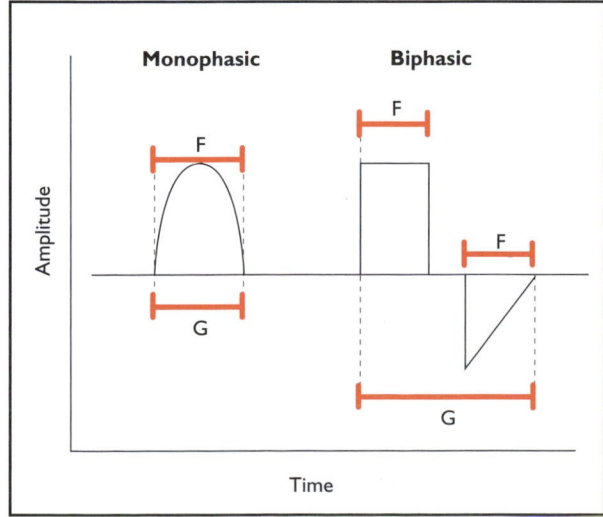

Figure 8-11 Characteristics describing the single pulse. (*F*) Phase duration. (*G*) Pulse duration.

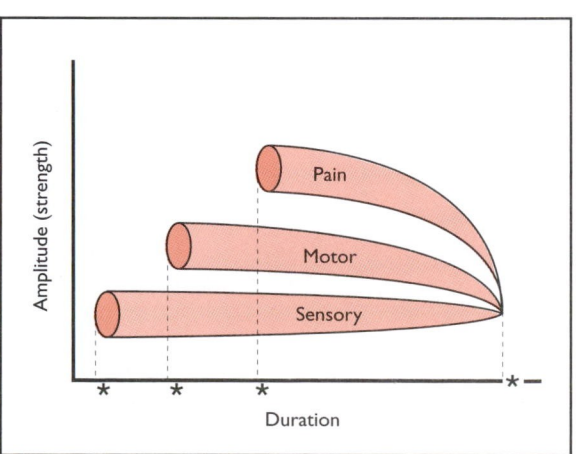

Figure 8-13 Discrimination of the excitatory responses in electrical stimulation. As the phase duration increases, the ability to selectively discriminate between the activation of sensory, motor, and pain nerve fibers decreases, and a point is reached where all the excitatory responses are evoked at the same time.

The magnitude of chemical changes in the tissue is directly proportional to the phase duration. Increased chemical effects occur as phase duration increases.

Short pulse and phase durations are associated with decreased impedance and better conductivity of current into the tissue.[16]

Phase duration can be fixed by the manufacturer or a variable control on the stimulation device. A variable phase duration permits custom fitting of the strength and duration of the current to the patient.

Charge

Phase charge is the amount of electrical energy delivered to the tissue with each phase of each pulse (microcoulombs per second). It is quantity of charge defined by amplitude and duration. Charge is represented by the area of the phase. Pulse charge is the sum of all the phase charges in the pulse. The phase charge equals the pulse charge in a monophasic pulse. Phase charge is illustrated in Figure 8-14.

Phase charge reflects the capable strength of the electrical stimulation unit. Machines are classified as weak, moderate, or powerful depending on the maximum phase charge that

the unit is capable of producing. The phase charge of the unit may be as weak as 12 μC or as powerful as 40 μC. Adequate phase charge determines tissue excitability. Excessive phase charge results in tissue damage.

The amount of charge necessary to evoke the three excitatory responses decreases as pulse and phase durations decrease.[36] This may be the result of reduced impedance at shorter pulse or phase durations lowering the charge needed for excitation.[16]

Describing the Pulse Train

All of the parameters related to the single pulse have been discussed. These characteristics are summarized in Figure 8-15. This section will detail the characteristics describing a series of pulses or the *pulse train*.

Interpulse and Interburst Intervals

The interpulse interval is the time period extending from the end of one pulse to the beginning of the next pulse and is measured in milliseconds. Bursts are separated by an interburst interval. The interburst interval is shorter than the interpulse interval because each burst contains more phases (Fig. 8-16). The interpulse interval decreases as phase or

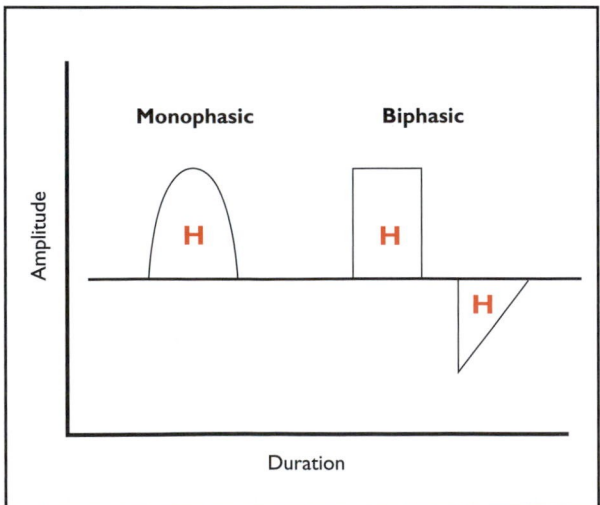

Figure 8–14 Characteristic describing the single pulse. *(H)* Phase charge.

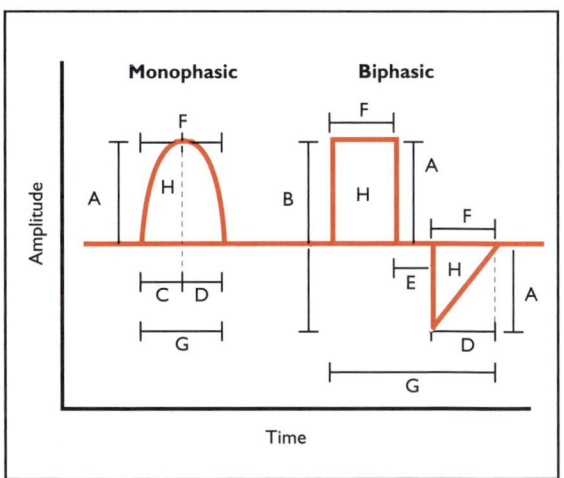

Figure 8–15 Summary of the characteristics describing the single pulse. *(A)* Peak amplitude. *(B)* Peak-to-peak amplitude. *(C)* Rise time. *(D)* Decay time. *(E)* Intrapulse interval. *(F)* Phase duration. *(G)* Pulse duration. *(H)* Phase charge.

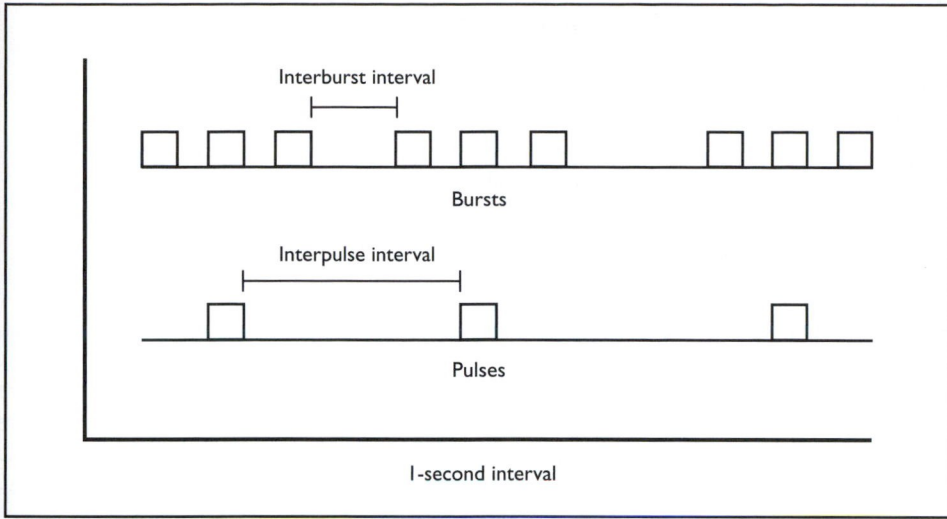

Figure 8-16   Characteristics describing the pulse train. The interburst and interpulse intervals. The interburst interval is shorter because the duration of the burst is longer than that of the pulse.

pulse durations increase (Fig. 8-17). Most stimulators produce relatively short pulse durations with long interpulse intervals. The interpulse interval, like the intrapulse interval, represents an interruption of current and results in less electrical stimulation fatigue. However, again like the intrapulse interval, there is no relaxation because the absence of current is too brief.[35] Any parameter decreasing the interpulse interval will increase the time of current flow and increase fatigue to electrical stimulation.

One reason polarity effects are less with pulsatile current than with DC is because of the intrapulse and interpulse intervals. Even though they are of extremely brief microseconds and milliseconds, respectively, they both shorten the period of time during which the current is on. The tissues have time to neutralize the chemical effects between phases

 Before You Begin

Remember that...
Interpulse interval relates to:

- Fatigue
- Chemical or polarity effect dependent on values of other parameters

or pulses and there is less residual electrical charge buildup in the tissues.

Frequency

Pulse frequency, which often is referred to as pulses per second (pps) or pulse rate, is the number of pulses delivered to the body in one second. The body responds to the number of pulses not the number of phases. A single monophasic, biphasic, or polyphasic pulse is "counted" as one pulse by the body. Carrier frequency is the base frequency of the AC sine wave produced before it is modified and delivered to the patient at a different frequency. The frequency of AC is expressed in hertz (Hz) or cycles per second (cps). Burst frequency is the number of *bursts per second*. Fatigue is greater at higher frequencies because the interpulse interval shortens (Fig. 8-18).

Whereas peak amplitude defines the intensity of the muscle response, frequency defines the quality of the muscle response dictating a twitch or tetanic contraction. Muscle response changes from twitch to tetany as frequency increases. The critical fusion frequency represents the point where the muscle twitch converts to a tetanic contraction.

Impedance is influenced by frequency. The capacitive reactance characteristic of tissue is inversely proportional to frequency.[37] Impedance will decrease as frequency increases.

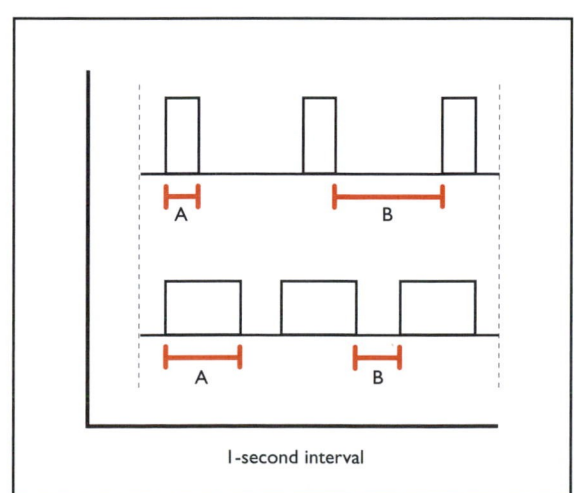

Figure 8-17   Relationship between (*A*) phase duration and (*B*) the interpulse interval. The interpulse interval shortens as phase duration increases.

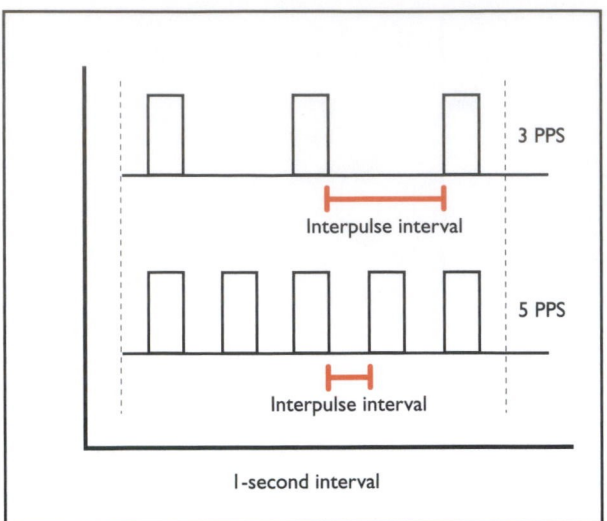

Figure 8-18   Characteristics describing the pulse train. Pulse frequency. The length of the interpulse interval decreases as frequency increases.

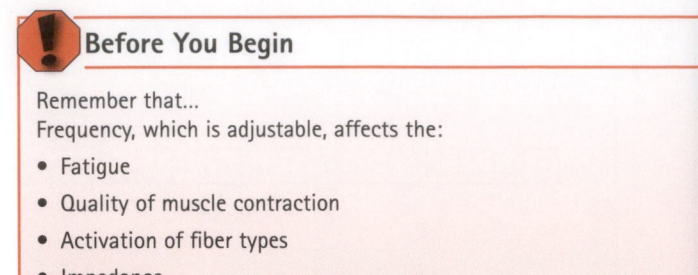

Before You Begin

Remember that...
Frequency, which is adjustable, affects the:

- Fatigue
- Quality of muscle contraction
- Activation of fiber types
- Impedance

Electrical stimulators are often referred to as low-, medium-, or high-frequency units, the low and medium frequencies having the ability to stimulate excitable tissue. Unfortunately, the classification of electrical stimulators into low and medium frequency has just resulted in confusion. Essentially all therapeutic electrical stimulation machines are low frequency. The "medium" frequency machines utilize a medium carrier frequency of AC that is delivered to the patient as a low-frequency current in the form of bursts. A carrier frequency of 2500 Hz has been found to be more comfortable than stimulation with 1000 or 5000 Hz.[25]

Frequency is a variable control on electrical stimulators and is usually labeled pulse rate. A frequency range of 1 to 120 pps is sufficient for most therapeutic goals.[35] Smooth muscle contractions occur at frequencies from 15 to 50 pps.[38] It has been found that stimulation at 50 pps is more comfortable than 35 pps.[9] Large-diameter nerves have higher firing rates than small-diameter nerves. Bioelectric investigations are providing some insight into the most appropriate frequency ranges for affecting both excitable and nonexcitable tissues. A frequency window has been postulated suggesting that cells may be receptive to certain frequencies and unresponsive to others,[39] an important concept for tissue and bone healing.

Duty Cycle

On time is the period of time the current is delivered to the patient. Off time is the period of time current flow stops. Both times are measured in seconds and are shown in Figure 8-19. The current must be on for at least one second and off for at least one second to be a true interruption of current with relaxation. Intrapulse, interpulse, and interburst intervals are much shorter than one second and therefore do not result in a true relaxation.

On time versus *off time* can be expressed as a ratio. If the current is on for 5 seconds and off for 20 seconds, the ratio is 1:4. Duty cycle is the percentage of time that the current is actually on. It represents the *on time* divided *by the sum of on and off time* expressed as a percentage. In the example above, the duty cycle would be 20%. The duty cycle must be known to calculate total stimulation time. Using the same example, if 5 minutes of contracting time was necessary, the total treatment time would have to be 25 minutes.

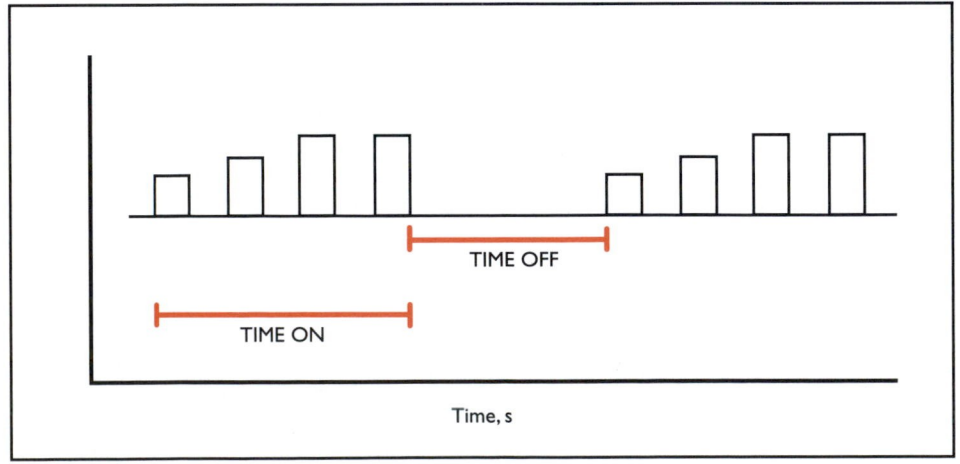

Figure 8-19   Characteristics describing the pulse train. On time/off time (duty cycle).

Muscle contractions generated by electrical stimulation are more fatiguing than those generated by the nervous system. The on-off time ratio plays an important role in circumventing muscle fatigue during stimulation. The longer the off time relative to the on time, the less the fatigue.

Ramp Time

Ramp time is the increase in amplitude to peak of the *pulse train*. It is how long it takes for the current to go from zero to peak amplitude and how long it takes for the current to go from peak amplitude back down to zero (Fig. 8-20). Ramp time is not synonymous with rise time. Rise time describes the change in amplitude in a single pulse. Ramp time describes the change in amplitude of the pulse train over a specific time period of current flow. *Ramp up* is an increase in amplitude over time. *Ramp down* is a decrease in amplitude over time. Both ramp times are measured in seconds.

Ramp time may be fixed or variable, depending on the stimulator. There may be one ramp feature, usually ramp up, or none at all. When variable, the adjustable range is generally 1 to 8 seconds.

Ramp time is associated with the comfort of stimulation, and a 2-second ramp is often adequate.[38] The ramp-up feature allows for more normal motor recruitment and smoother muscle contraction with slow buildup of current to peak amplitude. The ramp-down feature can increase patient comfort. An 8- to 10-second ramp-up is recommended when applying electrical stimulation to the antagonist of a spastic muscle.[38] Quick stretch and activation of the 1A afferents in the spastic muscle is then avoided.

The ramp time is added to the on time to ensure that peak contraction time is long enough. If a 10-second peak muscle contraction is desired with a 2-second ramp-up, the total on time is 12 seconds.

Total Current

Total current (average current) is the amount of current delivered to the tissue per second and is measured in milliamperes. Total current is very closely related to phase charge. Total current *equals* phase charge *times* number of phases *times* pulses per second.[16]

Total current determines safety of treatment and magnitude of the physiologic effect. Tissue damage is the result of thermal and electrochemical effects in the tissue and both are a function of total current.[40] Heat dissipation is generally not a problem with surface stimulation.[40] The tissues can be harmed if the total current is excessive and there will be no physiologic response if total current is too low. Most machines function within safe limits, but there are several commercial units with high total current outputs, such as Interferential and Russian stimulation.

Any parameter increasing the strength of the current stimulus or decreasing the length of the interpulse interval will increase the total amount of current to the patient. *Peak amplitude*, *pulse frequency*, and *phase duration* are all directly proportional to total current, as shown in Figure 8-21. Changes in peak amplitude and phase duration affect the strength of the pulse charge. Changes in phase duration and pulse frequency affect the length of the interpulse interval.

Total current is related to electrode size. A safe range of total current to the patient is considered to be 1 to 4 mA/cm² electrode area.[41] The lowest level of stimulation producing the desired response is the current level best used. Small electrodes should not be used with machines capable of delivering high total current. The strength of current is too concentrated and could cause tissue damage.

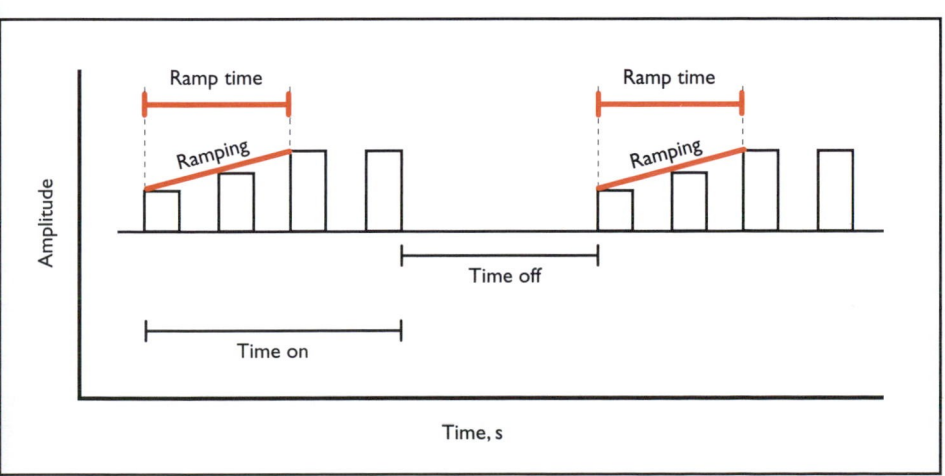

Figure 8-20 Characteristics describing the pulse train. Ramp time.

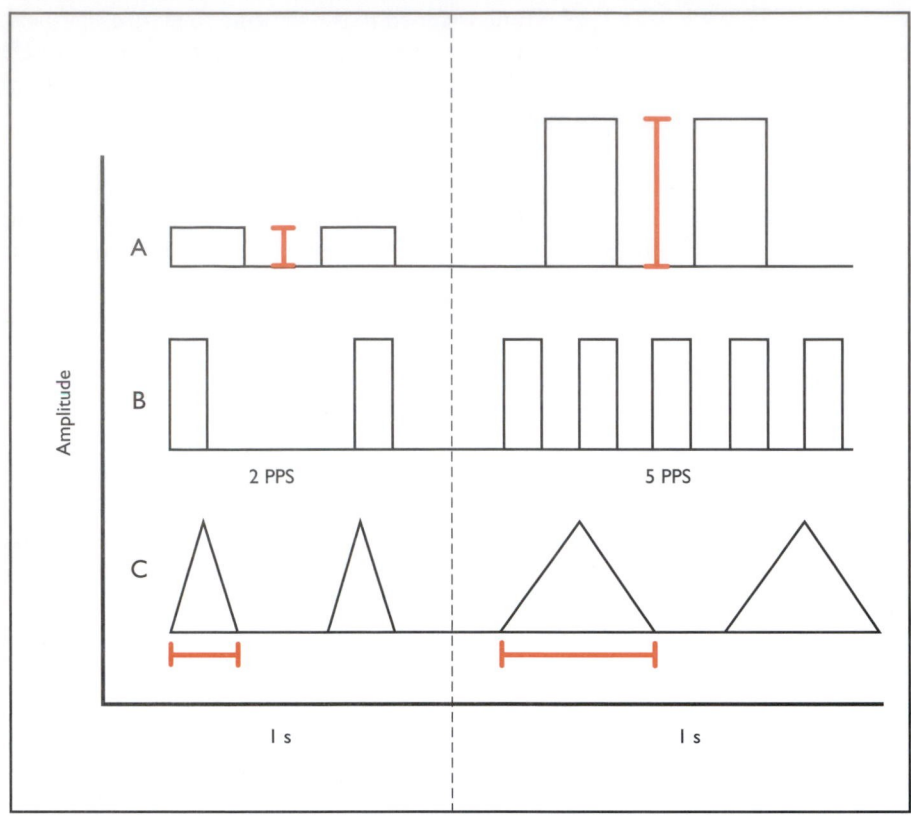

Figure 8–21   Total current can be increased by increasing (*A*) peak amplitude, (*B*) pulse frequency, and/or (*C*) phase duration.

Modulation

Modulation is varying one or more of the electrical parameters over time while delivering the stimulus. This prevents adaptation to the current. The single pulse or pulse train can be modulated. Amplitude and duration can be modulated in the pulse. Examples of modulation in the pulse train include frequency modulation, ramp time, on-off time, and bursting.

Amplitude, phase or pulse duration, and frequency can be modulated individually or in combination. Figure 8-22 illustrates the intermittent modulations of these parameters.

Sweep is a term used by manufacturers to denote sequential modulation of pulse frequency. This feature gives the option of a constant sequential modulation (sweep) of the entire available frequency range or portions of it.

Ramping is the sequential modulation of phase charge by changing the phase duration or amplitude. Ramp time has been discussed and it is an example of amplitude modulation.

Current can be delivered continuously or interrupted. The ability of the machine to do both is an important feature for versatility of treatment. On continuous mode, the current is delivered without interruption for the length of the treatment. On interrupted mode, the current ceases for specific periods of time of at least 1 second. The on-off time controls are used to set the periods of time. The interrupted mode can be set to activate all channels of the unit at the same time (simultaneous) or alternate between two channels (reciprocate).

"The Big Picture"

Each electrical parameter dictates a specific response in the body and intimately relates to many other parameters. The pulse and current variables form a delicate web of cause and effect, and it is important to choose the optimal parameters for treatment. The clinician who understands the basic concepts of electricity, terminology, relationships between electrical parameters, and effect on body tissue will be able to execute treatment confidently, safely, and effectively.

● **Why Do I Need to Know About...**

TOTAL CURRENT

Total current will affect:

- Patient comfort
- Magnitude of physiologic effect
- Tissue damage dependent on the values of other parameters and
- Modulation, which can be adjusted, will help decrease adaptation to the sensation

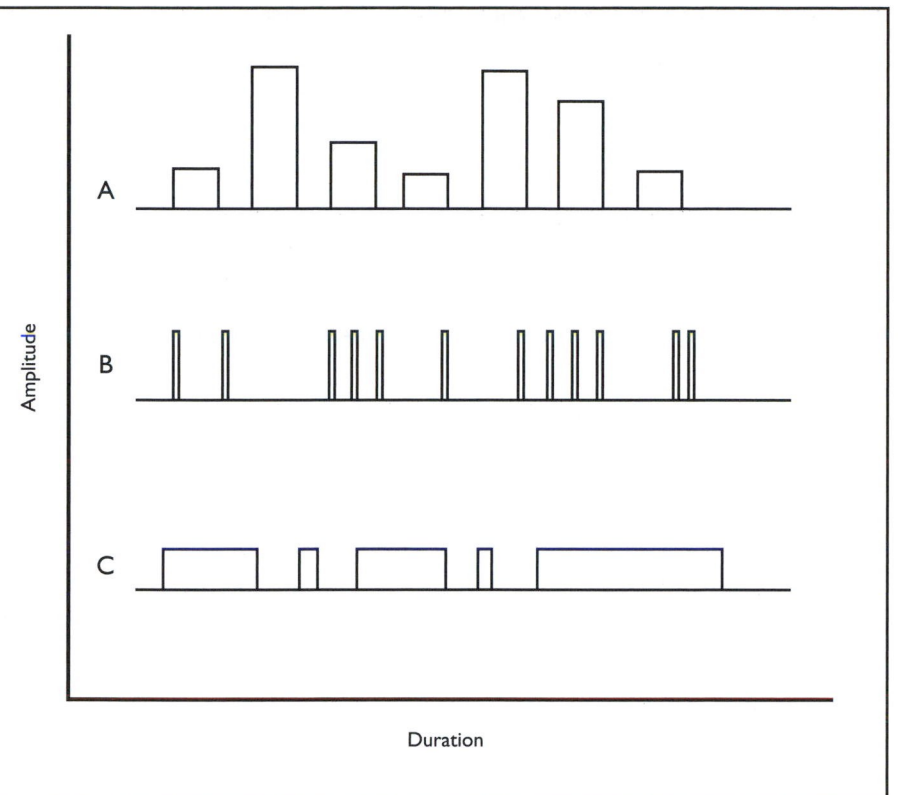

Duration

Amplitude

A

B

C

Figure 8-22   Modulation of current: (*A*) peak amplitude, (*B*) pulse frequency, and (*C*) phase duration.

Delivery of Electrical Stimulation

An electrical stimulation unit must be assessed in terms of its electrical features as "yes, effective to accomplish the goal" or "no, lacking the necessary features for this protocol."

Delivery of electrical stimulation can be either from a household-powered source (wall plug) clinical stimulator or a portable battery-operated stimulator. The battery-operated unit was found to be as effective as the wall-plug powered stimulator for generating contractions providing the parameters of intensity were available.[30] The current or voltage, depending on stimulator output, is converted from the power source current into the appropriate therapeutic current waveforms. Oscillator circuits within the machine allow independent control of the different treatment variables such as frequency, phase duration, and duty cycle.

Electrical stimulation is delivered to the body through electrodes. A lead wire connects the generator to the electrode. Electrodes have two functions. They can apply a stimulating current to the body tissue to excite, or they can record and detect the presence of an electrical signal in the body. The principles of electrode use and placement are discussed in detail in Chapter 9.

The electrical current can be introduced through transcutaneous electrodes in contact with the skin or through subcu-

taneous electrodes. The subcutaneous electrode is invasive and can be inserted through the skin via a wire or needle electrode percutaneously or surgically implanted on excitable tissue.[42] The percutaneous method is often used to assess the patient's response and reactions to the electrical stimulation prior to implantation.

Muscle and Nerve Physiology

An understanding of the physiological basis of nerve and muscle stimulation is essential for safe and effective delivery of electrical stimulation. The reader may find it helpful to review these concepts in more detail. Table 8-4 outlines the major concepts and important key terms.

Motor Unit Recruitment

There are several differences between a central nervous system generated muscle contraction (active) and one generated by an electrical stimulation unit (passive). The torque output or strength of a muscle contraction is determined by the number of motor units recruited. When a muscle is contracted by the central nervous system, small motor units are recruited first assuring development of smooth and gradual tension. Small motor units are usually made up of type I muscle fibers and tend to be fatigue resistant. The first motor units to be recruited can then sustain the longest contraction.

TABLE 8-4 Muscle and Nerve Excitation: Concepts to Review

- Resting membrane potential
- Action potential generation and propagation
- Nerve and muscle structure
- Synaptic structure and function
- Classification of peripheral nerves
- Muscle fiber type and recruitment pattern
- Muscle excitation and contraction
- Structure of the motor unit
- Motor unit recruitment

Key Terms: absolute and relative refractory periods, all or none phenomenon, accommodation, adaptation, saltatory conduction, nodes of Ranvier, orthodromic and antidromic conduction, sliding filament theory, size principle of recruitment

Large motor units are recruited as contraction strength increases. The order of motor unit recruitment is reversed with electrical stimulation. Large, superficial motor units are recruited first and these are usually made up of fatigable type II muscle fibers.

Another difference between the central nervous system and electrical stimulation (generated muscle contraction is the firing pattern of the motor units. During a voluntary contraction, motor units are activated asynchronously, constantly turning on and off in an alternate fashion. Asynchronous firing is highly energy efficient, delaying the onset of fatigue, and helps maintain smooth steady muscle tension. There is no asynchronous firing in electrical stimulation. The motor units that meet stimulus threshold fire and continue to fire until the electrical stimulus stops. This is called synchronous recruitment and, unlike asynchronous muscle contractions, is very fatiguing to the muscle.

A third difference between central nervous system and electrical stimulation generated action potentials is the direction of propagation. In the central nervous system, the action potential moves away from the nerve cell body in an orthodromic direction. Electrical stimulation results in the generation of an action potential in two directions, orthodromic and antidromic (back toward the cell body), from the stimulus site.

The combination of reversed recruitment order, synchronous recruitment, and bidirectional propagation of the action potential makes electrical stimulation very inefficient. Therefore, to avoid unnecessary fatigue, careful choice of stimulus parameters, such as frequency and on/off time, is important when designing neuromuscular stimulation programs.

Membrane Excitability

As previously discussed, there are three criteria for depolarization: the stimulus must be *strong enough* (amplitude), *long enough* (duration), and *fast enough* (rise time).

The resistive and capacitive reactance properties of nerve and muscle membranes allow these tissues to oppose current flow and store an electrical charge. If the membrane resistance is multiplied by its capacitance, it yields a value known as the time constant. The time constant sets the rate at which a charge across the membrane is altered by an electrical stimulus. The time constant of a membrane represents the minimum time that a stimulus must be applied before depolarization will occur.

If an infinitely long stimulus duration is applied, which is defined as 300 milliseconds, the minimum current amplitude that will produce excitation is called rheobase. If the rheobase intensity is doubled, the amount of time (pulse duration) that current must flow to achieve excitation is called chronaxie. If one gradually decreases the stimulus duration below 300 milliseconds and records the minimum intensity of stimulation required to generate a threshold response, a curve can be plotted representing the tissue's excitability, which is the SDC curve discussed earlier in this chapter.

Accommodation

There are conditions under which a nerve cell will not generate an action potential even in the presence of what would normally be considered a threshold stimulus. These conditions include subthreshold depolarization of the nerve prior to delivery of a threshold stimulus or presenting the nerve with a stimulus that has a slowly rising intensity (slow rise time). These situations raise the threshold of the nerve cell so that it now takes a suprathreshold stimulus to elicit an action potential. This property is called accommodation, and it is unique to nerve cells. The ability of muscle cells to accommodate is minimal. In addition to meeting certain minimal excitation requirements of the nerve, the current must reach its maximum intensity rapidly in order to avoid the effects of accommodation; otherwise, the stimulus will be ineffective in generating an action potential.

Use of Electrical Stimulation

APTA's *Guide to Physical Therapist Practice*[8] categorizes electrical stimulation under the procedural intervention *Electrotherapeutic Modalities*. This intervention has application across multiple practice patterns and is a valuable adjunct therapy in the treatment of musculoskeletal, neuromuscular, and integumentary system problems. The general indications, contraindications, and precautions will be discussed in this section.

Indications

Electricity can be applied to the body to treat (clinical stimulation) or to diagnose (nerve conduction velocity studies). Electricity from the body can be recorded to treat (biofeedback) or to diagnose (electromyography). Many indications have already been addressed in the section on therapeutic goals.

Electrotherapy has been long associated with pain management, muscle strengthening, and stimulation of denervated muscle. It also has a place in wound care, fracture healing, promotion of circulation, and edema management. It has been used to increase joint range of motion, deliver medications through the skin (iontophoresis), replace orthotics, reduce spasm and spasticity, and reduce scoliosis.

Contraindications

The contraindications of electrical stimulation are relatively few. Pregnancy should be considered a contraindication even when applied to an area distant from the abdomen. Pain management with electrical current during labor is occasionally used.

Electrical current can interfere with the functioning of a pacemaker. A demand pacemaker senses the heart activity and responds accordingly. A pulse from an external stimulator could deceive a demand pacemaker into suppressing needed rhythms or creating abnormal rhythms.[38] Fixed pacemakers could be affected by signals through the leads.

Electrical stimulation should not be used in the presence of other electrical implanted stimulators, in patients with cardiac arrhythmic instability, or in cases with cardiac conduction disturbances. A stable cardiac patient with a history of angina or myocardial infarction may receive electrical stimulation, but electrodes must be placed cautiously avoiding current flow across midline in the chest area. The patient should be monitored with an ECG initially and then closely monitored during treatment. Some therapists do not apply electrical stimulation to a patient with cardiac disease, whether stable or not.

Cancer is treated as a contraindication because of the risk of metastasis. This contraindication is sometimes waived in favor of the pain relief when patients are in advanced stages.

Stimulation should not be performed adjacent to or distal to an area of thrombophlebitis or phlebothrombosis because of risk of emboli. Many therapists treat these conditions as totally contraindicated for an electrical stimulation treatment.

Electrical stimulation should not be used in the presence of active tuberculosis. It should not be done over the carotid sinus or in areas of active hemorrhage.

Precautions

Electrical stimulation should be used cautiously in the presence of obesity. Fat is an electrical insulator and stimulation is generally not well tolerated. Greater-than-normal current levels are often required to achieve the desired physiologic effect.[38]

Caution should be exercised in areas of absent or diminished sensation. Areas of abnormal impedance should be avoided. Electrical currents can exacerbate eczema, psoriasis, acne, and dermatitis and can spread infections.[19] Patients including those with diabetes with thin fragile skin could be at risk for breakdown.

Peripheral neuropathies may prevent generation of muscle contractions at stimulation levels that are comfortable and safe.[38] Areas of denervation will not respond to any form of current other than DC.

In the presence of metal, either internal or external fixation devices, electrodes should be positioned with the metal well outside the pathway of current.

The patient should be cleared for active exercise in protocols requiring motor levels of stimulation. Care should be taken that the force of contraction is within a tolerated and permitted range of motion.[38]

Judgment is necessary to determine if electrical stimulation should be applied to any patient who is unable to follow instructions or provide feedback to the therapist. The treatment must be closely supervised if the decision is made to deliver the electrical stimulation.

Stimulation to patients with spinal cord injury may enhance an episode of dysreflexia.[38]

Electrical Safety

Equipment and User

Electrical shock is the response of the body to any electrical exposure that places the person within the circuit. This statement has just described treatment with electrical stimulation. The clinician must be aware of the potential dangers of applying electrical current and the measures ensuring safe treatment.

The magnitude of electrical shock depends on the amount of current (amperes) forced into the body. Currents between 100 and 200 mA are lethal.[43] Physiologic reactions to current intensities follow a progression of sensation, muscle contraction, fibrillation, defibrillation, and burns.[44] Electrical shock is first perceived as a faint tingling by sensory nerves around 1 mA, but current levels as low as several microamperes have been perceived by the finger tips.[45] Let-go current is the maximum current level allowing the voluntary release of the current source and emphasizes the danger of AC over DC. The motor response to DC is a twitch, whereas AC causes a holding or tetanizing contraction. The ability to *let go* may be lost at current levels of AC around 20 mA.[45] This value increases with pulsatile currents. The intrapulse and interpulse intervals provide current interruptions. Breathing can become labored at 20 mA of AC and cease before 75 mA.[43] Uncoordinated twitching of the heart's ventricles (ventricular fibrillation) occurs at levels greater than 80 mA.[42] The heart will maintain a sustained contraction (ventricular defibrillation) at 6 Å (6000 mA) and return to normal rhythm if exposure to current at that level is of short duration.[46] Burns occur at current levels above 12 Å.

Electrical shock is either *macroshock* or *microshock*. Macroshock is a perceptible current at levels of greater than or equal to 1 mA.[42] It occurs when current is introduced to the body through the skin and enters the body cavity. Microshock is below perceptible range and results from exposure to currents below 1 mA applied directly to the myocardium.[42] The current bypasses skin and enters the heart directly through cardiac catheter tips or myocardial electrodes. Pacemakers can be very susceptible to microshock through the pacemaker wires. The upper safety limit margin of current passing directly to the heart is 10 mA.[45]

As discussed earlier in the chapter, body tissues offer resistance to the passage of current. Skin resistance protects internal organs from shock and determines how much current enters. This resistance varies between people and varies within the individual depending on point of contact and skin hydration. Dry skin offers around 500,000 V of resistance, whereas moist skin offers approximately 1000 V.[43] This protective resistance is bypassed when an invasive electrode is used, but the use of this type of electrode is not common practice clinically.

Electric power is delivered to the machine through the ends of two wires having an electrical potential of 115 V between them. The *live* (hot) wire has the high electrical potential. The *neutral* wire has 0 potential and connects to the ground. The term ground refers to anything with an electrical connection to the earth. Earth is an inexhaustible source of electrons and is capable of accepting or donating large quantities of charge.[47] Generally, current flows from the live wire through the electrical unit back to the neutral wire and then to earth.[18] An exchange occurs between charged bodies and earth. A positively charged body will take electrons and a negatively charged body will give electrons to earth. Current flows. Grounded means there is no difference in potential between the conductor and earth, so current will not flow.

One potential clinical hazard is direct contact with the live wire circuit through a frayed power cord or an outlet problem.[45] Another possible hazard, earth shock, results from an indirect connection made between the live wire and the ground.[18] The live wire, possibly because of faulty or old insulation, makes contact inside of the machine with its casing. A person touching the casing and standing on the ground draws this current and completes a circuit between the live wire and the ground. Newer machines are now usually cased in plastic or other insulating material. Earth shock can also result from a phenomenon called leakage or *stray* current. It is an inherent flow of a small amount of current from the live circuit along an insulating surface such as the casing or accessories. Electric shocks can also result from contact with grounded objects such as water pipes, damp floor, and radiators during electrical treatments.

Earth shock can be avoided by a grounding wire that provides the path of least resistance from the machine casing to earth. The grounding wire, normally not conducting current,

triggers a fuse on the live wire when electrical problems cause current to flow through it. This stops current flow and alerts the operator to a problem. A polarized outlet and three-pronged plug provide this grounding circuit. The outlet receptacle has three slots, a small rectangular one for the live wire connection, a larger rectangular one for the neutral wire connection, and a round opening for the ground wire connection. This protective round pin is longer than the rectangular prongs, assuring that the ground wire is the first wire connected to the circuit and the last unplugged.[19]

Failure of the grounding wire to be connected in the building to a ground source or breaking of the ground wire in the receptacle can go undetected, creating a potential hazard. The electrical system is believed to be safe when in actuality the grounding circuit is nonfunctional. A ground fault interrupter (GFI) is a sensor shutting down the electrical circuit when it senses changes in electrical potentials, impedance, or an increase in normal leakage current levels.

Preventive maintenance is necessary to assure electrical safety in the treatment area. New equipment purchased should have the Underwriters' Laboratory (UL) approval seal, assuring the maximum degree of safety.[47] Table 8-5 outlines other safety guidelines that should be observed in the clinic. Electrical safety comes with awareness and knowledge. The clinician should always read the manufacturer's manual and be sure that he or she understands the limitations of the unit as well as its safety features.

Patient Factors

Patient Education   The public is familiar with electricity and the potential for shock and electrocution. Many patients

---

TABLE 8-5 Electrical Safety in the Clinic

Replacement of standard outlets with ground fault interrupters (GFI).
Replacement of plugs with hospital-grade UL (Underwriters' Laboratory) plugs with green dot.
Yearly maintenance checks of all electrical equipment by biomedical engineer.
Dated inspection sticker affixed to all electrical units.
Unplug equipment not in use.
Disconnect machines from outlet receptacles by plug not cord.
Frequently check the integrity of plugs, cords, and electrical stimulation leads for fraying or disruptions.
Report loose-gripping connections between plug and outlet receptacles.
Never use extension cords.
Never use cheater adapters allowing three-pronged plugs to be used in two-pronged receptacles.
Do not use electrical equipment near objects or environments that draw current.
Post sign notifying usage of equipment that may interfere with pacemakers.

may be initially fearful of treatment. A patient may be anxious or reluctant to place his or her foot in a tub of water containing two electrodes.

The key to successful treatment is patient education and cooperation. The questions concerning patient education that must be posed are *what* and *how much*. It has been shown that information can sometimes increase and develop stressful feelings that might not have been present ordinarily.[48] Two types of coping styles are identified. There are those people who seek information to get through an aversive event and there are those people who would rather not know anything. Patients treated according to their coping style exhibited increased tolerance levels to electrical stimulation.[48]

Certain safety instructions are necessary. Information that must be given includes the sensation of treatment and instructions concerning touching of controls, changing body position, and calling the therapist when there is a problem or change in sensation. Informational material includes the goal and expected outcome of treatment, number of expected treatment sessions, and the treatment time. Patients using the unit at home require more detailed instructions on how the unit works, application of electrodes, purpose and consequence of dial adjustments, how to protect the skin and inspect area before and after treatment, and under what circumstances to discontinue treatment. Written instructions should be given, especially diagrams of electrode placement.[49]

Equipment Positioning Electrical stimulation delivered by a line-powered unit (versus battery unit) should be administered in a predetermined area within the clinical setting where appropriate outlets (GFIs) have been installed. Electrical equipment generates heat and should be well ventilated. Equipment should not be placed next to water pipes, radiators, or other sources that may draw current, creating a shock hazard. The machine should be situated close to the wall outlet to avoid tension on the cord and possible tripping over cords. Positioning of the electrical stimulation unit must allow easy access to the therapist for adjustment of controls as well as avoiding excessive tension on lead wires or a situation where the patient is able to adjust parameters without supervision. The patient should be informed as to which dial controls the amplitude and how to turn it down. The current interruption switch should be easily accessed.

Skin Inspection The intensity of stimulation is guided by the patient's response and tolerance level. A sensory assessment of the treatment area is essential to establish patient reliability. The skin must be carefully inspected before electrodes are applied. Skin tone and color should be assessed for indications of circulatory impairment and fragility that could result in breakdown or tissue damage. The skin should be examined for conditions affecting skin impedance such as edema, ischemia, scars, skin lesions, and abrasions. Areas of abnormally high impedance require increased current levels for penetration. Areas of abnormally low impedance draw current and increase total current in a small area. Tissue damage could result from either situation. Abrasions and open areas that cannot be insulated with petroleum jelly should not be treated unless the treatment objective is wound healing.

Patient Positioning The basic tenets of positioning are patient comfort and accessibility to the treatment area. There are several considerations specific to electrical stimulation. Positioning should permit enough slack in lead wires from machine to electrodes so that connections will not disengage during treatment. Firm contact and securing of electrodes will influence choice of position. Some placement sites may require the patient's body weight on the electrodes. The patient must be in a position to use a call button or disengage the machine if a problem arises.

Patient Perspective

Remember that patients have had virtually no experience with electrical stimulation and there will be questions. Patients will need to know that it is safe, that you have felt it and what to expect when they feel it. The patient may not let you adjust the intensity to a high enough level to produce a motor response during the first visit. You will need to establish a level of trust with the patient before he or she will let you accomplish this. It is also important to remember that positive reinforcement is very helpful to the patient who is not quite sure what to expect when they feel a muscle contract with electrical stimulation.

PATIENTS' FREQUENTLY ASKED QUESTIONS

- Is it safe to use electrical stimulation during an electrical storm?
- Will I be "electrocuted" by the stimulator?
- What is the difference between the stimulators that are used in the clinic and a defibrillator?
- How long will the sensation of the stimulator continue after treatment?

The Treatment

A training period may be necessary with electrical stimulation, and required stimulation levels may not be achieved during the first session. Patient anxiety can sometimes be relieved by allowing the patient control of increasing the amplitude dial.

Muscle contraction time can be limited to 5- to 7-second peaks with low-level repetitions of 10 to 15 contractions the first treatment to prevent initial soreness.[35] On and off times have a high ratio initially (1:4; 1:5) but are reduced in subsequent treatments with conditioning.

The patient should be asked if he or she feels tingling in all areas of the electrode. The electrode could be secured improperly or losing its conductivity if the answer is no. If the patient is not feeling any sensation at all as amplitude is increased past a point where sensory fibers should fire, stop immediately and drop the amplitude control back down to zero before making any adjustments. Most contemporary machines have reset controls to protect against high levels of current surging into the patient when machines are energized with current levels up. These types of controls require that amplitude dials be clicked off prior to increasing the amplitude. Never increase amplitude during the off phase of the current cycle.

Clinical judgment must be exercised as to when a treatment should be discontinued because of physical or mental intolerance, preventing the safe achievement of intended goals.

The electrical stimulation treatment can be divided into *pretreatment*, *delivery*, *post-treatment*, and *documentation*. Patient comfort, tolerance, and safety are priorities. The manufacturer's instruction manual must be carefully read, understood, and followed. The following general guidelines will only assist with sequencing the treatment.

Pretreatment

- Machine wires and electrode check (inspection dates should be periodically checked) is performed.
- Patient education is given.
- Machine is plugged into the wall.
- Turn the machine power switch on.
- Patient is positioned.
- Skin in treatment area is inspected; gross assessment of sensation is made.
- Electrical stimulation machine is positioned.
- Electrode placement sites are determined.
- Treatment area is washed; electrodes are prepared and secured.
- Preset parameters on machine area adjusted such as frequency, phase duration, delivery mode (interrupted or continuous), on-off time, ramp, and choice of polarity, treatment timer.
- Make sure amplitude dials are on zero.

Delivery

- Increase amplitude to stimulation level but always within patient's tolerance.
- Ask patient *what do they feel* and *where do they feel it*.
- Adjust any parameters requiring modification.
- Stay with patient for several minutes to monitor reaction, tolerance, and appropriate amplitude level.
- Continue to monitor patient reaction and tolerance periodically through treatment.

Post-Treatment

- Turn amplitude to zero.
- Remove electrodes.
- Turn machine power off.
- Inspect treatment area.
- Note all variables set for treatment and document.
- Unplug unit from wall receptacle.

Documentation Documentation must be thorough and inclusive. Notes must stand up under close scrutiny in this age of liability and reimbursement. The written note ensures consistent replication of treatment; is a written record describing the patient's physical state, reactions, and progress; validates treatment success or failure to determine effectiveness; and justifies treatment for appropriate reimbursement.

The general elements of the electrotherapy note include the problem, therapeutic goal, type of application (e.g., ESTR), skin status, electrode technique, electrode size, number and placement of electrodes, commercial stimulation unit used, electrical parameters of treatment, treatment time, and response to treatment.

An electrical parameter that can be set on the machine or determined from a readout must be documented. Give specific settings for all parameters adjusted. Documented parameters may include, but are not limited to the following:

- Delivery mode (continuous, interrupted)
- Therapeutic stimulation level (subsensory, sensory, motor, noxious)
- Current type (AC, DC, pulsed)
- Waveform (monophasic, biphasic, polyphasic)
- Polarity of active electrode (monophasic waveforms)
- Peak amplitude (amperes or volts, phase charge is the readout)
- Frequency (pps, burst frequency, carrier frequency)
- Phase duration
- On-off/ramp times

A thorough note, reflecting all of the parameters, is essential for the first treatment. Changes in parameters and patient response will suffice for subsequent notes.

Clinical Decision Making

Clinical decision making is an ongoing process during patient/client management. In electrical stimulation, decisions may range from "*the choice to utilize electrical stimulation*" to "*the determination of the current parameters.*" Figure 8-23 outlines the components of the clinical decision-making process with electrical stimulation.

Electrical Stimulation Clinical Decision Making Tree

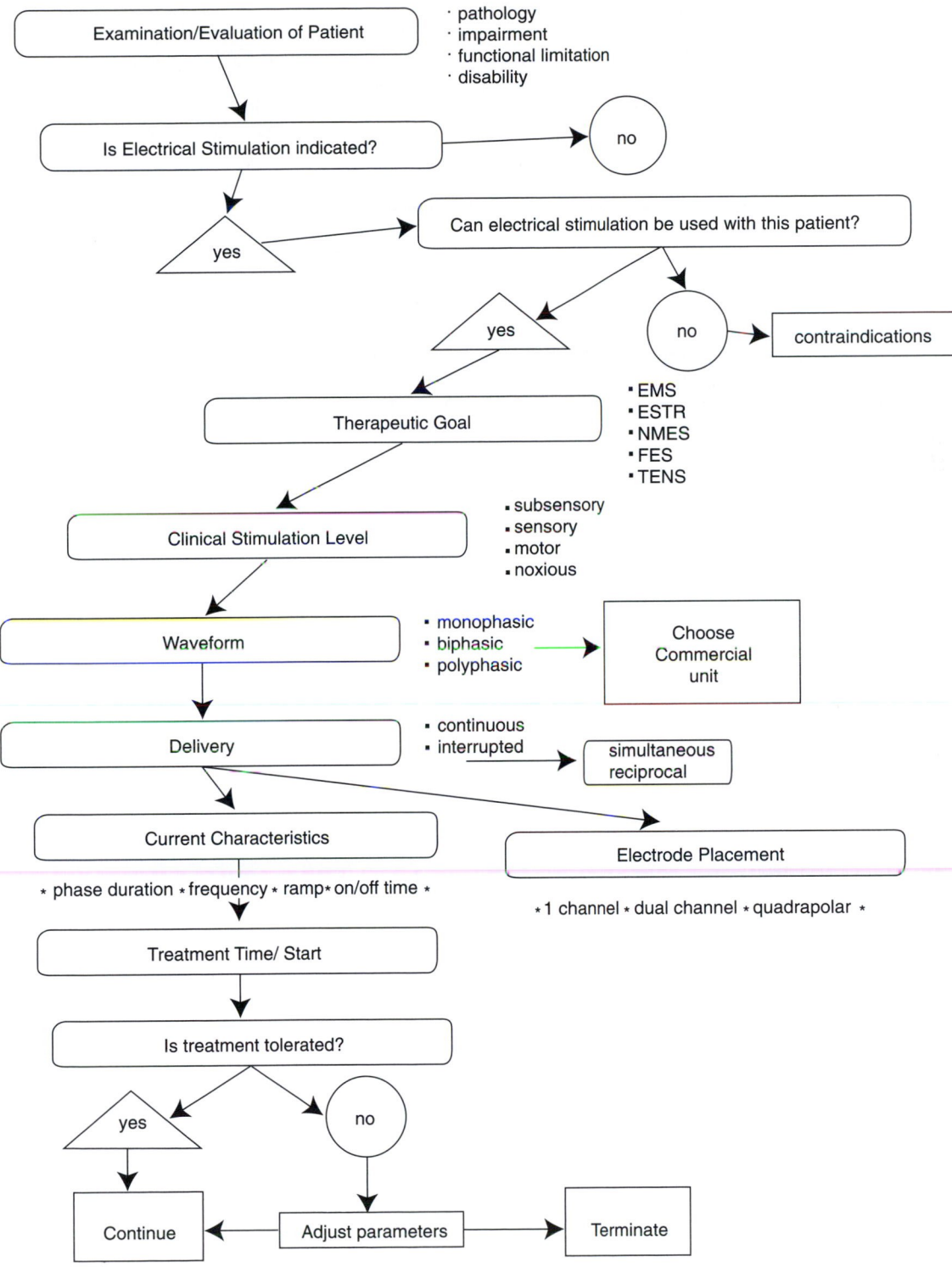

Figure 8-23 Clinical Decision Making Tree

Discussion Questions

1. How does Ohm's law relate to constant current and constant voltage outputs? And why would it potentially be important to know about the equipment that is being used?
2. Identify the three types of current and describe how they differ in structure and usage?
3. What are the differences between the different waveforms in terms of structure, chemical effects and usage?
4. What are the differences between a) ramp and rise time, b) intrapulse, interpulse, and off time, c) pulse and burst, d) phase charge and total current?
5. What are the indications, contraindications and precautions for the use of electrical stimulation and why are they so listed?
6. What are the differences between sensory, motor and pain fiber activation in terms of sensation, recruitment order and relationship of their strength duration curves?.
7. How does a central nervous system generated contraction differ from one generated by electrical stimulation?
8. What can be done to reduce fatigue when utilizing electrical stimulation to elicit a muscle contraction?

References

1. Watkins, A: A Manual of Electrotherapy. Lea & Febiger, Philadelphia, 1962.
2. American Physical Therapy Association: Electrotherapeutic Terminology in Physical Therapy. Section on Clinical Electrophysiology, 2001, Alexandria, VA.
3. Geddes, L: A short history of the electrical stimulation of excitable tissue. Physiologist (suppl) 27:S-1, 1984.
4. Licht, S: History of electrodiagnosis. In Licht, S (ed): Electrodiagnosis and Electromyography, ed 3. Elizabeth Licht, New Haven, CT, 1971.
5. Licht, S: History of electrotherapy. In Stillwell, G (ed): Therapeutic Electricity and Ultraviolet Radiation, ed 3. William and Wilkins, Baltimore/London, 1983.
6. Marcello, P: The Ambiguous Frog: The Galvani-Volta Controversy on Animal Electricity, translated by Mandelbaum. Princeton University Press, Princeton, NJ, 1992.
7. McNeal, D: 2000 Years of electrical stimulation. In Hambrect, T, and Reswick, J (eds): Functional Electrical Stimulation: Application in Neural Prosthesis, vol 3. Marcel Dekker, New York, 1977.
8. American Physical Therapy Association: Guide to Physical Therapist Practice. 2001: American Physical Therapy Association, Alexandria, VA.
9. Baker, L, et al: Effects of waveform on comfort during neuromuscular electrical stimulation. Clin Orthop Rel Res (233):75, 1988.
10. Bleese, P, et al: Implanted cardiac pacemakers: Clinical experience and evaluation. Med Progr Technol 1:69, 1972.
11. Ko, W: Instrumentation for neuromuscular stimulation. In Hambrect, T (ed): Functional Electrical Stimulation: Application in Neural Prosthesis. Marcel Dekker, New York, 1977.
12. Nashold, B, Somjen, G, and Friedman, H: The effects of stimulating the dorsal columns of man. Med Progr Technol 1:89, 1972.
13. Shealy, C: Electrical control of the nervous system. Med Progr Technol 2:71, 1974.
14. Mills, P, Deakin, M, and Kiff, E: Percutaneous electrical stimulation for ano-rectal incontinence. Physiotherapy 76:433, 1990.
15. Shelly, T: Implanted stimulators for the control of urinary incontinence: The physicians and patients standpoint. Med Progr Technol 1:82, 1972.
16. Alon, G, and DeDomenico, G: High Voltage Stimulation: An Integrated Approach to Clinical Electrotherapy. Chattanooga Corporation, Chattanooga, TN, 1987.
17. Binder, S: Applications of low- and high-voltage electrotherapeutic currents. In Wolf, S (ed): Electrotherapy. Churchill Livingstone, Edinburgh/London/Melbourne, 1981.
18. Forster, A, and Palastanga, N: Clayton's Electrotherapy: Theory and Practice, ed 8. London/Sydney/Toronto, Bailliere Tindall Books, 1981.
19. Wadsworth, J, and Chanmugam, A: Electrophysical Agents in Physiotherapy: Therapeutic and Diagnostic Use, ed 2. Science Press, Marrickville, 1983.
20. Killian, C: Basic electricity overview. Seminar on High Voltage Galvanic Stimulation. 1984.
21. Kahn, A, and Maveus, T: Technical aspects of electrical stimulation devices. Med Progr Technol 1:58, 1972.
22. Kukulka, C: Principles of neuromuscular excitation. In Gersh, M (ed): Electrotherapy in Rehabilitation. FA Davis, Philadelphia, 1992.
23. Patterson, R: Instrumentation for electrotherapy. In Stillwell, G (ed): Therapeutic Electricity and Ultraviolet Radiation. Williams and Wilkins, Baltimore, 1983.
24. Gracanin, F, and Trnkoxzy, A: Optimal stimulation parameters for minimum pain in the chronic situation of innervated muscle. Arch Phys Med Rehabil 56:243, 1975.
25. Baker, L, et al: Effect of carrier frequency on comfort with medium frequency electrical stimulation (abstract). Phys Ther 69:373, 1979.
26. Bowman, B, and Baker, L: Effects of waveform parameters on comfort during transcutaneous neuromuscular electrical stimulation. Ann Biomed Eng 13:59, 1985.
27. Delitto, A, and Rose, S: Comparative comfort of three waveforms used in electrically eliciting quadriceps femoris muscle contraction. Phys Ther 66:1704, 1986.
28. Baker, L, et al: Waveform and comfort of electrical stimulation in the upper extremity (abstract). Phys Ther 69(372), 1989.
29. Kantor, G, et al: The effects of selected stimulus waveforms on pulse and phase characteristics at sensory and motor thresholds. Phys Ther 74:951, 1994.
30. Laufer, Y, et al: Quadriceps Femoris muscle torques and fatigue generated by neuromuscular electrical stimulation with three different waveforms. Phys Ther 7:1307, 2001.
31. Alon, G: High voltage stimulation: Effects of electrode size on basic excitatory responses. Phys Ther 65(890), 1985.
32. Honert, C, and Mortimer, J: The response to the myelinated nerve fiber to short duration biphasic stimulating currents. Ann Biomed Eng 7(117), 1979.
33. Li, C, and Bak, A: Excitability characteristics of the A and C fibers in a peripheral nerve. Exp Neurol 50:67, 1976
34. Howson, D: Peripheral neural excitability: Implications for transcutaneous nerve stimulation. Phys Ther 58:1467, 1978.

35. Alon, G: Northeast Seminars: Electrosynthesis (lab course). Course Publication, 1993.

36. Alon, G: High voltage stimulation: Effects of electrode size on basic excitatory responses. Phys Ther 66:890, 1985.

37. Reilly, J: Electrical Stimulation and Electropathology. Cambridge University Press, 1992.

38. Benton, L, et al: Functional Electrical Stimulation: A Practical Guide, ed 2. Downy, Ranchos Los Amigos Rehabilitation Engineering Center, 1981.

39. Charman, R: Cellular reception and emission of electromagnetic signals. Physiotherapy 76(509), 1990.

40. Crago, P, et al: The choice of pulse duration for chronic electrical stimulation via surface, nerve and intramuscular electrodes. Ann Biomed Eng 2:252, 1974.

41. Ray, C, and Maurer, D: A review of neural stimulator system components useful in pain alleviation. Med Progr Technol 2:121, 1974.

42. Myklebust, B, and Kloth, L: Electrodiagnostic and electrotherapeutic instrumentation: Characteristics of recording and stimulation systems and principles of safety. In Gersh, M (ed): Electrotherapy in Rehabilitation. FA Davis, Philadelphia, 1992.

43. Clinic Notes: The fatal current. Phys Ther 46:968, 1966.

44. Sances, A, et al: Electrical injuries. Surg Gynecol Obstet 149:97, 1979.

45. Berger, W: Electrical shock hazards in the physical therapy department. Clin Management 5:24, 1994.

46. Bruner, J, and Leonard, P: Electricity, Safety and the Patient. Year Book Medical Publishers, Chicago/London/Boca Raton, 1989.

47. Buban, P, and Schmitt, M: Technical Electricity and Electronics, ed 2. McGraw-Hill Book Co, New York, 1977.

48. Delitto, A, et al: A study of discomfort with electrical stimulation. Phys Ther 72:11, 1992.

49. Lampe, G: Introduction to the use of transcutaneous electrical nerve stimulation. Phys Ther 72:11, 1978.

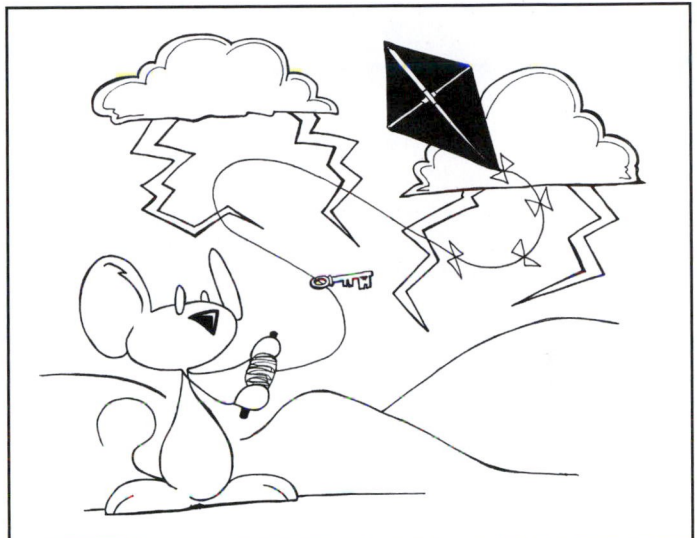

Objectives

- Describe the components and care of the electrode interface.
- Outline the process of electrode selection and placement.

Key Terms

Banana tip	Electrode	Monopolar	Quadripolar
Bipolar	Lead wire	Pin tip	

Barbara J. Behrens, PTA, MS

Electrodes: Material and Care

"Will I be electrocuted by what you are doing?"

Clinical electrical stimulation involves the passing of current through the skin via electrodes. An electrode is used to either deliver electric current or record electrical activity of muscle, such as in electromyography (EMG). The delivery of current is accomplished through a system of electrically conductive elements.[1] This includes the lead wire, two or more electrodes per circuit, a conductive substance such as referred to as the electrode interface, and the patient. Each of these components will affect the amount of electrical charge delivered to the patient. The influence of each of the components will either facilitate the flow of current, if the resistance is low, or inhibit the flow of current, if the resistance within the system is too high. Refer to Chapter 8 for a review of resistance and current flow.

Electrodes represent the "instrument" for current delivery from an electrical stimulation generator. Leads connect the electrodes to the stimulator. Each lead has both a jack and a pin to interconnect the electrode to the lead and the lead to the stimulator.[1] Each of these components will be discussed in terms of the structures themselves, their possible configurations, and appropriate handling techniques.

Electrodes vary in shape, size, and flexibility, to fit the needs of the therapeutic application of the electrical current to the patient. An electrode is made of an electrically conductive material that is housed in a nonelectrically conductive material. The purpose of the housing material is to inhibit the delivery of electrical energy to either the patient or the clinician if either should touch the back of the electrode.

Types of Electrodes

Metal Plate Electrodes

Early electrodes were composed of metal plates such as tin, steel, aluminum, and zinc, which are good electrical

Patient Perspective

Remember that your patient is curious about what you are doing with electrical stimulation. Some of the terms might be familiar, such as "stereo jack" or lead wire, but he or she will not know what you are going to do with them and why. Another key thing to remember is that you are deliberately moistening the electrodes, yet your patient may be fearful of the combination of water and electricity. It is the responsibility of the clinician to properly inform the patient about the rationale behind the "tasks" that are involved.

PATIENTS' FREQUENTLY ASKED QUESTIONS

1. Do you use tap water or distilled water? Why?

2. Why do you use water?

3. Will I be electrocuted by what you are doing?

4. Where will I feel that, and what will it feel like?

5. Why are you doing that to me?

6. Have you ever had this done to you?

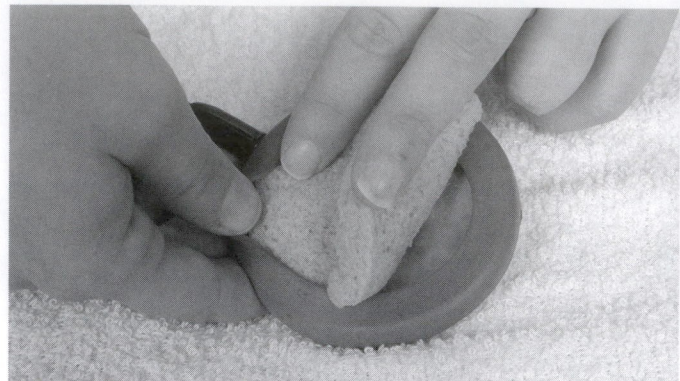

Figure 9–1   Metal plate electrode. The metal surface of the electrode is covered by a sponge that would be soaked in water. The left-hand corner of the sponge is folded back to reveal the metal plate. The electrode is encased in a nonelectrically conductive rubber cover.

conductors for therapeutic stimulation. The electrode was usually contained within a rubber casing with only one surface exposed to the patient. The interface between the metal electrode and skin was accomplished through a sponge or felt pad moistened with water. This served to reduce the skin—electrode impedance, because water is a good conductor of electricity. Distilled water should not be used; it contains no free ions, which are required for the transmission of electrical current,[1] and therefore would not be electrically conductive (Fig. 9-1).

Disadvantages of metal plate electrode systems include the following:

- Metal plates may not be flexible enough to maintain adequate contact with certain body parts.

- These electrodes may be difficult to secure comfortably to the patient.

- There are few sizes of these electrodes, making specific treatment goals for smaller treatment areas difficult to accomplish.

Carbon-Impregnated Rubber Electrodes

Electrodes composed of rubber, silicon, and polymer have mostly replaced the older metal plate electrodes and are typ-

ically used with clinical devices. Carbon-impregnated silicon rubber electrodes are commonly used in many clinics. They are backed with a nonconductive material to prevent unintentional current delivery. These electrodes are available in many shapes and sizes, and they can be trimmed or fitted to different locations of the body (Fig. 9-2).

Carbon-impregnated silicon rubber electrodes should be replaced when necessary. They degrade over time, resulting in nonuniformity of current delivery, or the presence of "hot spots." Hot spots represent those areas of the electrode that

 Why Do I Need to Know About...

APPLICATION OF ELECTRODES
You will be applying electrodes to patients and need to be familiar with the terminology and the purpose to be successful.

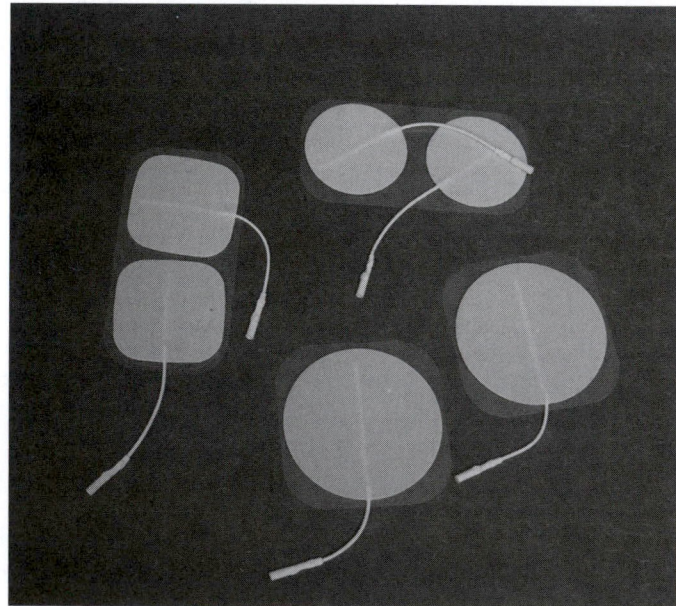

Figure 9–2   Several different sizes of self-adhering electrodes that have a mesh of electrically conductive material woven into them. This photograph depicts other self-adhering electrodes with smaller conductive surface areas and also illustrates the flexibility of the mesh electrodes. The mesh electrodes easily conform to irregular body surfaces.

continue to maintain their conductivity while other areas of the surface no longer conduct electrical energy. The result is analogous to 10 cars trying to merge onto an uncrowded highway versus those same 10 cars trying to merge onto a crowded highway. The 10 cars will get on the crowded highway, but if time was a factor, the amount of resistance that they would face in meeting their goal would be significantly higher when the traffic was heavy, or the window to merge was smaller. Carbon rubber electrodes should be rinsed off and dried after each use. Replace these electrodes every 12 months to ensure good conductivity. Again, if the goal is to have current pass through the electrodes, then they must be taken care of to maintain their conductivity.

Self-Adhering Single-Use or Reusable Electrodes

Self-adhering single-use or reusable electrodes are composed of other flexible conductors such as foil or metal mesh, conductive Karaya, or synthetic gel layered with an adhesive surface (see Fig. 9-2). The advantage of these electrodes is convenience of application. No strapping or taping is necessary to secure the electrodes to the patient.

Clinicians should carefully read the manufacturer's suggestions before utilizing these electrodes. Because of the potential for cross-contamination, use of a package of electrodes for each patient is prudent. The package can be marked with the patient's name and identification number so that they will only be used for a given patient.

Considerations for Electrode Selection

There are advantages and disadvantages with each type of electrode, including self-adhering electrodes. Often, the impedance of these electrodes is significantly higher than that of other electrode systems, resulting in reductions in potential current outputs of the stimulation device. These limitations may make it difficult or impossible to accomplish the desired clinical goal with a given stimulator, if the output of the stimulator is not sufficient to overcome the resistance of the electrodes.

The resistance of the electrode, which is listed in ohms, should be as low as possible when significant motor levels of stimulation are required. If the desired effect is a comfortable nonmotor level of stimulation, the impedance value of the electrodes is not as critical to success. If the impedance value of the electrodes is high, then the stimulator will need to overcome that value before the current is delivered to the patient. This may result in higher output levels of stimulation, which may be uncomfortable to the patient. The package of the electrodes may indicate the ohms of resistance, which will be lower with larger electrodes and higher with smaller electrodes.

Before You Begin

Ask yourself what types of electrodes are available and which ones would be the most economical and appropriate for the patient that you are treating. Not all clinics will have individual single-patient reusable electrodes. The insurance coverage for some patients does not permit this type of expense, so reusable carbon-impregnated rubber electrodes may need to be used.

The method of current delivery into the electrode will also affect the uniformity of the current delivery from the electrode. Some self-adhering electrodes have a metal wire that inserts into the center of a conductive-adhesive or adherent surface. The current delivery at the point of attachment of the wire to the surface will be relatively higher than the current delivery to the periphery of that electrode. This may result in a hot spot where the wire connects to the surface of the electrode. Optimally, the conductive surface of the electrode will have "uniform" conductivity. This potential for uniformity of conductivity is enhanced through foil or mesh surfaces within the electrode to spread out the delivered current.

Electrode Size and Current Density

Current density describes the amount of current concentrated under an electrode. It is a measure of the quantity of charged ions moving through a specific cross-sectional area of body tissue.

Electrode surface area is inversely related to total current flow. The same total current flow passing through large and small electrodes would result in lower current density at the larger electrode. The total current would be distributed over a larger surface area. Conversely, the smaller electrode would be delivering a high-current density because of its smaller surface area. Therapeutic electrical stimulation involves the active or stimulating electrode, the one that exhibits the greater current density, and the dispersive or inactive electrode, which delivers less current density. Electrodes should be appropriately sized for the desired result. If, for example, the treatment goal involved a motor response of one of the forearm muscles, an electrode that was 3 inches in diameter would produce a great amount of "overflow" of current into the surrounding muscles. It would be more appropriate to utilize a small electrode that more closely approximates the size of the target tissue, such as a $1\frac{1}{2}$-inch diameter electrode (Fig. 9-3). The reverse is also true. If the treatment goal involved a tetanic contraction of the rectus femoris, then the electrode size that would afford the greatest comfort would probably be 3 inches in diameter or greater. Smaller electrodes may provide too great a current density, but not enough current flow to elicit a tetanic contraction (see Fig. 9-4).

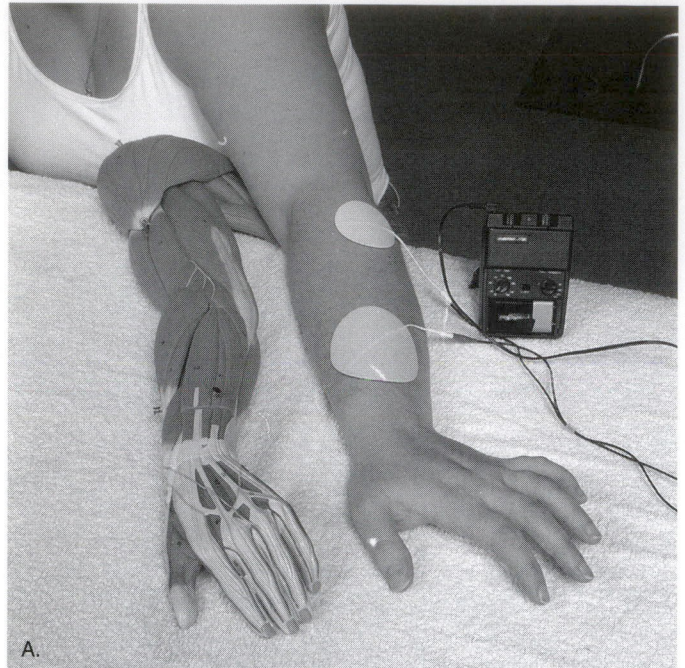

A.

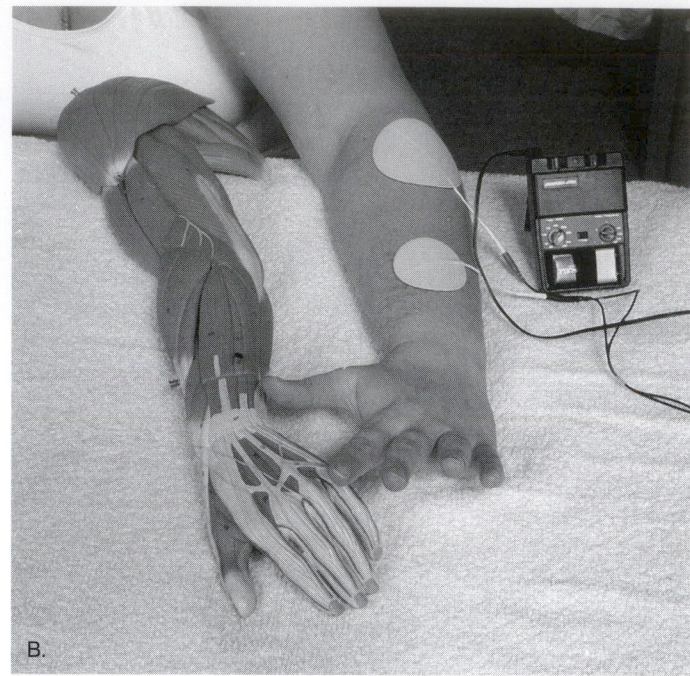

B.

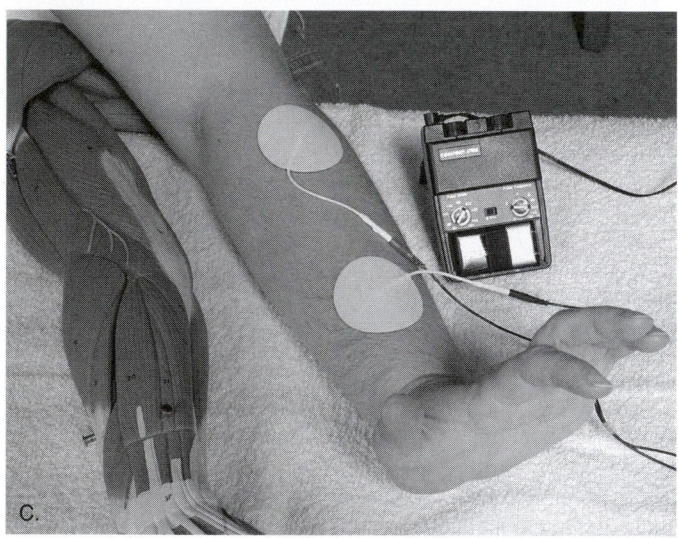

C.

Figure 9-3   Each of the photographs depicts identical electrode placement sites with identical electrical stimulation parameters. The goal for the stimulation was wrist extension. However, in **A**, the distal electrode is larger than the proximal electrode, causing ulnar deviation. In **B**, the proximal electrode is larger than the distal electrode, causing radial deviation. In **C**, wrist flexion is accomplished this time with equally sized electrodes.

Coupling Media and Attachment

Surface-stimulating electrodes require the use of a coupling medium. This medium can be water via soaked sponges,

 Why Do I Need to Know About...

ELECTRODE SIZE
Remember that Ohm's law states that the delivered energy is directly related to the amount of resistance encountered. If you use small electrodes, the resistance will be higher and the sensation potentially more uncomfortable, making it impossible to accomplish a treatment goal.

or electrically conductive gel. The coupling medium reduces the impedance at the interface between the electrode and the skin. This results in less current amplitude needed to produce the desired effects of stimulation.[2,3]

Pliability of the electrode to conform to the body part is necessary. Rigid metal electrodes do not conform well to contoured anatomic regions. Poor conformity can also result in hot-spot delivery of the electrical energy. In this case a high concentration of electrical energy over a small area, for example, the "hot spot," is a factor of not having all of the conductive surface of the electrode in contact with the patient's skin. Patient responses indicative of this would be noticeable after several minutes of treatment: the patient moved, he or

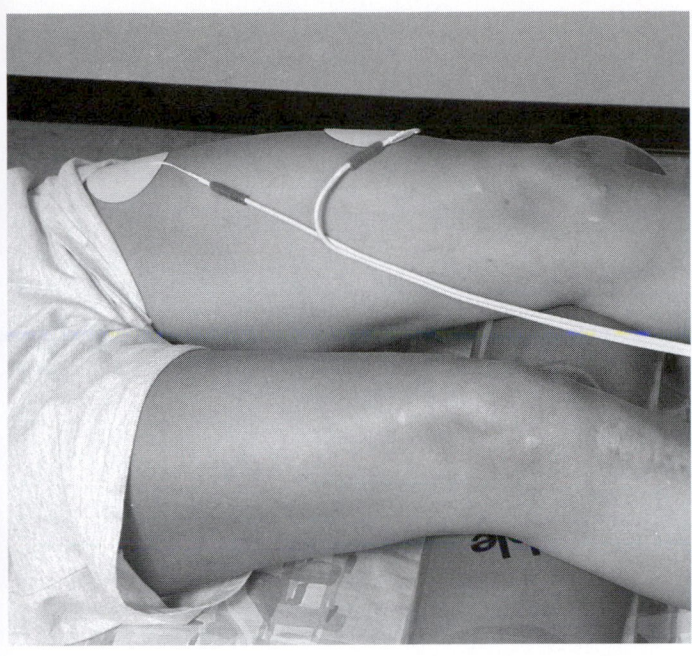

Figure 9-4 Contraction of the rectus femoris with the use of electrical stimulation delivered through two 3-inch-round electrodes placed on the muscle.

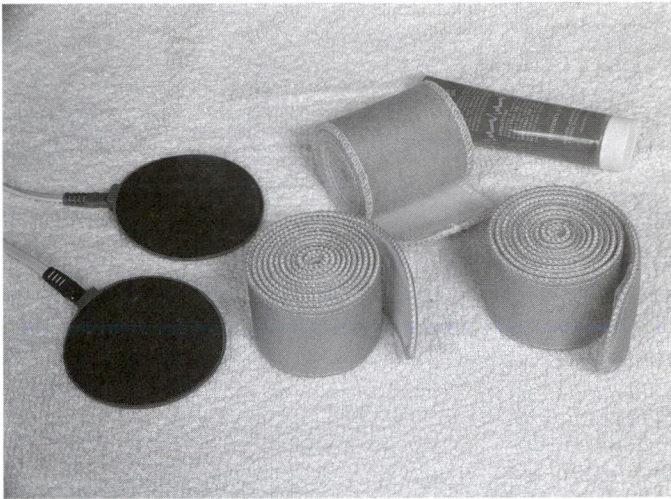

Figure 9-5 Straps used to hold carbon rubber electrodes with sponges or gel, in place during treatment.

she now feels a prickling sensation ("hot spot") and is afraid to move back to the original position. To remedy this, the concentration of the energy will diminish if the patient returns to the original position, because the uniformity of the contact between the electrode and the patient will have been restored. It is often difficult to convince a patient that if he or she leans back on the electrode that is causing the prickling sensation, that the degree of prickling will subside. Explanations for the phenomenon can reduce the patient's anxiety regarding the electrical stimulation and potentially offset increased muscle guarding as a result of that fear.

Caution should be exercised to make sure that the electrode interface has not dried out during the treatment. If so, repositioning the patient will not remedy his or her complaint, but rehydration of the electrode may do so. This is yet another reason to check on a patient after treatment with electrical stimulation has been initiated.

The electrode should conform to the anatomic region to obtain optimal stimulation. Electrode attachment methods to maximize surface contact include the use of straps, tape, and self-adhering electrodes.

Straps or Tape for the Attachment of Electrodes

Straps have been commercially manufactured to be easy to use, inexpensive, and versatile. Many of the commercially available straps have rubber-backed stretch "eyed" surfaces, with one end of the reversed side of the strap covered with "hooks." These straps should be used to secure either the carbon-impregnated rubber electrodes or the metal-plate electrodes. Proper utilization involves strapping circumferentially around the limb with sufficient pressure to maintain good uniform contact between the electrode and the patient's skin. The pressure should be centered so that the electrode remains flat against the surface of the skin. Once the strap is secured, it should be checked for positioning that may have changed slightly once the strap has been stretched. Straps come in a variety of lengths for different areas of the body and different strapping configurations (Fig. 9-5).

Tape can also be used to attach electrodes to the patient, and it has several distinct disadvantages. For example, it can be costly and patients may be allergic to the adhesive. If the electrodes are not properly cleaned after use, the adhesive may migrate to and collect on the conductive surface of the electrode. This decreases both the conductive surface area and increases the potential for skin irritation.

Leads

Leads provide a conductive path for current flow. Electrical stimulators will always have a pair of leads emerging from them. They are the intermediary between the generator and electrodes. The electrodes are connected to the electrical stimulation generator by lead wires. A lead wire has several parts: the point of exit from the stimulator, the wire itself, and the point of attachment to the electrode, known as the tip. The point of exit is referred to as the "jack," which, if it contains two leads, is referred to as a "stereo jack."

The jack plugs into the stimulator and is typically encased in hard plastic. The jack is the portion of the lead that is meant to be handled, and it is constructed to maintain its

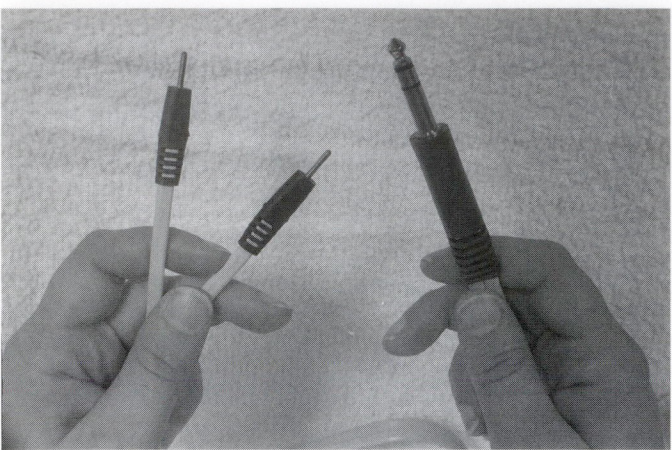

Figure 9–6 The lead wire to an electrical stimulation device connects to the device via a "stereo jack" and is divided into two leads, which are usually pin leads as pictured.

integrity even with multiple plugging and unplugging of the lead into the stimulator. In order for the lead to be able to deliver electrical energy, the jack must be securely plugged into the stimulator so that there is no metal showing between the jack and its plug or receptacle. Each lead wire will usually have two electrodes attached to it by a metal tip that inserts into the electrode (Fig. 9-6). There are different types of electrode/lead wire configurations, such as the pin tip lead and the banana tip lead, which are attempts to standardize the lead–electrode interface and ease the attachment of the electrode to the lead for the clinician (Fig. 9-7). Regardless of the type of tip, it is prone to corrosion and should be cleaned regularly. Scheduled maintenance of the tips should prevent potential problems with current delivery. Steel wool can be used to clean a tip. Gentle rubbing with the steel wool should

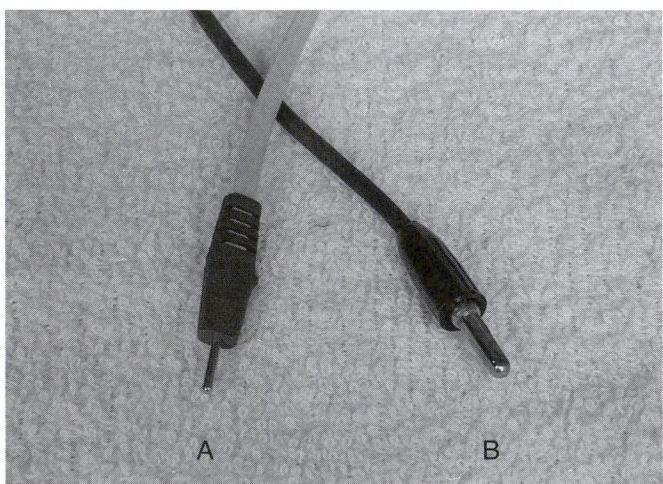

Figure 9–7 **(A)** "Pin" tip. **(B)** "Banana" tip. Banana tips are adjustable. If the tip no longer fits tightly in an electrode, then the sides of the tip may be spread apart slightly.

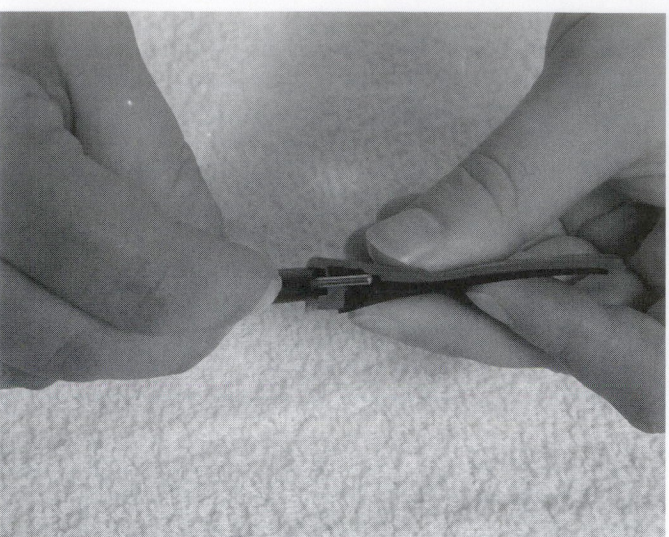

Figure 9–8 The tip must be fully inserted into the electrode so that the metal pin tip touches the conductive surface of the electrode. Failure to insert the pin into the electrode fully will result in poor current delivery to the electrode.

restore the shiny metal surface of the tip, which will maintain its conductivity.

The tip can assist in the delivery of electrical energy only if it is in contact with the conductive surface of the electrode. There is a small housing that surrounds the tip opening within every electrode. The tip must be pushed as far as possible into the opening so that it does come in contact with the conductive surface of the electrode. There should be no metal showing between the plastic-coated pin housing and the electrode. Failure to insert the electrode properly will result in poor clinical results because current cannot be delivered to the patient (Fig. 9-8).

Many electrical stimulation devices have multiple lead wires that have one stereo jack with two leads and pins for two electrodes. If the intended result is to cover a larger area and there are not any additional channels of electrodes available, then each lead may be "split" through the use of a bifurcator. A bifurcator is an attachment that fits on the pin of the lead wire and has two smaller leads coming off of it. Use of a bifurcator will split the output from that lead into the two electrodes attached to it, thereby decreasing the total amount of current flow through each independent electrode. (Current density is reduced or dispersed). If a patient perceives too much sensation underneath one of the electrodes from a channel, then either the size of the electrode can be in-

● **Why Do I Need to Know About...**

TIP MAINTENANCE
Sometimes the reason that the current is not being perceived is as simple as the point of attachment to the electrode. BEFORE checking to see if this is a problem, make sure that the intensity is at ZERO.

TABLE 9-1 Channel Setups and Lead Management

TREATMENT GOAL	NO. OF LEADS AND ELECTRODES	MONOPOLAR	BIPOLAR	QUADRIPOLAR
Muscle (motor) stimulation	One lead per muscle with both electrodes on the same muscle, two leads if it is a larger muscle or if the device has more than one head		X	
Sensory stimulation	One or two leads depending upon the size of the area; use as many electrodes as possible for sensory stimulation			X
	One lead if only one lead and two electrodes fit into the treatment area		X	
	One lead with one electrode at the spinal nerve root and the other in the sensory area	X		
Delivery of medication	One lead and one electrode in the treatment area and the other more proximally placed on soft tissue	X		

creased or a bifurcator can be used, which would then split the output delivered to that electrode.

Neither lead should be considered a "ground" but rather part of the electrical circuit. If there are not at least two points of contact between the electrical stimulation device and the patient, the patient will not have any electrical stimulation. A circuit has not been completed. Some older sources for electrical stimulation may use the term "ground" for the dis-persive electrode but this is a misnomer. Each electrical stimulation device will have its own set of peculiarities with respect to the management of leads. Examples of the channel setups and lead management can be found in Table 9-1. Potential causes and remedies for patient complaints of prickling or itching sensations underneath the electrodes are listed in Table 9-2.

TABLE 9-2 Potential Causes and Remedies for Patient Complaints of Prickling or Itching Sensations Underneath the Electrodes

COMPLAINT	POTENTIAL CAUSE	REMEDY
Prickling or itching underneath the electrodes during treatment	The patient is moved off of one of the electrodes during treatment.	Restoring contact with the electrode will restore the sensation; however; you may need to decrease the intensity of the unit first before a patient will let you do this.
	One of the electrodes is not making good contact.	Restoring contact with the electrode will restore the sensation; however, you may need to decrease the intensity of the unit first before a patient will let you do this.
	One of the electrodes has dried out.	Restoring the moisture necessary for good conduction can be as easy as re-wetting the electrode.
	The patient has dry skin.	Restoring the moisture necessary for good conduction can be as easy as re-wetting the electrode. If the patient has dry skin, his or her skin may absorb the moisture rapidly. Sponges may work better for these patients.
	The patient's skin is oily.	This patient may not be receiving the appropriate current density due to his or her own skin condition. Cleansing the skin with alcohol can remove the oil from the surface of the skin.
	The patient's skin is soiled under the surface of the electrode.	This patient may not be receiving the appropriate current density due to his or her own skin condition. Cleaning the skin with alcohol can remove the oil from the surface of the skin.
	The electrode is losing its conductivity.	The electrode may need to be replaced. The patient is NOT always the problem.
	A strap has come undone.	Restoring contact with the electrode will restore the sensation. You may need to resecure the straps. However, you may need to decrease the intensity of the unit first before a patient will let you do this.
	Water dripped out from the sponge when the straps were applied.	Restoring the moisture necessary for good conduction can be as easy as re-wetting the electrode. Restoring contact with the electrode will restore the sensation; however, you may need to decrease the intensity of the unit first before a patient will let you do this.

Transcutaneous and Percutaneous Electrodes

Electrodes that are applied to the surface of the skin are termed transcutaneous electrodes. Transcutaneous refers to the delivery of electrical energy or recording of electrical energy across the skin. Percutaneous electrodes are inserted into the skin. Percutaneous electrodes are commonly used for invasive EMG procedures, or they may be used for the application of electrical stimulation for patients with quadriplegia or paraplegia. Of the two types of electrodes, transcutaneous electrodes are more common in therapeutic delivery of electrical stimulation.

Terminology for Configurations of Electrode Setups

Electrodes can be oriented in monopolar, bipolar, and quadripolar manner, meaning one, two, or four electrodes in the treatment area, respectively. Placement across body tissues can be longitudinal and parallel, such as when stimulating quadriceps muscles of the thigh to facilitate a stronger contraction, or they may be criss-crossed, as when administering electrical stimulation treatment for pain management.

Monopolar Application of Electrodes

The monopolar technique involves a single electrode from a channel, usually smaller in size, placed over the target area called the active electrode. The greatest stimulation perception will be in the target tissue area. The larger dispersive electrode or second electrode is placed at a distance from the target electrode to complete the circuit. Its placement is usually over the nerve root supplying the target treatment area. The size differential between the electrodes ensures a greater current concentration in the treatment area (Fig. 9-9A).

Bipolar Electrode Setup

The bipolar electrode technique requires two electrodes from one channel within the target treatment area. They are usually of equal dimension and shape. Current flow through tissue is usually confined to the problem area. When using the bipolar placement, the patient will experience an excitatory response and/or sensation under both electrodes. One can be smaller if the intention is a more effective activation of excitable tissues. This would be an appropriate electrode setup for eliciting a motor response.[4] One of the electrodes will be placed over the motor point, and the other electrode, which may be slightly larger, will be placed somewhere else over the muscle belly (Fig. 9-9B). Occasionally, a clinician may bifurcate the leads when a situation requires a larger target area, such as with a combination of back and lower ex-

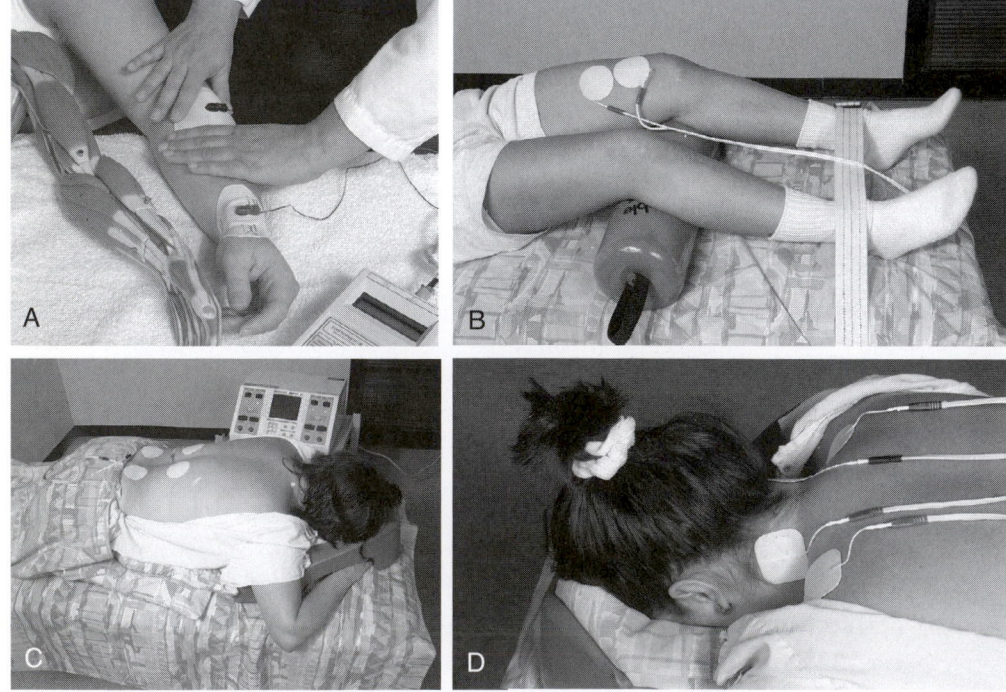

Figure 9-9 Various electrode setups. (A) Monopolor electrode placement setups with only one electrode from the channel in the target of treatment area. (B) A bipolar electrode setup, with both electrodes from the same channel in the target or treatment area. (C) A quadripolar treatment setup in the low back and (D) a dual bipolar setup for the cervical musculature.

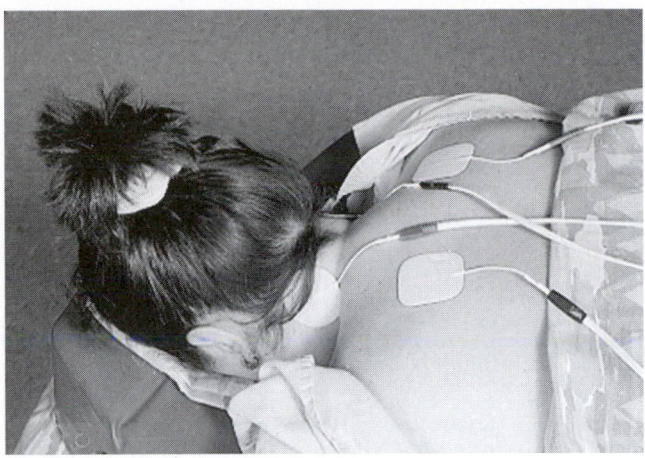

Figure 9-10 A quadripolar electrode setup in the cervical region to help provide analgesia and relieve muscle guarding as a secondary response to pain reduction.

tremity radicular pain. Bipolar techniques are well suited for stimulation of a large muscle.[5–9] Monopolar techniques are better suited for stimulation over a motor point or a wound.[10–13]

Quadripolar Electrode Placement

The quadripolar method of electrode application involves electrodes from two or more channels, each lead with two electrodes. The electrodes can be positioned in a variety of configurations. Quadripolar electrode placement occurs with an interferential device; however, it also occurs when there are four electrodes within the treatment area, regardless of the type of stimulator utilized to deliver the current.

Quadripolar electrode setups are often used to deliver the electrical stimulation to a larger area, such as in pain management techniques that rely on sensory stimulation of larger fibers for analgesia[14,15] (Figs. 9-9C,D and 9-10).

Application Guidelines

- Make sure that all connections are tight.
  Stereo jack into the stimulator
  Pin or banana into the electrode
  Electrode interface onto the skin
- Make sure that electrode interfaces are moist.

● Why Do I Need to Know About...

PROPER TERMINOLOGY
The terminology for electrode setups is verbally communicated between clinicians. Knowing what is meant by the terms helps you to understand what other clinicians are referring to and decreases the confusion in an already terminology-laden intervention.

Self adhering

Sponges
- Gel must be electrically conductive.
- Water must NOT be distilled water as there are NO ions present for the conduction of electrical current.
- Make sure that your patient does not move the electrodes once they are positioned.
- Make sure that your patient knows how to contact you if he or she needs to during treatment.

 ## Care of Electrodes

Because electrodes represent the point of delivery of therapeutic electrical stimulation, the proper care for and cleaning of electrodes are essential. The impedance of carbon-impregnated silicon rubber electrodes can be significantly altered if the surface is allowed to dry or cake with gel. Carbon-impregnated silicon rubber electrodes can easily be cleaned in mild soap and warm water to remove gels. Cracking or "polished" appearance of the electrode surface may indicate that the surface is no longer uniformly conductive. This may result in the formation of spots of high current density on the electrode and poor current delivery. Harsh disinfectants can damage both carbon rubber and metal electrodes. Excessive alcohol use can cause carbon rubber electrodes to lose conductivity. An early sign of electrode wear is a stinging sensation under the electrodes. If there are cracks or uneven surfaces, the electrodes may need to be replaced.

"Hot spots" represent an increase in current concentration or current density within the electrode area, which could result in skin irritation. Patients who complain that they feel a biting or stinging sensation when receiving therapeutic current are probably describing an electrode with uneven conductivity. It is time to replace the electrode, or at least have it checked with an ohmmeter for resistance to determine whether use of the electrode should be continued.

If they are not cleaned on a regular basis, sponges soaked with water may be a source of potential cross-contamination from patient to patient. Germicidal soaps can be used to rinse through the electrodes before their application on a patient. Soap residue must be removed because soap acts as an insulator to the passage of electrical energy. It is usually easier, though, to replace the sponge electrodes with new ones.

 ## Summary

Proper care and selection of electrodes could represent the success or failure of a treatment intervention with electrical

CASE STUDY

Susan is an athletic trainer for the local community college women's field hockey team. She spends a great deal of time kneeling while taping the ankles of the team members. She fell down on her knees and has now been diagnosed with chondromalacia of the patella in both knees. There is marked weakness of the vastus medialis, edema superior to the patella, and a palpable painful crepitus in both knees when descending stairs.

The treatment goals include pain relief, edema reduction, and muscle strengthening.

Electrical stimulation was applied in a quadripolar setup for each of Susan's knees, which initially felt "very comfortable." Susan is now complaining that it feels as if "ants are crawling around" on her knees.

- What probably happened, and what could be done to improve the situation?

stimulation. The electrodes, leads, and electrode interface must be appropriate for a treatment intervention to have a chance of being effective. If a patient is not feeling electrical stimulation where he or she is supposed to be feeling it, due to an unpleasant sensation, clinicians must understand enough to know what to do to remedy the problem. This chapter provided a sampling of what to look for and what to do when problems arise. Familiarity with the equipment that is being used must include all of the peripherals, such as the leads and electrodes.

Discussion Questions

1. Of what significance is the choice of electrodes for a given patient?
2. If the patient complained of a prickling sensation underneath one of the electrodes, what would be the potential causes and potential remedies?
3. If a patient stated that he or she was not feeling the sensation underneath all of the electrodes, what might be the cause for this and what could you do?
4. Using terminology that a patient would understand, how would you explain electrical stimulation to him or her?
5. Your patient decides to lift up the corner of one of the electrodes; what would happen and why?

Recommended Reading

Baker, LL, et al: Electrical stimulation of wrist and fingers for hemiplegic patients. Phys Ther 59:1495, 1979.

Halstead, LS, et al: Relief of spasticity in SCT men and women using rectal probe electrostimulation. Paraplegia 31:715, 1993.

Kloth, LC, and Feedar, JA: Acceleration of wound healing with high voltage, monophasic, pulsed current. Phys Ther 68:503, 1988.

Melzack, R, and Wall, DW: Pain mechanisms: A new theory. Science 150:971, 1965.

Melzack, R: Myofascial trigger points: Relation to acupuncture and mechanisms of pain. Arch Phys Med Rehabil 62:114, 1981.

Melzack, R, Stillwell, DM, and Fox, EJ: Trigger points and acupuncture points for pain: Correlations and implications. Pain 3:3, 1977.

References

1. Buban, P, Schmitt, ML, and Carter, CG Jr: Electricity and Electronics Technology. Glencoe/McGraw-Hill, 1999.
2. Nolan, MF: Conductive differences in electrodes used with transcutaneous electrical nerve stimulation devices. Phys Ther 71:746, 1991.
3. Lieber, RL, and Kelly, MJ: Factors influencing quadriceps femoris torque using transcutaneous neuromuscular electrical stimulation. Phys Ther 71:715, 1991.
4. Benton, LA, et al: Functional Electrical Stimulation—A Practical Clinical Guide, ed 2. Downey, CA, Rancho Los Amigos Rehabilitation Engineering Center, 1981, 34–36.
5. Snyder-Mackler, L, Delitto, A, Bailey, S, et al: Strength of the quadriceps femoris muscle and functional recovery after reconstruction of the anterior cruciate ligament. A prospective, randomized clinical trial of electrical stimulation. J Bone Joint Surg Am 77:1166–1173, 1995.
6. Fitzgerald, GK, Piva, SR, and Irrgang, JJ: A modified neuromuscular electrical stimulation protocol for quadriceps strength training following anterior cruciate ligament reconstruction. J Orthop Sports Phys Ther 33:492–501, 2003.
7. Snyder-Mackler, L, Ladin, Z, Schepsis, AA, et al: Electrical stimulation of the thigh muscle after reconstruction of the anterior cruciate ligament. Effects of electrically elicited contraction of the quadriceps femoris and hamstring muscle on gain and on strength of the thigh muscles. J Bone Joint Surg Am 73:1025–1036, 1991.
8. Lewek, M, Steven, J, and Snyder-Mackler, L: The use of electrical stimulation to increase quadriceps femoris force in an elderly patient following a total knee arthroplasty. Phys Ther 81:1565–1571, 2001.
9. Gotlin, RS, Hershkowitz, S, Juris, PM, et al: Electrical stimulation effect on extensor lag and length of hospital stay after total knee arthroplasty. Arch Phys Med Rehabil 75:857–959, 1994.
10. Paternostro-Sluga, T, Fialka, C, Alacamliogiu, Y, et al: Neuromuscular electrical stimulation after anterior cruciate ligament surgery. Clin Orthog 368:166–175, 1999.
11. Kloth, LC, and McCulloch, JM (eds): Wound Healing: Alternatives in Management, ed 3. FA Davis, Philadelphia, 2002.
12. Feedar, JA, et al: Chronic dermal ulcer healing enhanced with monophasic pulsed electrical stimulation, Phys Ther 71:639, 1991.
13. Feedar JA, Kloth, LC, and Gentzkow, GD: Chronic dermal ulcer healing enhanced with monophasic pulsed electrical stimulation. Phys Ther 71:639, 1991.
14. Fitzgerald, GK, and Newsome, D: Treatment of a large infected thoracic spine wound using high voltage pulsed monophasic current. Phys Ther 73:355, 1993.

15. Hurley, DA, Minder, PM, and McDunough, SM, et al: Interferential therapy electrode placement technique in acute low back pain: A preliminary investigation Arch Phys Med Rehabil 82:485–493, 2001.

16. Jarit, GJ, Mohr, KJ, Waller, R, et al: The effects of home interferential therapy on post-operative pain, edema, and range of motion of the knee. Clin J Sport Med 13:16–20, 2003.

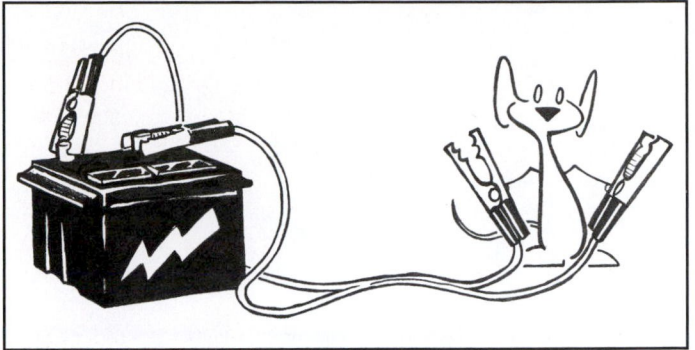

Objectives

- Discuss the specific clinical applications for neuromuscular electrical stimulation (NMES) for strengthening and endurance, range of motion, facilitation of muscle function, management of muscle spasms and spasticity, edema reduction, and orthotic substitution.
- Outline treatment techniques for patient problems.
- Discuss the factors that determine whether NMES would be appropriate for a patient.
- Discuss the clinical decision-making process for determining the effectiveness of the use of NMES and whether modifications should be made.

Key Terms

Functional neuromuscular electrical stimulation (FNS or NMES)	Partial denervation Intact peripheral nerve Stimulation parameters	Waveform Amplitude Pulse duration Duty cycle Ramp	Balanced contraction

Joy C. Cohn, PT, Cecilia Mullin, PTA

Neuromuscular Electrical Stimulation

Outline

"The stimulation seemed so scary when you suggested it but I can see the muscle working!"

The purposes of this chapter are to demonstrate the clinical use of surface electrical stimulation (ES) to accomplish a variety of therapeutic goals and to explore the guidelines for clinical decision-making and intervention.

Technological development of ES devices and the treatment of human ills have progressed hand in hand to the present day, but not without confusion. To utilize ES devices effectively, it is important to focus on the outcome expected. Although the technology for ES may change over time, the goal of the intervention will probably remain the same.

This chapter considers the use of neuromuscular electrical stimulation (NMES) in physical therapy interventions. NMES is defined as "the use of electrical stimulation for activation of muscle through stimulation of the intact peripheral nerve."[1] Functional electrical stimulation (FES) and functional neuromuscular stimulation (FNS) are forms of NMES. They are used as a substitute for an orthosis to activate muscle contractions in paretic or paralyzed muscles to assist in functional activities, such as standing or grasping an object. Other potential uses of electrical stimulation, such as wound healing, are covered in other chapters of this text.

Identifying Appropriate Patients

NMES requires an intact, or at least partially intact, peripheral nerve to respond to the stimulation. A stimulated muscle contraction will always be generated via the innervating peripheral nerve, if intact. In the case of partial denervation because of a peripheral neuropathy of metabolic or neurologic origin (e.g., diabetes or Guillain-Barré), it may not be possible to stimulate a contraction of any more strength than the patient is able to produce voluntarily as a result of diffuse denervation commonly associated with these diseases. Electrical muscle stimulation (EMS) is pulsed monophasic current that is used to activate denervated muscle directly. EMS is considered to be of questionable value[2] and will not be covered in this chapter. Innervation status, if in doubt, is determined via history, physical examination, and a strength-duration test (S-D test) or an electroneuromyographic (EMG) evaluation. There is a questionable role for NMES in the presence of primary muscle disease such as muscular dystrophy. Further study is required.

There are a few contraindications to NMES.[3] The presence of a cardiac demand pacemaker is an absolute contraindication because of the possibility that the electrical current will interfere with the electronics of the pacemaker. Use of NMES with any other pacemaker should be undertaken with great caution, and the supervising physician should be contacted prior to use if ES is seen to be an essential part of the intervention plan. Precautions for NMES include the following[4,5] (Box 10-1):

- Elderly patients should be monitored closely for heart rate and blood pressure responses during initiation of a stimulation program to rule out unknown cardiac problems in response to exercise.
- The effect of NMES during pregnancy on the fetus is unknown. It may induce labor in a woman in her third trimester, and therefore should be avoided.
- Superficial metal (e.g., staples, pins, external fixation devices) will be a site of concentration for the current delivered to the skin in the vicinity and can cause discomfort. Orthopedic metal implants (e.g., total hip replacement) are generally located too deep beneath the skin surface to be cause for concern.
- Absent or impaired skin sensation is not a contraindication but requires close monitoring of the skin response, careful choice of and application of electrodes, and in general, use of biphasic and short-duration waveforms

BOX 10-1 Contraindications to Electrical Stimulation

Absolute
- Presence of demand cardiac pacemaker

Relative
- Any other type of cardiac pacemaker
- Pregnancy in the third trimester
- Broken or irritated skin at electrode site

Precautions for Electrical Stimulation
- Older or cardiac patients monitor blood pressure and heart rate
- Superficial metal (i.e., staples, pins, external fixation)
- Absent or impaired skin sensation

to avoid the potential tissue damage associated with direct current. Safety issues in the use of electronic equipment will be considered later in the chapter and have been thoroughly discussed in Chapter 8.

Therapeutic Current Characteristics

Individuals may respond negatively when first introduced to a stimulation program because of an innate fear of electricity or discomfort with stimulation. However, careful explanation of the goals of an intervention, gradual introduction of the stimulation amplitude, and readiness to consider a change in stimulation waveform or parameters can lead to success in most cases. This chapter contains a brief review of therapeutic interventions. The reader is urged to refer to Chapter 9 for a more detailed description of terminology.

The two main concerns in planning a program of NMES are

1. The quality of the stimulated muscle contraction
2. Patient comfort leading to cooperation with the intervention plan

! Before You Begin

Ask yourself the following questions:
1. What size electrode should I use?
2. How do I get the best possible muscle response?

Both are greatly affected by the stimulation parameters. The success of the intervention program is not based on the stimulator chosen; many different stimulators have been used effectively. It is a knowledge of the "features" (i.e., parameters) of a particular stimulator that should most affect intervention planning (Box 10-2).

Waveforms

Patient comfort has been investigated in many studies. Three studies of note investigated comparative comfort with differing waveforms. Delitto and Rose[6] found that there was no clear choice among three symmetrical biphasic waveforms, and that different preferences existed for different patients. In a comparison of symmetrical and asymmetrical biphasic waveforms, Bowman and Baker[7] found that normal female subjects preferred the symmetrical waveform when a large muscle group (quadriceps) was stimulated. But in another, similar study,[8] it was found that when the target muscle groups were small (wrist flexors and extensors), normal subjects preferred an asymmetrical biphasic waveform. In a study comparing current frequencies with a symmetrical biphasic waveform,[9] the authors demonstrated a preference for higher frequencies when 30, 50, and 100 pulses per second (pps) were tested in stimulation of a tetanic contraction of the quadriceps muscle.

Different waveforms have also been investigated for the degree of torque and fatigue produced. In a study of quadriceps stimulation, monophasic and biphasic waveforms produced greater torque and less fatigue than polyphasic waveforms.[10]

Amplitude

Current amplitude (intensity) must be gradually increased when first introducing a stimulation program to a patient. A patient will become comfortable with the sensation of stimulation within the first 15 minutes of a gradually introduced stimulus amplitude, thereby becoming able to tolerate an increase in amplitude to achieve the desired muscle response. The desired muscle response can usually be accomplished within one or two sessions.

The quality of a stimulated muscle contraction is determined by a combination of many parameters, including stimulus amplitude, pulse duration, stimulus frequency, and duty cycle. Increasing the stimulus amplitude causes recruitment of additional nerve fibers (smaller fibers and fibers further from the electrode), leading to increased force of muscle contraction. There is a limit to the force increase observed once most of the muscle fibers have been recruited. Because most portable electrical stimulation devices use an arbitrary 0-to-10 scale for the amplitude control, it is difficult to quantify the amount of current delivered to the patient, and the therapist must rely on the muscular response seen and the patient's sensory tolerance. The amplitude of current needed to achieve the desired response will also vary from patient to patient because of differences in resistance (impedance). In obese patients, it may not be possible to achieve the desired muscle response because the motor nerve may be too "insulated" by the intervening layer of fatty tissue to allow sufficient stimulation without painful stimulation of the sensory nerves in the skin.

Pulse Duration

The pulse duration has a corresponding relationship with stimulus amplitude. This relationship can be seen by examination of a strength-duration curve. A short pulse duration (below 40 milliseconds) requires a much higher stimulus amplitude. A high stimulus amplitude is necessary to elicit a muscular response until a pulse duration over 40 milliseconds is chosen. When the pulse duration is set between 40 and 500 milliseconds, an increase in amplitude between 15 and 40 mA (a relatively small range) will give you the full range of muscular responses. Increasing the pulse duration above 500 milliseconds will not improve muscular responses (Fig. 10-1).

One of the primary differences between stimulators lies in the pulse duration available for use. High-voltage pulsed-current stimulators have short and usually fixed-pulse durations (generally not above 200 milliseconds). Most other units appropriate for NMES have generally pulse durations between 20 and 500 milliseconds. Whether the pulse duration is adjustable varies from unit to unit. A unit that has a pulse duration between 200 and 400 milliseconds will be more than adequate for NMES applications.

Pulse Rate

On many NMES units, the primary controls regulate amplitude and pulse rate (frequency). As pulse rate increases, the rate of motor nerve firing rises and the overlapping twitch response leads to a stronger contraction. However, one must recognize the difference between voluntary and an electrically induced contraction (see Chapter 8). An electrically induced contraction results in reverse motor unit recruitment (large superficial motor units are usually recruited first) with synchronous activity of nerve and muscle fibers. This relationship causes action potentials of nerve and muscle to be dependent on frequency; higher frequency leads to more rapid fatigue. To minimize fatigue, lower the pulse rate.

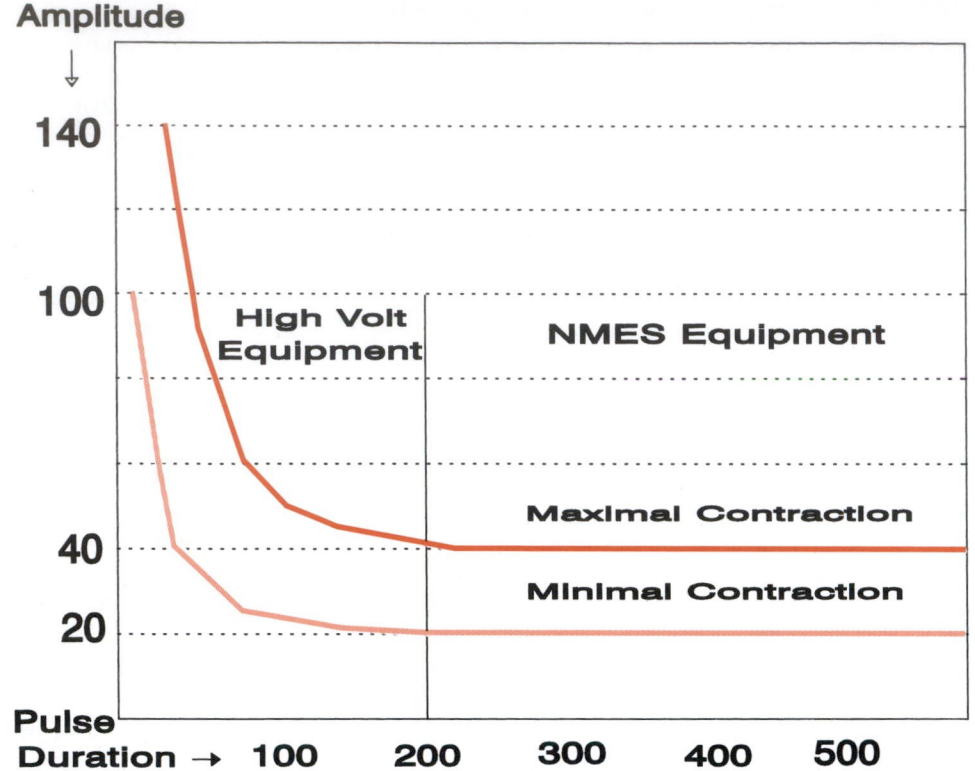

Figure 10-1 This annotated strength-duration curve demonstrates the inverse relationship between the amplitude of current and the pulse duration. The range of pulse duration available is one of the primary determinants of different classes of clinically available stimulation units.

Fused tetany can occur at frequencies as low as 12 pps, depending on the muscle.

Timing Modulation Duty Cycle On/Off Ratio

Another stimulus parameter that affects fatigue is the duty cycle or on/off ratio. Duty cycle is defined as "the ratio of on time to the total time of the trains of pulses or bursts."[11] Duty cycle is expressed as a percentage and calculated by dividing the on time by the total cycle time (on time + off time) and multiplying by 100. The on/off ratio is expressed in seconds and is calculated by dividing the on time by the off time. An example of a 1:3 ratio is where the on time is 4 seconds and the off time is 12 seconds (4/12 = 1:3).

The off time of the stimulation program represents the time during which a muscle is able to recover from the previous contraction and rest. Insufficient rest leads to rapid fatigue and limited success in achieving various intervention goals. The majority of clinical intervention paradigms utilize a 1:3 or 1:5 on/off ratio with the typical on time being 2 to 10 seconds. Total contractions for a typical 30-minute intervention session when a 1:5 on/off ratio is chosen are reduced by one half. Knowledge of this fact should influence the length of the intervention session.[11] The on time chosen can often affect patient comfort as well. Because there is a range of on times from 2 to 10 seconds, documentation should include both the ratio and the actual on time. Patients generally find

a contraction of 8 to 12 seconds in length to be very uncomfortable, sometimes likening it to a "charley horse" or cramp.

Ramp Modulation

A ramp is another possible modulation of the therapeutic current chosen. The current is gradually increasing or decreasing with a "plateau" of stimulation.[13] The ramping of the current can be achieved by

- A gradual increase of the amplitude, or
- Increase of pulse duration from zero to the maximum setting over a set time interval.

The perceived difference between a ramp of amplitude or pulse duration is "virtually indistinguishable"[13] and therefore is determined by the manufacturer in most devices and not often clearly identified for the user. The user must be aware that many devices include ramp time within the chosen on time. Therefore, to ensure that the stimulus reaches peak amplitude, the ramp time must be less than the on time. The usefulness of a ramp lies in the ability to "grade" the muscular response as it begins and ends with stimulation. Rarely do muscular movements occur abruptly. They are more commonly graded in intensity as the muscle fibers are recruited. This type of stimulated contraction is usually much more comfortable for a patient. A "ramp down" of the stimulation allows a more controlled return of the limb to its resting position than would a sudden drop that occurs if the stimulation ends abruptly. When determining the on/off ratio of a stimulation program, the on time is considered to be only the time of the "plateau" of maximum stimulation and the off time should be set accordingly. In most clinical paradigms, a ramp of 2 or less seconds is sufficient. Ramps of greater than 2 seconds are generally chosen when there is a very high level of stimulation required or with a spastic muscle that is sensitive to a rapid stretch.

General Guidelines for Clinical Applications

Patient Positioning

The patient should be positioned for comfort. A comfortable patient is best able to attend to the intervention program and can participate in reaching the therapeutic goals established. It is always worth the few extra minutes taken to achieve a comfortable starting position. Whenever possible, position a patient to allow him or her to see the results of a stimulated contraction. Visual feedback for the patient enhances sensory information and learning. Varying the patient's position during the course of an intervention will also enhance learning. For example, if the goal of an intervention is to achieve independent ankle dorsiflexion, the muscles for dorsiflexion might be stimulated first in a supported long sitting position; progress to sitting with feet on the floor; and then progress to standing. Finally, the contraction could be timed to coincide with the correct phase of the gait cycle.

When stimulating weakened muscles, careful attention to limb position can take advantage of the length-tension relationship to enhance muscular performance. For example, a quadriceps contraction would be enhanced with stimulation if the patient was positioned semireclined with a bolster under the knee. In this position, the quadriceps is mildly stretched and more likely to achieve a visible limb movement.

The intervention program must take into account range-of-motion (ROM) limitations either imposed by a joint instability or dictated by a surgeon following a reconstruction. For example, in the early phase of rehabilitation following an anterior cruciate ligament reconstruction of the knee, patients may not actively or passively extend the knee beyond a position of 45° of flexion to avoid stressing the newly repaired ligament. Patients can safely perform stimulation augmented quadriceps and hamstring exercises by using isokinetic equipment, which allows for range limitations and/or "locking" the limb into fixed positions for isometric exercise (Fig. 10-2).

Electrodes

Three decisions must be made with regard to electrodes: type, size, and placement. These issues are discussed in Chapter 9.

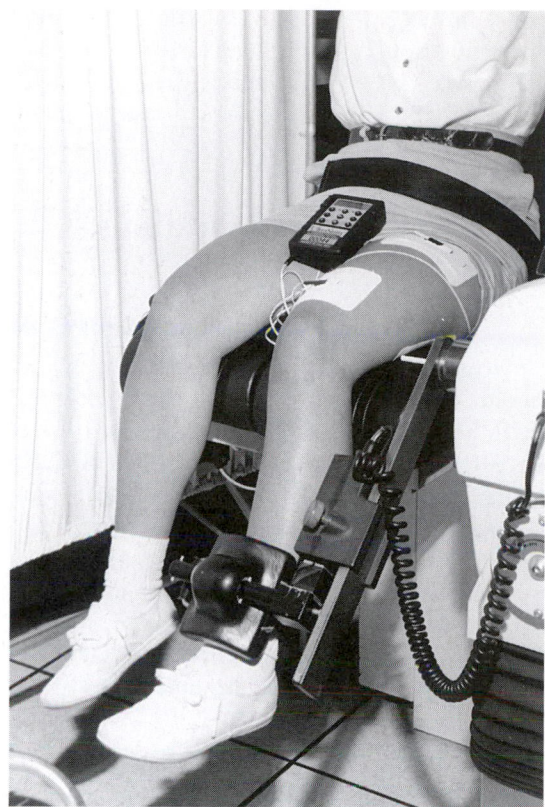

Figure 10-2   This patient setup illustrates how to exercise the quadriceps isometrically without endangering a recent anterior cruciate ligament repair. This setup can be used for isometric quadriceps contractions or co-contractions of the hamstrings and quadriceps. Note the carbon rubber electrodes secured by self-adhesive foam patches over the quadriceps muscle. Hamstring electrodes are not visible. *(Ultra Stim model 650-01; Neuromedics, Inc., Clute, TX.)* (Photograph courtesy of Kathy Goodstein, Shriners Hospital, Philadelphia Unit.)

A stimulated contraction will be most effective in meeting your goals if it closely approximates a "normal" contraction. In addition to the current modulations already discussed, it is important to attempt to achieve a "balanced" movement at the joint most affected by the muscle contraction. For example, in stimulating the wrist extensors, the goal is extension of the wrist without excessive ulnar or radial deviation. A balanced contraction most closely approximates a functional movement in most cases and provides the patient with the best opportunity to reexperience normal movement. Careful electrode placement with a small negative electrode over the (small) target muscle and an asymmetrical biphasic waveform will offer the best chance of success.

Duration and Frequency of Intervention

Clinical decision making becomes most difficult when considering the duration and frequency of an intervention. It is very dependent on the short-term goals, expected outcome, and patient response to an intervention. Frequent reexaminations will guide the decision to continue an intervention. The duration of an intervention will vary from as much as 6 weeks if the goal is muscle endurance, to as little as one intervention for muscle facilitation. A patient with an orthopedic injury and a "normal" nervous system will generally respond more quickly than will the patient with a neurologic disease or injury.

 ## Specific Clinical Applications

Strengthening and Endurance

The interest in using NMES to increase muscle strength was sparked after Russian athletes were observed being treated with ES during the 1976 Olympics. In 1977, a USSR physician, Dr. Kots, gave a series of lectures in Canada and made claims that ES with a "Russian current" stimulation protocol could lead to a 10% to 30% increase in muscular strength above what an athlete could achieve by conventional exercise regimens.[14] The Russian current he described has been investigated with mixed results. However, Kots's claims led to renewed interest in using other more familiar NMES devices and protocols to achieve strength gains in normal as well as patient populations.

Conventional exercise programs to increase strength are based on the overload principle of eliciting a small number of high-intensity contractions (at least 70% of a maximal contraction 3 to 10 repetitions or less) in an intervention session performed three to five times per week for 2 to 3 weeks. The same parameters of exercise apply when using NMES to augment strength in healthy and healthy-but-injured patient populations. There is compelling research evidence that NMES adds to the strength gains that normal individuals can achieve through conventional training programs alone.[15,16] However, in an intervention following limited traumatic or orthopedic injuries, NMES has been shown to lead to greater strength gains than those achieved with conventional exercise.[17-19]

Candidates for NMES can be any patients with multiple areas of weakness and deconditioning. These patients frequently benefit from a program that emphasizes endurance of the muscle or muscles of interest. This emphasis on endurance spotlights the other major function of a muscle, the ability to produce a force repetitively. Conventional endurance exercise programs consist of a decreased force of contraction and high repetitions (a Fair to Fair Plus contraction and a total of "30 to 60 minutes of stimulated contraction per day"[20]) in intervention sessions five to seven times per week for 2 to 10 weeks. Several shorter sessions during the course of the day make the exercise programs more manageable, but the total time of cycled stimulation must take into account the total on time (in this instance, including the ramp time).

An example of a patient with a musculoskeletal injury could be a woman with a reconstruction of her anterior cruciate ligament (ACL) because of a skiing injury. This patient

may not be allowed to fully extend her knee through an ROM against resistance in the early weeks of rehabilitation. One example of an intervention plan to enhance muscle performance could be as follows:

- Conventional exercise program to maintain right hip and ankle strength and overall aerobic capacity.
- NMES to increase isometric strength of the right quadriceps and hamstring muscles. Large rectangular electrodes should be used over large muscles like the quadriceps and hamstrings. Placing the proximal quadriceps electrode over the course of the femoral nerve near the femoral triangle will generally improve the muscular response.
- Ice to the right knee to control edema after exercise.

Results of studies using NMES have shown that superior isometric strengthening can be achieved in comparison to conventional isometric exercises.[20,21] The NMES program can be carried out in two ways: simultaneous stimulation of the quadriceps and hamstrings to achieve co-contraction with no net extension force or NMES to the quadriceps with the knee held in 45 degrees or more of flexion. In both instances, the use of an isokinetic machine to limit ROM and monitor the force produced by the stimulation program allows for safe exercise and quantitative information regarding improvement in force production (Fig. 10-2).

If the hamstrings and quadriceps are both stimulated, the two channels of stimulation must be synchronized and balanced for comfort and force production. Stimulation of the quadriceps alone requires only one channel of stimulation. Amplitude is adjusted to achieve a maximally tolerated isometric contraction.

An example of a patient with a neurological deficit is a woman with a left middle cerebral artery infarct who had a flaccid right hemiplegia initially but progressed to walking with a straight cane and molded ankle-foot orthosis (MAFO) on the right leg. She is able to ambulate without the MAFO, but her ankle dorsiflexors on the right fatigue within 20 feet. A typical intervention plan may include

- General conditioning exercises to improve overall fitness level
- Traditional strengthening exercises for all right leg muscle groups
- Closed-chain exercises, including use of a biomechanical ankle platform
- NMES endurance program for the right ankle dorsiflexors

It is important to achieve a "balanced" response in the foot (Fig. 10-3) and an ankle with a neutral position relative to inversion and eversion without clawing or hyperextension of the toes (Fig. 10-4). Trimming a 2 × 2-inch electrode down to a 1-inch circle will increase the current density over the

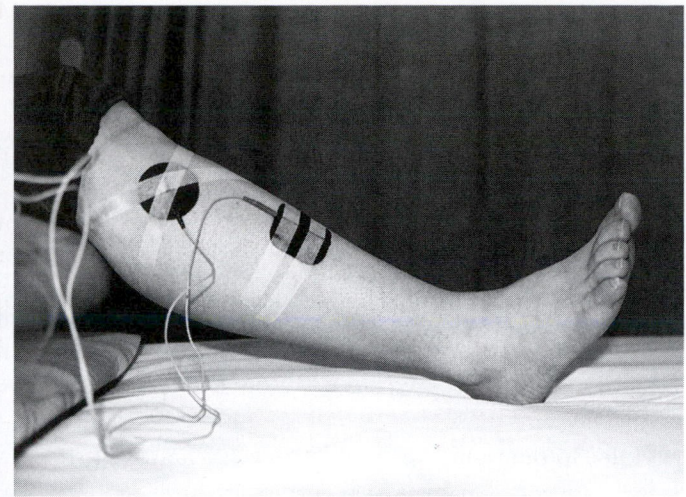

Figure 10-3   A balanced dorsiflexion response to NMES. Note electrode placement and extremity positioning.

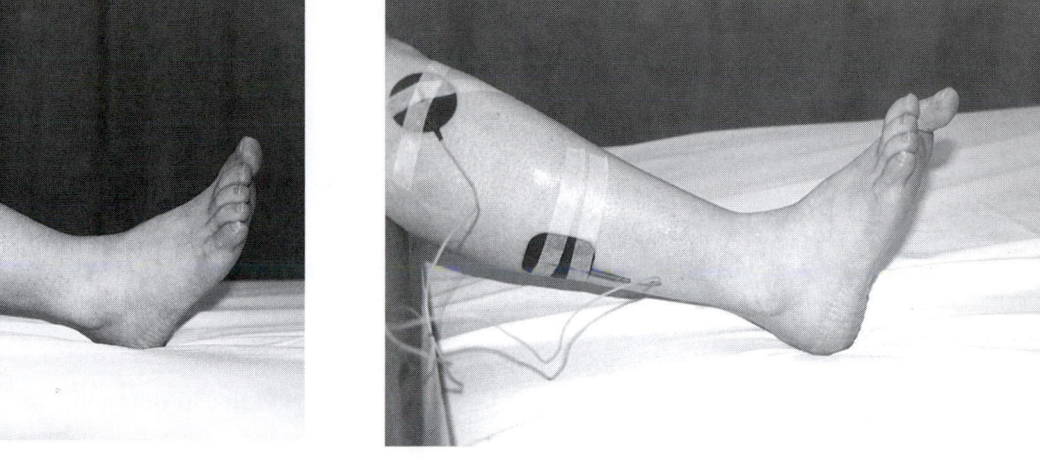

Figure 10-4   An unbalanced dorsiflexion response with excessive toe extension.

peroneal nerve proximally and usually improve the stimulated response. A portable NMES unit would be ideal to allow this patient to continue stimulation at home on a daily basis because endurance training requires an extended intervention protocol. See Box 10-3 for a suggested patient educational handout.

BOX 10-3   Educational Instructions for Home Use of Stimulator

Instructions for Home Use of Stimulator

Your treatment time is _____ minutes _____ times per day.

Your response to the treatment is dependent on your effort to adhere to the suggested program.

Preparing to Use the Stimulator

Clean the skin with mild soap and water in the area where you will place your electrodes.

Prepare your electrodes as instructed by your therapist and apply securely to the designated areas.

Connect the electrodes to the stimulator—be sure to insert all plugs completely so that there is no exposed metal.

Preparing to Exercise

Position yourself comfortably as instructed by your therapist.

Adjust the intensity control(s) until you experience a sensation and muscle response similar to your supervised exercise with your therapist.

Exercise for the length of time designated above.

Ending your Exercise Session

Turn the intensity control(s) to OFF.

Disconnect all of the wires by pulling on the plugs. (Do not pull on the wires!)

Remove the electrodes and clean/store as instructed by your therapist.

Precautions for Stimulator Usage

The stimulator is preprogrammed for your personal use only and should not be used on another part of your body or any other person.

It is recommended that the patient also be given a diagram of electrode placement or preferably a photograph.

Carefully inspect your skin in the electrode area before and after you apply the electrodes. Do not apply the electrodes to broken or irritated skin. Slight reddening of the skin under the electrodes is normal after stimulation. If you experience persistent skin irritation, stop using the stimulator until you see your therapist.

Do not bathe or shower while wearing the stimulator.

Troubleshooting

No stimulation felt—

- Recheck all connections.
- Recheck electrode contact with skin.
- Recheck or replace batteries.

Stimulation uncomfortable—

- Recheck electrode contact with skin.
- Readjust intensity controls.
- Check skin under electrode for irritation.

Stimulation intermittent—

- Check wires for a break.
- Check connections.
- Check electrode contact to skin.

Range of Motion

Methods to maintain ROM for some neurologically impaired and orthopedic patients are often taught to patients and their families. Passive ROM for neurologically impaired patients with mild spastic tone often has a good outcome. However, patients with moderate to severe spasticity tend to have difficulty making gains with passive ROM that may limit their daily functions. Patients with musculoskeletal impairments differ in that they have limited ROM as a result of immobilization of a muscle and/or a joint or pain.

A case example of a patient with a musculoskeletal impairment could include a male who has just had a cast removed because of a tibial fracture and is unable to fully extend his knee. An example of an intervention plan would be as follows:

- NMES of quadriceps muscle to achieve increased knee extension
- Home exercise program

It is important to avoid excessive knee joint compression when initiating this program to prevent increased joint irritation.

An example of a patient with a neurologic deficit would be a young woman with a closed head injury. The patient exhibits bilateral biceps spasticity with elbow flexion contractures. An example of an intervention plan is as follows:

- Serial casting
- NMES to the triceps muscle to restore elbow extension

In order to not limit her daily functions, such as self-feeding, the nondominant arm is treated first. The patient is casted in the available extension range, blocking flexion but not limiting extension while using NMES (Fig. 10-5). The time of ramp-up must be extended in this instance because of the spasticity present in the opposing muscle group. A ramp-up time of 6 to 8 seconds may be necessary to achieve a slow, effective stretch without increasing spasticity in the biceps by a quick stretch. Each week the serial cast should be removed and ROM measurements taken to document improvement. The serial cast is again applied in the available extension range, blocking flexion but not limiting extension to continue NMES sessions. In some instances a fabricated splint is preferred.

Facilitation or Retraining of Muscle

Following a neurologic injury or surgery (especially orthopedic surgery), a patient may have difficulty in initiating movement in a muscle group. This is especially the case if the patient has been unable to use the muscle for any length of time, leading to disuse atrophy, weakness, or pain. The central nervous system (CNS) relies heavily on the many forms of sensory feedback received to modulate performance. In the case of a neurologic injury, that feedback can be greatly affected by sensory loss or distortion and/or change in available movement strategies and tone. In the case of surgery, the motoneuron pool can be directly inhibited by the pain efferents, and it has been suggested that cutting of a joint capsule during surgery can affect the normal proprioceptor activity.[21]

The desired response is a voluntary contraction that is enhanced by the NMES to increase CNS feedback and motor learning. Timing and coordination are crucial to the relearning of motor skills. Therefore, it is important that the NMES

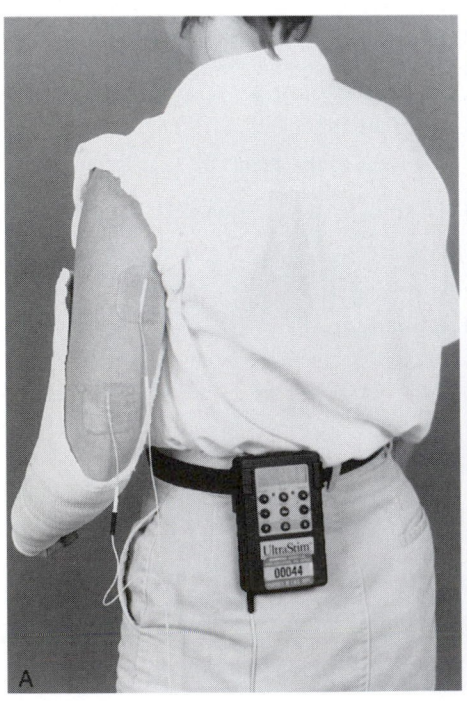
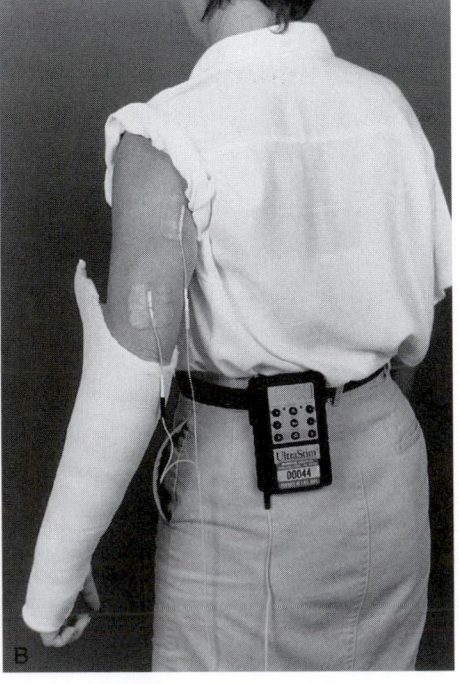

Figure 10-5 The "drop-out" cast required to achieve improved elbow extension range of motion. On the left side of the figure, elbow flexion is blocked by the front of the cast. On the right side of the figure, elbow extension is stimulated with the electrode placements illustrated to gain additional extension range. (*Ultra Stim model 650-01; Neuromedics, Inc., Clute, TX; Pals Reusable Neurostimulation Electrodes, Axelgaard Mfg. Co., Ltd, Fallbrook, CA.*) (Photograph courtesy of Kathy Goodstein, Shriners Hospital, Philadelphia Unit.)

occurs at the correct time in the anticipated motor response. The timing of the stimulus must be controlled by the therapist or patient by use of an external trigger that is generally a foot or hand switch.

Sometimes the contraction must be initiated by NMES, but in other situations the stimulation is used to augment a weak voluntary response or to allow stabilization via stimulation of a related muscle group. This type of NMES program is not generally used by patients independently, but it represents a powerful adjunct for the therapist during an intervention session. Facilitation, to be most effective, requires patient cooperation and timing of stimulation within functional tasks.

An example to emphasize these concepts would be a female who is status post a left total knee replacement (TKR). In attempting to teach the woman quadriceps isometric exercises, you realize that she, despite a strong effort, is unable to activate her quadriceps effectively. One example of an intervention plan is as follows:

- NMES to facilitate quadriceps activity
- Conventional exercises to maintain ipsilateral hip and ankle strength and prevent circulatory stasis
- Protected weight-bearing and gait training with appropriate assistive device when indicated
- Ice to the left knee to control edema after exercise

The location of the distal electrode over the quadriceps may have to be modified if staples are still present at the incision site because electrical current can concentrate around superficial metal and cause pain. The distal electrode should be moved more proximally (leaving a gap of at least 1 inch between the electrode and staples) so that the staples are not within the main current path. An alternative is to use an asymmetrical biphasic waveform and place the anode posteriorly on the hamstrings. This should ensure a comfortable stimulus for the patient. If not, NMES should be reconsidered, if needed, once the staples are removed. Close observations of the incision site is called for with an intervention to ensure that there is not excessive pull on a healing incision. If there is, a decreased amplitude may still be effective in giving a sensory cue for a quadriceps contraction. It is expected that this type of facilitation will be needed for only a short period of time because this patient has a normal CNS requiring possibly only one or two sessions of 15 to 20 minutes each before the patient is able to continue strengthening exercises on her own.

An example of a patient with a neurologic deficit would be a woman who had a left middle cerebral artery thrombosis 3 months prior to her initial examination. She has returned for additional therapy because she states that she has begun to move the fingers of her right hand. As part of a complete evaluation, it is found that she can actively flex and extend her fingers (although not through a complete range), but she cannot actively extend and stabilize the wrist, limiting her ability

to produce a functional grasp. One example of an intervention plan is as follows:

- Conventional rehabilitation to maximize motor learning for functional independence
- NMES to facilitate voluntary movement in right wrist extensors
- Functional training in conjunction with NMES as appropriate

It is important to cue this patient visually so that she can receive visual, kinesthetic, and cutaneous feedback and coordinate stimulation with volitional prehension activities.

The wrist and finger muscles are very close in the forearm and careful placement can include or eliminate activity in the fingers as desired. "Balanced" wrist extension without excessive ulnar or radial deviation is optimal. Trimming electrodes to small patches can help limit spread of the stimulus to other muscles. Also, carefully consider the path of the current between the electrode placements to limit spread of stimulation. This patient has an abnormal CNS and may have increased difficulty in recruiting some muscle groups, although the electrically stimulated response in this group can approach the torque achieved in an unimpaired muscle group.[22] Therefore, she may require more experience with NMES to be capable of activating her wrist extensors independently and appropriately and can then achieve close to normal torque. The intervention time could be as limited as 15 to 20 minutes per session, but the duration of an intervention might be as long as a week or two, especially if an effort is made to vary the motor learning experience by attempting functional activities such as grasp and release or different upper extremity positioning during wrist extension activation. If a patient is not successful with a trial of NMES because of her evolving neurologic status, it may be appropriate to try again at another time in the intervention course.

Management of Muscle Spasms (Guarding) and Spasticity

NMES is widely used to address pain by reducing the tension in a muscle in spasm because of injury. However, if the mechanism of improvement is not clear, high-frequency stimulation can lead to rapid muscle fatigue in a constantly active muscle. It is possible to break the so-called pain-spasm-pain cycle with relief of pain for up to several hours postintervention. This allows one to improve ROM and treat the particular areas of injury effectively.

In a patient with neurologic impairment, stimulating a spastic muscle causes relaxation similar to that of a muscle in spasm; however, the relaxation period is brief because of the continued underlying abnormality in the CNS. During this brief relaxation period, the extremity can be repositioned to allow casting or bracing to be applied effectively.

An example of a patient with musculoskeletal impairments would be a secretary who has been spending hours upon hours at the computer and has neck pain with muscle spasms of the right upper trapezius and rhomboids and limited rotation and forward flexion of the cervical spine with pain upon movement. When evaluated, the patient demonstrates acute muscle spasms with limited rotation and forward flexion because of pain with movement. One example of an intervention plan is as follows:

- Pulsed current (see Fig. 10-6 for an example of this application) to trapezius muscles
- Heat or ice is frequently used in conjunction with stimulation
- Home exercise program
- Patient education on sitting posture

This patient could benefit from either a bipolar or monopolar electrode placement (see Chapter 9). Documentation of the time frame of pain relief after an intervention will assist in determining the necessity to continue the electrical stimulation intervention.

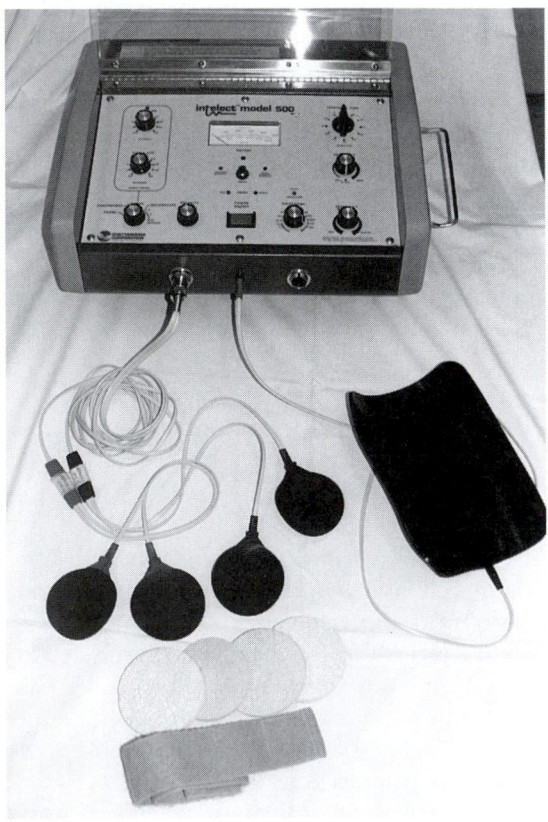

Figure 10-6 This unit illustrates the available adjustable parameters and electrode selection with one version of a clinical High Volt Pulsed Current Stimulation Unit (Intelect model 500; Chattanooga Corp, Chattanooga, TN).

Edema Reduction

Acute edema develops because of trauma to the blood vessels with leakage of blood cells and plasma proteins into the interstitial space. These blood components are negatively charged and, when exposed to a negative polarity, they are repelled from the area.[23] As a result, the excess fluid, because of its attachment to the negatively charged proteins, is also shifted from the area.[24] Chronic edema requires venous and lymphatic drainage that is enhanced by cyclic muscle contractions. Treatment of edema (both chronic and acute) typically includes ice application or cool water immersion, elevation, and compression. NMES can be an effective adjunct to these standard interventions.

An example of a patient with edema could be a construction worker who sustained a crush injury to the left hand 3 days ago. There were no fractures, but the patient has severe edema with limited ROM. An example of an intervention plan is as follows:

- NMES to the hand with the hand in elevation
- Elevation for exercising and rest
- Active ROM exercises as tolerated

Electrodes would be placed over the volar and dorsum of the hand with the hand in elevation. The reduction of edema will be most effective if the muscles within the hand (the intrinsics) contract, so the active electrode should be moved to maximize the intrinsic activity. The current should be adjusted to elicit a brief but effective contraction of the local muscles (frequency of 20 to 50 pps). Continuation of an intervention is based on edema reduction.

Orthotic Substitution

The ability to activate innervated but inactive, paretic, or paralyzed muscle has proved to be an effective replacement for orthotics in the management of deformity, or to assist purposeful movement. Beginning in the 1960s, a great deal of research took place with what has come to be called functional electrical stimulation, or FES. This continuing research explores many areas, including the restoration of standing and ambulation in paraplegic patients (Fig. 10-7), a dorsiflexion assist for hemiplegic patients, and surface stimulation to substitute for bracing in idiopathic scoliosis.[25-27] Many of the functional activities in which FES offers promise are complex activities (such as walking) requiring multiple channels of stimulation and feedback to allow the stimulation to be modulated to meet varying conditions. These crude systems are experimental presently.

Electrical stimulation to activate the ankle dorsiflexors in the swing phase of the gait cycle is widely used in the clinic because of the repetitive, rarely varying nature of the movement (Fig.10-8). The system requires a portable electrical stimulator with an external switch under the heel and one

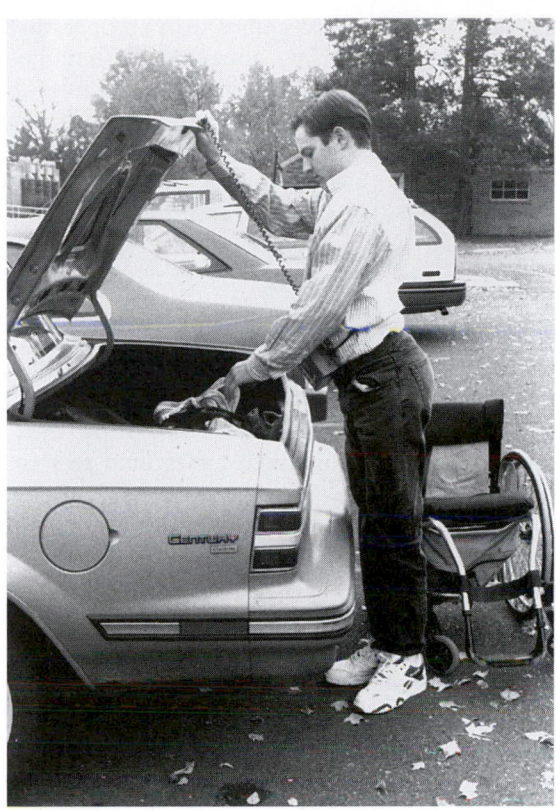

Figure 10-7   This research participant is a T4 level paraplegic who is pictured using an experimental, multichannel neuromuscular stimulator (worn at his waist) to achieve standing without bracing. *(Photograph courtesy of Kathy Goodstein, Shriners Hospitals, Philadelphia Unit.)*

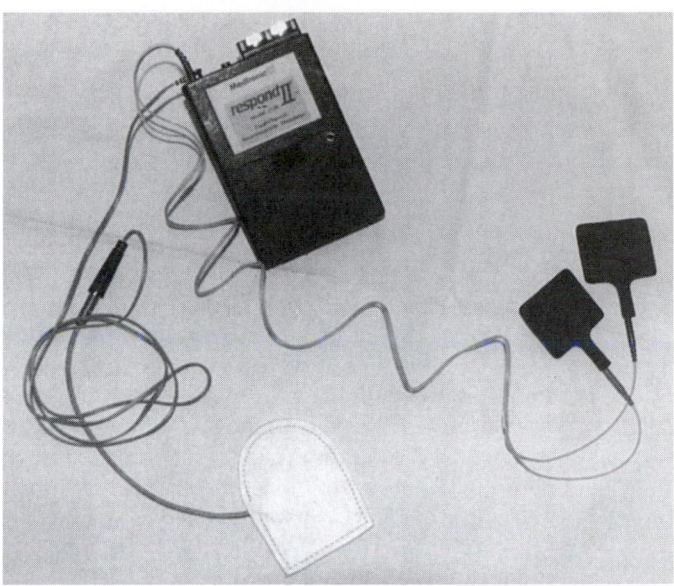

Figure 10-9   This unit is a commonly available portable unit for NMES with two channels of stimulation and an optional external heel switch to time the stimulated contraction with the gait cycle. *(Respond II FES Unit, model 90003108; Medtronic Corp, San Diego, CA.)*

clinical application of NMES as an orthotic substitute first requires the development of muscular endurance described earlier in this chapter. Baker and associates[28] have clearly described an FES program to address shoulder subluxation, which can accompany the flaccid paralysis of a cerebrovascular accident.

Partial Denervation

NMES can be effective in retraining a muscle that is recovering its innervation following a peripheral nerve injury. The reinnervation process following a nerve injury is slow, unpredictable, and seldom complete. The degree of expected

channel of stimulation (Fig. 10-9). The stimulation is activated by the heel rising off the floor at the end of stance leading to stimulation of the ankle dorsiflexors to allow toe clearance during swing.

Because of the repetitive nature of the muscular activity necessary to achieve long-term substitution for orthotics, any

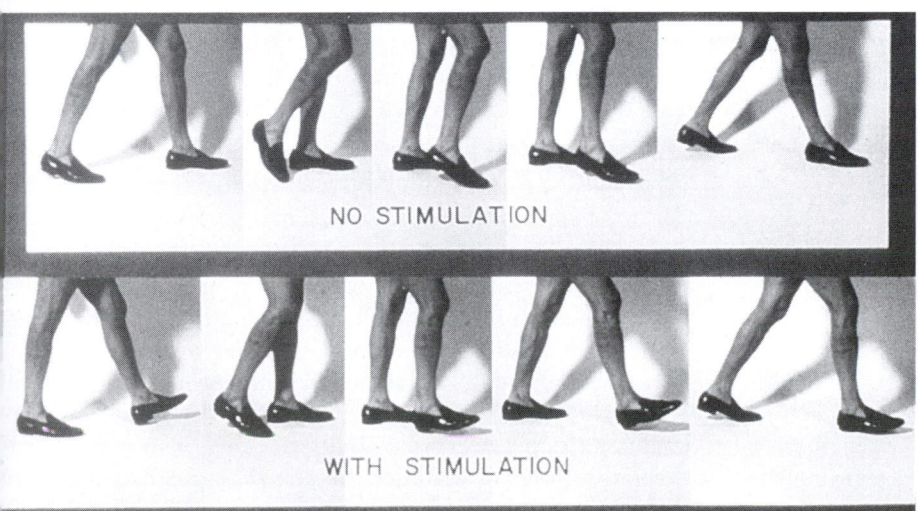

Figure 10-8   This is a comparison of the swing phase of the right lower extremity with and without the aid of timed NMES. The patient seen here had experimental implanted electrodes instead of the clinically used surface electrodes. *(From Los Amigos Research and Education Institute, Downey, CA, with permission.)*

function is difficult to predict and depends on many factors, including the

- Degree of atrophy
- Mechanism and extent of the nerve injury
- Time since the injury

With the paresis or paralysis associated with a peripheral nerve injury comes a "disconnection" of the CNS to the particular muscle(s).

With reinnervation, many patients find that they are no longer able to activate the muscle without the sensory cues associated with NMES: cutaneous, kinesthetic, and visual. The otherwise normal CNS readily accommodates allowing the patient to begin to "reconnect" and initiate movement. In addition the muscle strength can increase, usually within only a few sessions. It is difficult, however, to predict the muscular response achievable, given limited knowledge of the innervation status.

An example of a patient with partial denervation would be a man who experienced a peroneal nerve injury during a right total knee replacement 9 months ago. The patient has needed an ankle-foot arthrosis (AFO) on the right because of a foot drop since surgery, and he is unable to actively dorsiflex the right ankle. According to the results of an EMG, the tibialis anterior muscle is reinnervating; however, the patient is unable to perform a volitional contraction. An example of an intervention plan is as follows:

- NMES to reeducate reinnervating muscle
- Conventional strengthening exercises if patient learns to contract voluntarily
- Gait training with externally triggered NMES if appropriate to progress to ambulation without AFO

In the presence of partial denervation, the motor point placement is difficult to predict with motor points moving more distally in most instances.[29,30] A stimulus with a longer pulse duration is preferable in the presence of partial denervation. The patient may have to be followed monthly or quarterly to assess reinnervation status until a Fair Minus or Fair contraction can be generated volitionally. Reinnervation is difficult to predict and requires frequent reexamination.

Safety Considerations

Equipment

It is the clinician's responsibility to ensure the safety and proper operation of all equipment. Inspection of equipment before use is an important safety measure that should be implemented as routine. A professional inspection of equipment should be scheduled yearly with a sticker clearly showing the date of the last inspection.

Every piece of equipment comes with an operating manual. Take the time to read the manual, which should be readily available. Equipment should never be operated if the user is not thoroughly familiar with its operation. Although the clinician's safety is an important factor when using electrical equipment, the patient's safety is obviously paramount. Refer to Chapter 8 for details on safety conditions.

Patient Factors

Medical History

It is recommended that before an intervention the patient should be questioned relative to the indications and contraindications of the modality being used. At the time of the examination, the patient may have forgotten to mention a possible problem or may have developed a problem that could make the application of the modality questionable. Thus, it is good practice to interview the patient prior to all interventions.

Skin Condition and Sensation

A visual inspection of the area to be treated will identify both normal and abnormal skin conditions. Normal findings may include birthmarks or other skin discolorations that will remain after an intervention is given. Observations should be clearly documented in the patient's medical chart to inform other therapists who may provide the intervention and to enable the treating therapist to identify any change in skin conditions that may result from an intervention.

After an intervention, the stimulated skin area may be pink as a result of an increase in the superficial blood flow that results from an intervention. These changes should resolve within 30 to 60 minutes following the treatment. If the area remains quite red and/or color changes do not resolve, an electrical burn may have occurred and the patient must be treated immediately with the appropriate first aid. Maintenance of a good interface between the electrode and the patient by using an adequate amount of gel, complete contact of the electrode with the skin, and adequate fixation will prevent tissue damage.

Your communication with and observation of the patient and the area being treated are critical. Careful selection of waveform, pulse duration, and electrodes will prevent tissue damage from stimulation electrodes.

Cognitive Issues

Cognition, psychologic abilities, and neuromuscular performance are interdependent. Impairment of cognition may be identified during the examination and relayed to you, or you may identify cognitive impairment through your careful observations and good communication. Cognitive impairments include a decreased ability to learn or understand instructions or an inability to translate instructions into expected outcomes. Clear and concise communication is essential. The use of visual and tactile cues will be beneficial. Demonstration and feeling a normal muscular contraction on an unaffected body part may be one way to explain the goal of muscle reeducation clearly. Remember that most patients do not have medical backgrounds. The use of laypersons' terms to describe procedures is important.

Cognitive dysfunction can be incorrectly translated to poor motivation. Clinicians must continuously encourage and reinforce positive results throughout the intervention. Patient understanding can be determined by asking the patient to repeat the instructions, the process, and the expected outcomes. Most important, help the patient understand why the intervention is needed and how it will relate to his or her everyday activities.

Lack of cognition does not prohibit the use of electrical stimulation. Electrical stimulation has been found to be very effective in decreasing spasticity and improving ROM in comatose patients.[31] Careful observation is mandatory for safety in this application.

Patient Education

Expected Outcomes

Expected outcomes are directly related to the patient's education and understanding before, during, and after an intervention. Patients must understand the reason for the intervention, the process of the intervention, and the outcomes and benefits of the intervention. Explaining the rationale for intervention will allow the patient the opportunity to communicate his or her needs, which then can be incorporated into the intervention plan. The reason for intervention is usually identified or most understood in functional terms. Electrical stimulation for muscle reeducation to the quadriceps may benefit the patient in transfers or ambulation potential. It is important to communicate the expected outcome and not provide false hope to the patient.

Explaining procedures used during the intervention process and the expected sensations will reduce the patient's fears and anxieties. Education and understanding of these procedures and sensations will allow the patient to better communicate and give the therapist feedback with which to maximize the intervention.

Proper education of the expected outcomes and benefits is crucial. Clinicians must understand these outcomes prior to the initiation of an intervention and appropriately utilize them with each patient. Electrical stimulation has many uses in physical therapy as was previously discussed. Electrical stimulation may be used for muscle relaxation as in the case of spasticity. Achievement of this relaxation may assist antagonist muscles to function, or improve mobility through increased ROM. Muscle reeducation is commonly seen

with the use of electrical stimulation. Increased strength and utilization of extremities are often seen as volitional control is redeveloped. Reduction of swelling and edema through the utilization of electrical stimulation can also enhance ROM and use of extremities in all facets of activities of daily living.

Clinical Decision Making

Evaluating Intervention Effectiveness and Modifying the Intervention

Goals should be realistically and reliably achieved. A thorough understanding of the application of electrotherapy is very important to its use, especially because it is not a modality that is readily understood by many physicians or insurance companies, much less the patients who will experience it. It is equally important to be able to assess the outcome of the intervention once initiated. It is impossible to do so without timely, appropriate, and reliable measurements of the patient's physical status before, during, and after the intervention. On a daily basis, it is important to assess skin integrity, patient's response to the last intervention, and any complaints of discomfort or change in symptoms.

Documenting an Intervention

At examination and subsequent regular reexaminations, other measurements of status are made. Although the issue of reliability of clinical measurements is beyond the scope of this chapter, certain types of measurement have been accepted as generally reliable. Isokinetic examinations of strength are frequently used and in many cases have been shown to be very reliable for the examination of strength and endurance.[32] Active and passive ROM measurements are very useful in documenting progress in contracture management and motor control. It is frequently important to measure both active and passive ROM. In the examination of edema and hypertrophy, girth measurements at reproducible landmarks with a nonstretch measuring tape are frequently used. Volumetric measurements of the amount of water displaced by a limb are also reliable though rarely used. Accurate descriptions of gait or movement patterns and measurement of the temporal aspects of gait with a stopwatch are all useful, and when available, videotaping of the patient's performance is especially helpful.

The use of NMES to address the wide variety of patient scenarios presented in this chapter requires a familiarity with the equipment available in your facility and the characteristics of the available waveforms and stimulation parameters available with that equipment. Portable equipment in general will be less powerful, have fewer adjustable parameters, and can be more prone to damage. Clinical models will be potentially more versatile (for applications such as iontophoresis and wound healing, which are beyond the scope of this chapter), but less portable and more powerful, with a greater likelihood of causing tissue damage.

As stated previously, patient comfort is of primary importance because an intervention that cannot be tolerated is an ineffective treatment. It is very important for the patient to be monitored closely during the initial intervention sessions to assess comfort and whether a change in parameters should be considered.

Summary

In this chapter, the application of NMES as a clinical modality has been briefly reviewed. Understanding the rationale for using NMES when making clinical decisions for your patients will ultimately be reflected in their progress. This broad topic merits additional study through further reading.

Acknowledgments

The authors would like to thank Jean Scofield from Rancho Los Amigos for her assistance with photograph permission; Kathy Goodstein from Shriners Hospitals, Philadelphia Unit, for photography; Shriners Hospitals, Philadelphia Unit, Research Department for their support; and Elizabeth R. Gardner, MS, PT, NCS, Linda Baird-Jansen, MS, PT, Betsy Butterworth, PTA, Vicki Vanartsdalen, PTA, and Sophia Mullin Selgrath for their editorial recommendations. Most important, thanks to Andy, Alex, and Ellen for their understanding, love, and support.

Discussion Questions

1. What are the sensory and motor effects of altering current, amplitude, and pulse duration?
2. When stimulating a patient, what is the importance of the current path?
3. If a patient has external metal on his or her skin such as staples, can electrical stimulation be used, and why should your placement of the electrodes be carefully considered?
4. When stimulating the ankle, should you be concerned with deviations such as inversion and eversion? What can you do to address these deviations produced by the electrical stimulation?
5. What size surface electrode would you choose when stimulating the gluteus maximus, and why is the size of the surface electrode important?

Researching The Literature

An essential reference is Electrotherapeutic Terminology in Physical Therapy—Revision 2000, which is available from The American Physical Therapy Association at their website: www.apta.org.

References

1. Electrotherapeutic Terminology in Physical Therapy. Section on Clinical Electrophysiology: American Physical Therapy Association, Alexandria, VA, 1990, p 29.
2. Nelson, RM, and Currier, DP: Clinical Electrotherapy. Appleton and Lange, Norwalk, CT, 1987, p 110.
3. Baker, LL, et al: Neuromuscular Electrical Stimulation: A Practical Clinical Guide, ed 3. Los Amigos Research and Education Institute, Downey, CA, 1993, p 73.
4. Baker, LL, et al: Neuromuscular Electrical Stimulation: A Practical Clinical Guide, ed 3. Los Amigos Research and Education Institute, Downey, CA, 1993, p 75.
5. Snyder-Mackler, L, and Robinson, AJ: Clinical Electrophysiology—Electrotherapy and Electrophysiologic Testing. Williams & Wilkins, Baltimore, 1989, p 131.
6. Delitto, A, and Rose, SJ: Comparative comfort of three waveforms used in electrically eliciting quadriceps femoris muscle contractions. Phys Ther 66:1704, 1986.
7. Bowman, BR, and Baker, LL: Effects of waveform parameters on comfort during transcutaneous neuromuscular electrical stimulation. Ann Biomed Eng 13:59, 1974.
8. Baker, LL, Bowan, BR, and McNeal, DR: Effects of waveform on comfort during neuromuscular electrical stimulation. Clin Orthop Related Res 233:75, 1988.
9. McNeal, DR, et al: Subject preference for pulse frequency with cutaneous stimulation of the quadriceps. Proc Rehabil Eng Soc North Am 9:273, 1986.
10. Laufer, Y, Ries, JD, Leininger, PM, and Alon, G: Quadriceps femoris muscle torques and fatigue generated by neuromuscular electrical stimulation with three different waveforms. Phys Ther 81:1307–1316, 2001.
11. Electrotherapeutic Terminology in Physical Therapy. Section on Clinical Electrophysiology: American Physical Therapy Association, Alexandria, VA, 1990, p 25.
12. Baker, LL, et al: Neuromuscular Electrical Stimulation: A Practical Clinical Guide, ed 3. Los Amigos Research and Education Institute, Downey, CA, 1993, p 87.
13. Electrotherapeutic Terminology in Physical Therapy. Section on Clinical Electrophysiology: American Physical Therapy Association, Alexandria, VA, 1990, p 21.
14. Ward, AR, and Shkuratova, N: Russian Electrical Stimulation: The Early Experiments. Phys Ther 82:1019–1030, 2003.
15. Currier, DP, and Mann, R: Muscular strength development by electrical stimulation in healthy individuals. Phys Ther 63:915, 1983.
16. Robinson, AJ, and Snyder-Mackler, L (eds): Clinical Electrophysiology—Electrotherapy and Electrophysiologic Testing, ed 2. Williams & Wilkins, Baltimore, 1995, pp 129–130.
17. Delitto, A, et al: Electrically elicited co-contraction of thigh musculature after anterior cruciate ligament surgery. Phys Ther 68:45, 1988.
18. Selkowitz, DM: Improvement in isometric strength of the quadriceps femoris muscle after training with electrical stimulation. Phys Ther 6:186, 1985.
19. Lewek, M, Stevens, J, and Snyder-Mackler, L: The use of electrical stimulation to increase quadriceps femoris muscle force in an elderly patient following total knee arthroplasty. Phys Ther 81:1565–1571. 2001.

20. Baker, LL, et al: Neuromuscular Electrical Stimulation: A Practical Clinical Guide, ed 3. Los Amigos Research and Education Institute, Downey, CA, 1993, p 51.

21. Draper, V, and Ballard, L: Electrical stimulation versus electromyographic biofeedback in the recovery of quadriceps femoris muscle function following anterior cruciate ligament surgery. Phys Ther 71:455, 1991.

22. Landau, WM, and Sahrmann, SA: Preservation of directly stimulated muscle strength in hemiplegia due to stroke. Arch Neurol 59:1453–1457, 2002.

23. Sawyer, P (ed): Biophysical Mechanisms in Homeostasis and Intravascular Thrombosis. Appleton-Century-Crofts, New York, 1965.

24. Nelson, RM, and Currier, DP: Clinical Electrotherapy. Appleton and Lange, Norwalk, CT, 1987, p 176.

25. Phillips, CA: Functional electrical stimulation and lower extremity bracing for ambulation exercise of the spinal cord injured individual: A medically prescribed system. Phys Ther 69:842, 1989.

26. Baker, LL: Neuromuscular electrical stimulation in the restoration of purposeful limb movements. In Wolf, SL (ed): Clinics in Physical Therapy—Electrotherapy. Churchill Livingstone, New York, 1981, p 25.

27. Eckerson, LF, and Axelgaard, J: Lateral electrical surface stimulation as an alternative to bracing in the treatment of idiopathic scoliosis. Phys Ther 64:483, 1984.

28. Baker, LL, and Parker, K: Neuromuscular electrical stimulation of the muscles surrounding the shoulder. Phys Ther 66:1930, 1986.

29. Richardson, AT, and Wynn-Parry, CB: The theory and practice of electrodiagnosis. Ann Phys Med 4:3, 1957.

30. Wynn-Parry, CB: Strength duration curves. In Licht, S (ed): Electrodiagnosis and Electromyography, ed 2. Elizabeth Licht, 1961, p 241.

31. Baker, LL, Parker, K, and Sanderson, D: Neuromuscular electrical stimulation for the head injured patient. Phys Ther 63:1967, 1983.

32. Farrell, M, and Richards, JG: Analysis of the reliability and validity of the kinetic communicator exercise device. Med Sci Sports Exer 18:44, 1986.

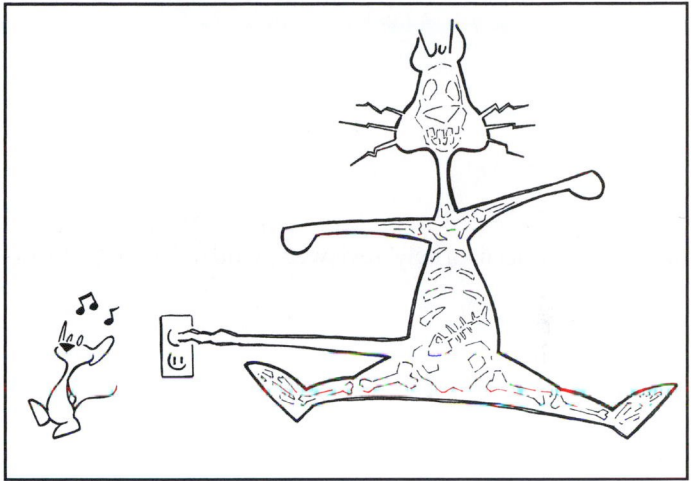

Objectives

- Describe the use of electrical stimulation for medication delivery.
- Outline the medications used and their polarity.
- Discuss the classifications of wounds.
- Discuss the electrical potentials of normal and injured tissues.
- Outline the application of electrical stimulation to promote tissue repair.
- Discuss documentation of or electrical stimulation for wound care.

Key Terms

Alternating current	Autolytic debridement	Diabetes mellitus	Pressure
Antimicrobial	Bipolar	Direct current	Pulsed current
Arterial insufficiency	Blood flow	Galvanotaxis	Venous insufficiency
	Current of injury	Monopolar	
		Polarity	

Ute H. Breese, PT, MEd, OCS   *Peter C. Panus, PT, PhD*   *Elizabeth Buchanan, PT*

Electrical Stimulation for Tissue Repair

Outline

Physical therapy…"The science of healing. The art of caring"

The use of electrical stimulation as a therapeutic intervention has its beginning in the 1700s. Work during this time included the discovery of direct current by Luigi Galvani in 1791, the invention of the alternating current induction motor by Nikola Tesla in 1882, and demonstration of the "current of injury" by Carlo Matteucci in the 1800s. This "current of injury" is the production of an electrical current by injured tissue, and is believed to activate the body's healing response to the wounded tissue.[1-3]

Electrical stimulation for wounds has been defined as "…the use of a capacitive coupled electrical circuit to transfer energy to a wound."[4] A complete description of electrical stimulation devices, terminology, and definitions is beyond the scope of this chapter; for greater detail, the reader is advised to consult additional sources of information and previous chapters in this text.

Although electrical stimulation has been used to promote healing of bone and other musculoskeletal injuries, this chapter will focus on how electrical stimulation has been used in the healing process of wounds. The first part of this chapter will review the cascade of wound repair, and then center on the proposed mechanisms by which electrical stimulation may affect tissue repair. The next part of the chapter will discuss the conclusions of research studies on the effectiveness of electrical stimulation in healing wounds. The final part of the chapter will review the literature on the protocols for clinical procedures using electrical stimulation for tissue healing. While stimulation parameters and mechanism of tissue healing have yet to be completely defined, the underlying

Patient Perspective

Remember, your patient will be very cautious and curious about what you are going to do. It is important to thoroughly explain what you are going to do and what would be reasonable for your patient to expect. This type of application is very "new" to most patients and some might be skeptical about the potential benefits. Explain them to your patients.

PATIENT COMMENTS

The wound seems to be healing a lot better since starting the electrical stimulation.

 Why Do I Need to Know About...

INFLAMMATION

Inflammation is an important step in the healing process that must take place in preparation for tissue repair.

conclusion of many studies is that electrical stimulation may be of benefit in tissue repair.[2, 5-15]

 ## Cascade of Injury Repair: How Do Wounds Heal?

The healing model that is discussed in this section is that of an acute full-thickness integumentary wound. Chronic full-thickness wounds are thought to heal by a similar process, but these wounds may be hindered in their progression toward healing due to various factors that are yet to be fully identified.[4] For a more detailed discussion, the reader is referred to wound care texts.[4,16,17] When damaged, wound tis-

sue healing generally follows three phases of repair that coincide and overlap to some extent (Fig. 11-1). The following description characterizes the three phases.

When the integument is damaged, an inflammatory process occurs that allows the body to seal off the area, prevent the spread of a potential infectious process, and halt the bleeding of tissues. This process lasts for 3 to 7 days[4] and is defined as the inflammatory phase. In this phase, hemostasis occurs during the first hours, and vasoconstriction is followed by a localized vasodilation and arrival of cells, including polymorphonuclear cells and macrophages. The process of migration of these cells to the site of injury by way of a chemical signal is called chemotaxis.[18] These cells help rid the injury site of the associated tissue debris or pathogenic organisms.[16] When the wound is clean, the second phase of injury repair may begin.

The second phase is termed the proliferative phase, and this phase is characterized by several events, including the formation of new blood vessels (angiogenesis or neovascularization), and the production of an extracellular matrix to fill the defect within the tissues. The matrix repair occurs through

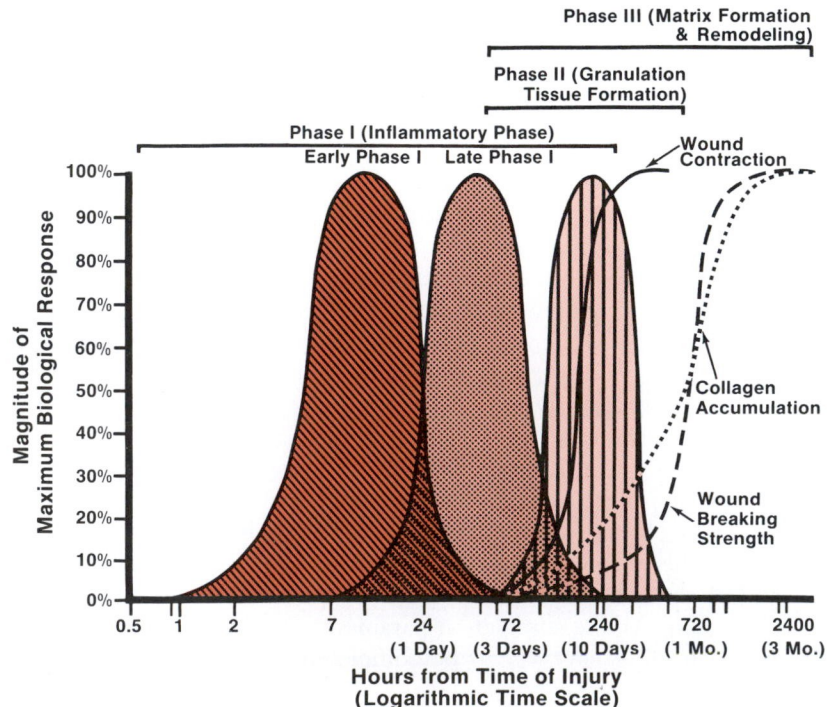

Figure 11-1 The phases of wound healing. (Reprinted with permission from Kisner, RS, and Bogensberger, G: The normal process of healing. In Kloth, LC, and McCulloch, JM [eds]: Wound Healing Alternatives in Management, ed 3. FA Davis, Philadelphia, 2002, pp 3-34.)

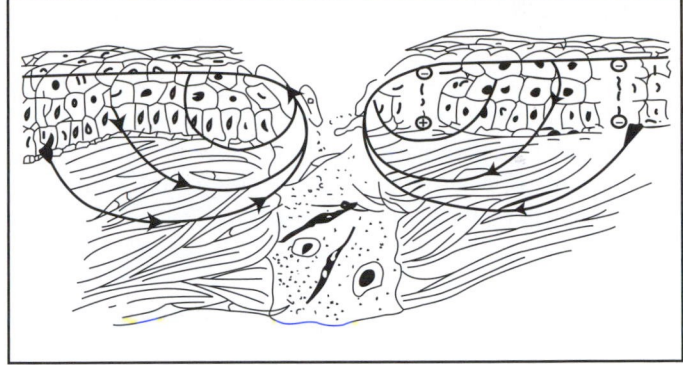

Figure 11–2 The "current of injury" flows out from the wound, and returns to the battery via the sodium ion pump. (Reprinted with permission from Sussman, C, and Byl, NN: Electrical stimulation for wound healing. In Sussman, C, and Bates-Jensen, BM [eds]: Wound Care, ed 2. Aspen Publishers, Gaithersburg, MD, 2001, pp 497–545.)

the formation of granulation tissue that acts as the foundation for scar tissue development.[19] The main cell involved in this process is the fibroblast. Another event that occurs during the proliferative phase is that of wound contraction. Wound contraction consists of myofibroblast activity within the wound bed acting to pull the edges of the wound together.[17] Additionally, throughout the first two phases of healing, and especially in the second phase, epithelial cells regenerate and migrate from the margin to the center of the wound.[19]

The third phase is the remodeling phase. This process can last for as long as 2 years following wound closure.[17] In this phase, the amount of collagen in the healing tissue increases, and there is a gradual conversion from type III collagen to type I collagen.[16] During the remodeling phase, the initial highly disorganized and weak scar is transformed into a more organized and stronger scar, with progression from a raised and reddened scar to a thinner, less bulky, and more elastic scar.[4,16,17,20]

Electrical Stimulation for Tissue Repair: What Are the Findings?

There are many theories as to how electrical stimulation can promote the healing of tissues. Some of the main concepts and proposed mechanisms of healing are described in this section, but it is important to note that definitive explanations for the effect of electrical stimulation on healing tissues have yet to be fully defined.

The Current of Injury

Injured tissue has been found to produce a measurable "current of injury."[21–23] This current applies to the presence of the skin battery potential, in which negative potentials exist in the stratum corneum with respect to the underlying dermis.[24] Normally, intact skin creates a barrier that results in a transepithelial potential between the dermis and epidermis of the skin. The transepithelial potential is believed to be produced by the sodium (Na^+) ion pump.[23,25] When the skin is damaged, the difference in potential is believed to be the source of the "current of injury" that occurs as a result of an interruption in the barrier,[22] and a lateral voltage gradient exists in the skin at the edge of the wound[23,26] (Fig. 11-2).[23,26] A flow of current with a positive polarity occurs within the wound.[22,23]

This current has been suggested as a trigger to wound healing[1–3] and also appears to be associated with the moist wound-healing process.[3] Experimental research has shown that wounds that are permitted to dry cease demonstrating a postwounding current of injury, while wounds that are kept moist maintain a postwounding current of injury.[23] The value of the moist wound healing process has been described,[17,27,28] and the association between the current of injury and the moist wound-healing process has been proposed as one reason why the rate of healing in dry wounds is reduced compared with moist wounds.[4,25] Further support for the beneficial effect of the current of injury is supported by an experimental study in which transepithelial sodium transport was inhibited, resulting in a reduced current of injury and reduced wound healing.[29]

Scientists have suggested that the use of exogenous electrical stimulation influences the current of injury and the lateral electric field that exists in areas of skin disruption.[22] Electrical stimulation may mimic the body's own bioelectric currents, and thus reinitiate or facilitate the wound-healing process,[4,24,25,30] although the actual contribution of the Na^+ current of injury to wound healing has not been determined.[16]

The positive wound potential is believed to serve as an indicator of healing: when the wound closes over, the positive potential disappears.[22] However, an experimental study has reported changes in the polarity of wounds as healing progresses.[21] In this study, the current within the wound was initially positive during the first 3 to 4 days following injury, and then became negative during the subsequent days of healing. This finding is of interest in view of electrical stimulation protocols in which the polarity of the treatment electrode is alternated during the healing process. Several clinical studies have used such protocols,[2,7,8,14,31] whereas others have used the same polarity for the treatment electrode throughout the study's duration.[9,10]

Galvanotaxis

Galvanotaxis describes the process in which cells possessing a positive or negative charge are attracted to an electric field of opposite polarity.[16] As a result, the positively or negatively charged cells that normally respond to injury may be attracted to the positive or negative pole of the stimulating electrode, depending on the cell's polarity.[16,17,30] This concept is supported by the findings of several in vitro studies in which the cells involved in tissue repair were found to be preferentially attracted to one pole of the stimulating electrode.[32,33] Neutrophils are attracted to the positive pole of the stimulating electrode at pH 8.0 to pH 6.8, and to the negative pole at pH 4.9.[32] Macrophages are attracted to the positive pole,[33] whereas fibroblasts have maximum stimulation of protein and DNA synthesis when in proximity to the negative pole.[34] Isolated epidermal cells, cell clusters, and cell sheets migrate toward the negative pole in DC electric fields of 0.5 to 15 V/cm.[35] However, basic science research results show enhanced epithelialization of partial thickness wounds by a regimen of an initial day of negative polarity followed by 7 days of positive polarity using monophasic pulsed current.[36] These results were found in comparison to other regimens consisting of only negative polarity; only positive polarity; or daily alternating negative and positive polarities. Results from another study, using high-voltage monophasic pulsed current, suggested a higher rate of epithelialization (compared with a control group) in dermal wounds stimulated using a regimen of three days negative polarity followed by 4 days positive polarity of the treatment electrode.[37]

Antimicrobial Effects

Electrical stimulation has been demonstrated to have a bacteriostatic or bacteriocidal effect on various pathogenic organisms that are commonly found to infect wounds.[38–43] Caution is recommended in applying the results of these studies to predict the effectiveness of electrical stimulation on pathogenic organisms in the clinical treatment of wounds. This is because of the difficulties inherent in applying the results of in vitro studies[38–41,43] to predict in vivo behavior, and in the use of studies with acute wounds in animals[42] to predict the behavior of chronic wounds in humans.

Studies vary in the type of electrical stimulation used. Antimicrobial effects have been demonstrated with the use of microamperage direct current,[3,41,42] milliamperage direct current,[39] and high-voltage pulsed current.[40,43] However, the range of high voltages such as those found to be effective with high-voltage pulsed current are unlikely to be well tolerated if applied clinically.[16,40]

The effects of electrical stimulation against pathogenic organisms may be affected by factors such as electrode polarity and electrode composition. The cathode is associated with antimicrobial effects against *Pseudomonas aeruginosa*,[42] whereas both the anode and the cathode are associated with action against *Staphylococcus aureus*.[38–40,43] Electrode composition may also be an important factor; one study[38] demonstrated that electrodes consisting of silver wire showed superior antimicrobial effects when compared with stainless steel, platinum, or gold wire electrodes while using anodal stimulation in the 0.4 to 4.0 microampere range.

For clinical application, these studies indicate there may be a possible antimicrobial effect with the use of low-intensity direct current, although further research is needed in this area.

Effects on Blood Flow

One of the proposed mechanisms by which electrical stimulation is believed to accelerate wound repair is by enhancing blood circulation. In studies of electrical stimulation and blood flow, various assessment measures have been used to determine blood flow, including skin temperatures,[44–46] transcutaneous oxygen ($TcPO_2$) levels,[47–51] venous occlusion plethysmography,[52,53] photoplethysmography,[54] ultrasonic Doppler flowmetry,[55,56] and laser Doppler flowmetry or imaging.[57–60] Comparison of study results is difficult due to the differences in the outcome measures, as well as in methodologies, electrode placement sites, study populations, and other factors.

Electrical stimulation using alternating square wave pulses at 80 Hz was found to increase blood flow in ischemic skin flaps.[59] Blood flow was also noted to increase with the application of low-frequency transcutaneous electrical nerve stimulation (TENS) to the forearms of healthy volunteers[58] and to the lower legs of nine healthy female volunteers.[60] However, there was great individual variation in the latter study[60] results, with two individuals showing marked responses, and the rest demonstrating less obvious responses. Another study[57] using low-frequency TENS was found to increase blood flow in chronic leg ulcers and in the intact skin surrounding the ulcer. In this study, the electrical stimulation unit delivered constant biphasic square wave pulses at 2 Hz, and electrodes were placed 5 cm proximal, and 5 cm distal, to the ulcer.

Several other studies have reported changes in blood flow associated with the use of electrical stimulation. Studies using motor level stimuli have reported increases in blood flow[52,53,55] or no effect on blood flow.[56] In contrast to these studies, which primarily assessed the effect of electrical stimulation on blood flow in the same extremity in which the electrodes were placed, another study[44] assessed the effect of electrical stimulation on blood flow in all four extremities. This study found that motor level stimuli, using stimulation

---

● **Why Do I Need to Know About...**

GALVANOTAXIS

Using the information from these studies, the theory of galvanotaxis may be used as a basis for the selection of polarity in the treatment electrode.[16]

of a distant point (electrodes were placed on one hand), resulted in a skin temperature rise in the extremities. In contrast, a study that used sensory level stimuli with pulsed galvanic stimulation over arterial blood vessels in the upper extremity was found to have no effect on blood flow.[54]

The circulatory system allows oxygen and nutrients to reach tissues,[61] and sufficient oxygen is required for all phases of wound healing.[4] Diminished oxygen levels, as determined by transcutaneous oxygen ($TcPO_2$) levels, show a trend of being associated with the presence of pressure ulcers in individuals with spinal cord injury.[62] Additionally, low $TcPO_2$ levels have been tied to a reduced potential for the ability of ulcers to heal.[4,16] The use of electrical stimulation has been associated with increases in $TcPO_2$ levels in individuals with spinal cord injury,[50] normal adults,[47] and individuals with diabetes.[46,47,50] However, at least one other study has shown conflicting results when assessing the effect of electrical stimulation on $TcPO_2$ levels in individuals with diabetes.[49] In this study, cathodal high-voltage pulsed current was applied to the foot or leg at the most distal site where the 5.07 Semmes Weinstein monofilament could be felt. $TcPO_2$ levels were found to decline following treatment. However, the study authors reported there was a subgroup of patients that had increased skin blood flow in response to electrical stimulation, and suggested the need for further research.

Several studies have examined the effect of electrical stimulation on skin temperatures. Wong and Jette[46] found that the use of TENS over acupuncture points in the forearm and hands was associated with decreases in index finger skin temperature in healthy subjects. Scudds et al.[45] found that high- and low-frequency TENS had no effect on finger skin temperature in asymptomatic subjects, while high-intensity, low-frequency TENS was associated with a rise in mean hand temperature as measured by infrared thermography. As noted previously, a study by Kaada[44] reported that the use of low-frequency TENS on the hands of individuals with Raynaud's phenomenon or diabetic polyneuropathy was associated with an increase in skin temperatures in the extremities.

Some researchers have suggested that skin temperature is not a reliable measure of skin blood flow,[54,60] and newer, more precise methods such as laser Doppler imaging are suggested.[60] Support for this concept is seen in a study that assessed the effect of TENS on cutaneous blood flow.[58] This study concluded that low-frequency TENS applied to the skin overlying the median nerve resulted in significant increases in blood perfusion as measured by laser Doppler flowmetry, while concurrent measures of skin temperature were found to have no significant changes. Other discrepancies have been noted, in which skin temperatures were found to have little or no relationship with photoplethysmography,[54] laser Doppler imaging,[57,60] or laser Doppler flowmetry.[58] Researchers have suggested that the laser Doppler technique may be a more sensitive measure of microcirculation in the skin.[60]

Other study findings for the effect of electrical stimulation on blood flow suggest that results may be affected by factors such as the electrode placement sites,[63] the presence of impaired peripheral perfusion,[51] the use of motor level versus sensory level stimuli,[47] the stimulation frequency,[52,55,58,60] and, as noted previously, the outcome measure that is used. Further research in this area would be beneficial.

Effects on Necrotic Tissue

A suggested use for electrical stimulation is to facilitate autolytic debridement via the galvanotaxis theory.[30] Using the theory of galvanotaxis, a treatment electrode of positive polarity is placed over the wound to attract the negatively charged neutrophils and macrophages to promote autolysis.[30] Conversely, autolytic debridement may be supported by the use of polar effects to produce an alkaline pH to solubilize the necrotic wound tissue.[16] Production of an alkaline pH is more likely to occur with the use of cathodal direct current, as compared to the use of pulsed currents.[16]

Electrical stimulation for autolytic debridement of necrotic tissue is supported by observations in two studies, although no randomized controlled studies that have specifically examined this effect have been found. In one study,[2] the wounds of 30 hospital inpatients were treated with 2 hours of electrical stimulation twice daily using low-intensity direct current. Negative polarity was used for the first 3 days, then positive polarity until the wound healed or a plateau in healing was reached. All wounds were debrided prior to admission to the study. However, only the treated wounds did not require any further debridement during the duration of the study. In another, more recent study,[10] 42 chronic leg ulcers of varying etiology were treated with cathodal high-voltage pulsed current or sham treatments. These wounds were also debrided, primarily on a single occasion for removal of excess callus from foot ulcers during a 1- to 2-week period of conventional wound care at the initiation of the study. Only the treated ulcers showed improvement based on scores using the Photographic Wound Assessment Tool (PWAT), and these improvements were attributed to the loss of necrotic tissue and an increase in granulation tissue.

Does Electrical Stimulation Work?

In 1994, the Agency for Health Care Policy and Research[64] recommended that clinicians "consider a course of treatment with electrotherapy for Stage III and IV pressure ulcers that have proved unresponsive to conventional therapy. Electrical stimulation may also be useful for recalcitrant Stage II ulcers." The strength of evidence rating was as-sessed at a "B" rating, indicating that "results of two or more controlled clinical trials on pressure ulcers in humans provide support, or when appropriate, results of two or more controlled trials in an animal model provide indirect support."

Clinical studies have reported beneficial results associated with the use of electrical stimulation in the healing of wounds,[2,5–13,15] although at least two recent reviews have concluded that there were difficulties in reaching conclusions[65] or insufficient reliable evidence[66] about the effectiveness of electrical stimulation. The first of these publications was a critical review of electrical stimulation for pressure ulcers. The study authors determined that conclusive results could not be drawn for the efficacy of electric currents in relation to wound healing, and that further study using clinical trials are needed. The second was a technology assessment that was published in 2001, and included a review of 16 randomized controlled trials that examined effectiveness of electrical therapies on chronic wounds. The conclusions of this study were that there was "…insufficient reliable evidence to draw conclusions about the contribution of…electrotherapy…to chronic wound healing." The study also concluded that electrotherapy for the treatment of pressure sores was one of the most promising physical therapies for further investigation.

Two meta-analyses of electrical stimulation and tissue healing have recently been published.[67,68] Gardner et al.[68] reviewed studies that included ulcer or periulcer electrical stimulation of chronic wounds in human subjects. Chronic wounds were defined as pressure ulcers, venous ulcers, arterial ulcers, or neuropathic ulcers. For inclusion in the meta-analysis, the studies had to report quantitative data of baseline and post-treatment wound size, or the percent of wound healing per week. Results of this meta-analysis showed the rate of healing per week to be 22% for the electrical stimulation samples, and 9% for control samples. The electrical stimulation healing rate represents an increase of 144% over the control rate. The authors stated that study findings supported "…the merits of electrical stimulation for treating chronic wounds… ." The study authors also called for additional research to examine factors such as the optimal-dose response and factors related to the electrical stimulation device or wound.

The second meta-analysis[67] reviewed the results of randomized controlled trials (RCTs) for the effect of electrical or electromagnetic field stimulation on musculoskeletal tissues that included both bone and soft tissues. Twenty-nine RCTs were identified for soft tissues and joint; 16 of these studies used end points that were sufficient for calculation of a combined effect in the meta-analysis. The overall statistical analysis for the 16 studies demonstrated support for the effectiveness of electrical stimulation. In interpreting this information, clinicians should note, while the majority of the studies (10 of the 16) used electrical or electromagnetic field stimulation to treat wounds, the rest involved the treatment of various musculoskeletal disorders such as osteoarthritis. The authors also noted that, while the results of this meta-analysis did not constitute conclusive evidence that electrical

> ● **Why Do I Need to Know About...**
>
> **CURRENT TRENDS IN HEALTH CARE POLICY**
>
> Without reimbursement for electrical stimulation for chronic wounds and pressure ulcers, these beneficial physical therapy treatment interventions would no longer be used.

stimulation has specific effects on health, the statistically significant results of the pooled data could not be ignored.

The Centers for Medicare and Medicaid Services (CMS) issued a decision of coverage of electrical stimulation for chronic wounds in July 2002.[69] This decision of coverage was limited to chronic wounds such as Stage III and Stage IV pressure ulcers, arterial ulcers, diabetic ulcers, and venous stasis ulcers. The decision was based on a systematic review of published clinical trials and input from a number of sources, including the American Physical Therapy Association, the Emergency Care Research Institute, the Association for the Advancement of Wound Care, the Agency for Health Care Policy and Research, and the Medical and Surgical Procedures Panel of the Medicare Coverage Advisory Committee.

Current Type: Does It Matter Which Type Is Used?

Various types of electromedical currents exist and have been classified by the section on Clinical Electrophysiology of the American Physical Therapy Association (see Fig. 11-3).

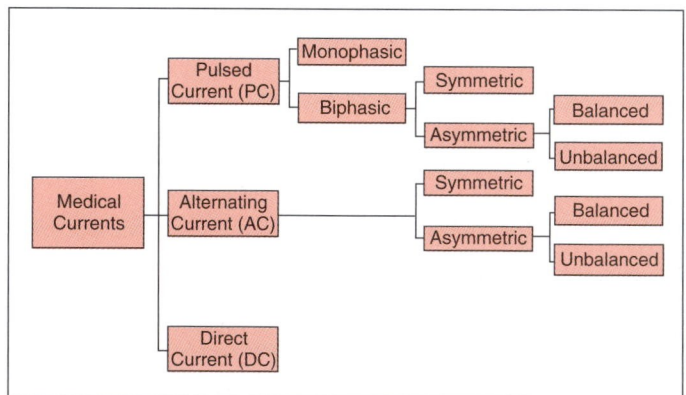

Figure 11–3 Classification of Electrical Currents, Clinical Electrophysiology Section of the American Physical Therapy Association (2001). With this classification model, the various types of pulsed current that are used with the majority of electrical stimulation devices have been classified under the heading of "pulsed current." Pulsed currents are actually a subdivision of the main two types of current, alternating current and direct current. The separate and additional classification for "pulsed current" is intended to ease the interpretation of the various types of electromedical currents that exist. (Reprinted with permission from Kloth, LC: Electrical stimulation for wound healing. In Kloth, LC, and McCulloch, JM [eds]: Wound Healing Alternatives in Management, ed 3. FA Davis, Philadelphia, 2002, pp 271–315.)

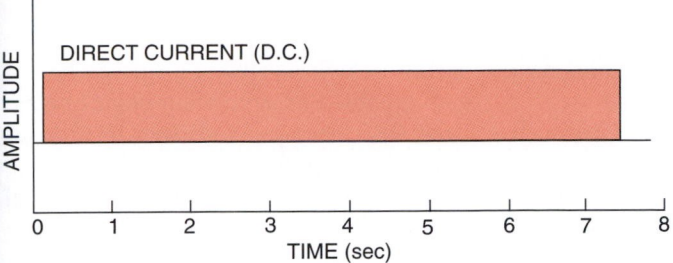

Figure 11–4   Illustration of the waveform for direct current. (Reprinted with permission from Kloth, LC: Electrical stimulation for wound healing. In Kloth, LC, and McCulloch, JM [eds]: Wound Healing Alternatives in Management, ed 3. FA Davis, Philadelphia, 2002, pp 271–315.)

Researchers have reported beneficial results with the use of low-intensity direct current (Fig. 11-4),[2,14,31,70] pulsed current,[5–11,13,15] and alternating current.[12] Further differentiation between the different pulsed current characteristics shows beneficial results with the use of low-voltage monophasic pulsed current (for an example of this current type, see Fig. 11-5),[27,32] high-voltage monophasic pulsed current (for an example of this current type, Fig. 11-6),[9–11] and low-voltage asymmetric biphasic pulsed current (for examples of this current type, see Figs. 11-7 and 11-8).[5,6,13] The asymmetric biphasic pulsed current waveform, in studies by Baker and colleagues,[5,6] was found superior to a symmetric biphasic pulsed current waveform when wounds were differentiated into those demonstrating "good responses" among ulcers in patients with spinal cord injury,[6] and into those requiring more than 8 days of treatment among ulcers in patients with diabetes.[5] Both studies had three stimulation groups (asymmetric biphasic stimulation; symmetric biphasic stimulation; microcurrent stimulation) and a control group. Significantly improved healing rates were found for the asymmetric bipha-

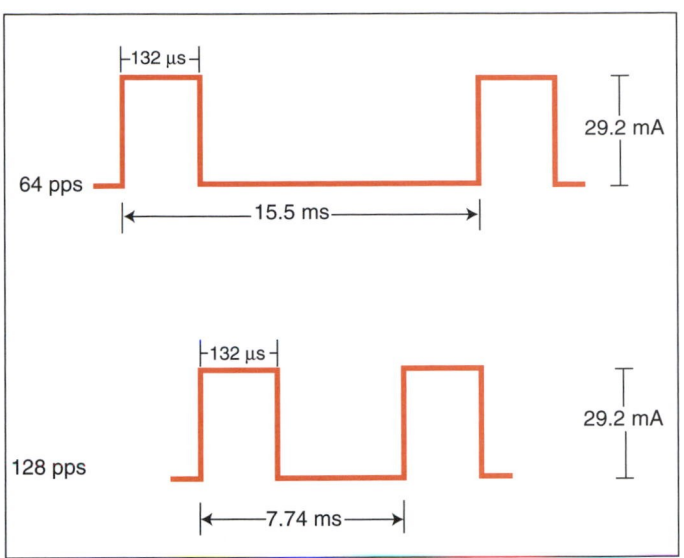

Figure 11–5   Illustration of the low-voltage monophasic pulsed current waveform used in the study by Feedar et al. (Reprinted with permission from Feedar, JA, Kloth, LC, and Gentzkow, GD: Chronic dermal ulcer healing enhanced with monophasic pulsed electrical stimulation. Phys Ther 71:639–149, 1991.)

sic waveform when compared to the microcurrent or control group in the first study, and when compared to the combined results from the microcurrent and control groups in the latter study. The study by Stefanovska and colleagues[13] concluded that an asymmetric biphasic pulsed current waveform seemed to be more effective than low-density direct current, but that comparisons regarding the size of the difference were premature. The current type used in a study by Wood et al.[15] is reported as a pulsed low-intensity direct current. However, according to the electrotherapeutic terminology adopted by the Clinical Electrophysiology section of the American

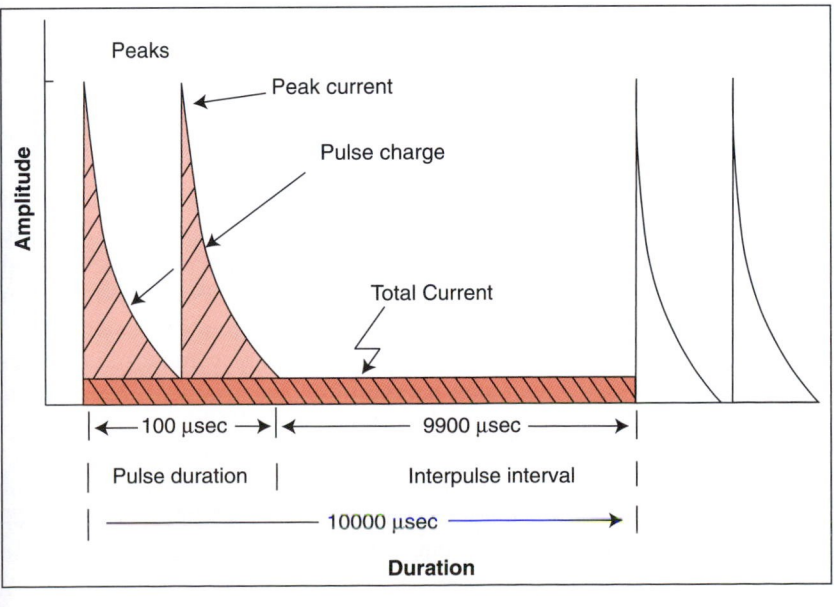

Figure 11–6   Illustration of high-voltage monophasic pulsed current waveform. (Reprinted with permission from Nelson, RM, and Currier, DP [eds]: Clinical Electrotherapy. Appleton & Lange, Norwalk, CT, 1987.)

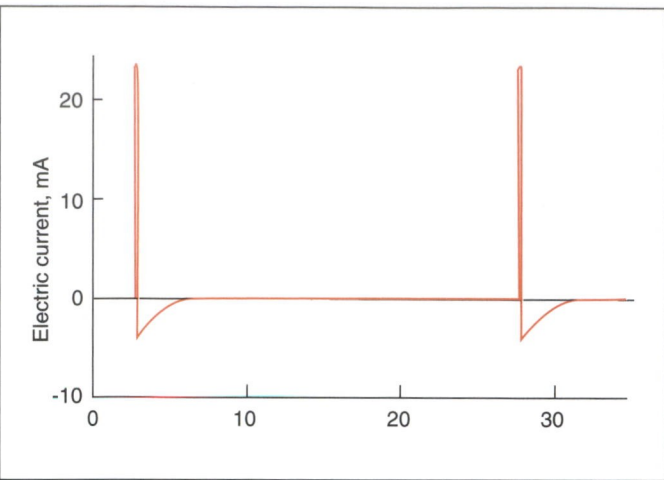

Figure 11–7 Illustration of low-voltage asymmetric biphasic pulsed current used in the study by Stefanovska et al. (Reprinted with permission from Stefanovska, A, Vodovnik, L, Benko, H, and Turk, R: Treatment of chronic wounds by means of electric and electromagnetic fields. Part 2. Value of FES parameters for pressure sore treatment. Med Biol Eng Comput 31:213–220, 1993.)

Physical Therapy Association in 1991,[71] the stimulation characteristics reported in the study by Wood et al. may be classified as low-voltage, monophasic pulsed current.[16] Review of these studies demonstrates that various electrical stimulation current types have been reported as beneficial in enhancing the healing of chronic wounds.

Does Polarity Matter?

Treatment protocols that use concepts such as galvanotaxis, enhancement of the current of injury, and potential bacteriocidal effects may incorporate the use of polar effects. The use of currents that are capable of producing polar effects may be a factor in facilitating a healing response. Experimental evidence suggests that wounds possess a specific polarity, usually positive, although an experimental study has reported changes in the polarity of wounds, from positive to negative, as healing progresses.[21] These findings imply that

	A	B	MC
Amplitude	Below contraction	Below contraction	4 mA
Phase duration (μs)	100	300	10
Frequency (pps)	50	50	1
On:off times (s)	7:7	7:7	7:7
Waveform	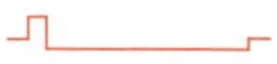	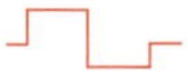	

Figure 11–8 Illustration of low-voltage asymmetric biphasic pulsed current used in the studies by Baker et al. (Reprinted with permission from Baker, LL, Chambers, R, DeMuth, SK, and Villar, F: Effects of electrical stimulation on wound healing in patients with diabetic ulcers. Diabetes Care 20:405–412, 1997.)

shifts in potential may be involved in the natural healing process of wounds.[26]

Studies have reported beneficial effects on tissue healing for the use of currents capable of introducing polar effects.[2, 5–14, 31] Polar effects may be introduced to tissues by a variety of current types, including monophasic and unbalanced or asymmetric biphasic waveforms. The potential for polar effects may be further modified by the selection of continuous versus pulsed current, the use of a specific polarity for the treatment electrode, and by varying the treatment electrode polarity during the episode of care.

Experimental evidence exists for beneficial effects with the use of electrical stimulation protocols in which treatment electrode polarity is varied during the episode of care. In basic science research, one study[36] found that the use of negative polarity for one day followed by the use of positive polarity on subsequent days resulted in the highest percentage of wounds healed. Another study[72] found increased rates of wound closure with positive alternating with negative currents on 3-day cycles. Several clinical studies have reported successful results for tissue healing using protocols in which the treatment electrode polarity was changed throughout the healing process.[2,7,11,14,31]

The results from these studies suggest that polar effects may be an important factor in the healing process. Further support for this concept may be noted in the results of studies by Baker and colleagues, who found the use of an asymmetrical biphasic waveform superior to a symmetric biphasic waveform.[5,6] The asymmetric waveform may have allowed chemical changes in the tissues as a result of the charge asymmetry. These chemical changes would then account for the enhanced healing of the asymmetric waveform.

Electrode Placement: Which Protocol Is Best?

Electrode placement can vary, and methods include the direct technique and the periwound technique.[17] Studies have reported beneficial effects for both the direct technique[2,7,9–11] and the periwound technique.[5,6,13] The direct technique used in these studies is with placement of the stimulating electrode directly over the wound, with a dispersive electrode located on intact skin peripheral to the wound. This method has also been described as a monopolar technique.[4] The periwound technique used in these studies is with placement of two electrodes on intact skin surrounding the wound. This method has also been described as a bipolar technique.[4] In general, research studies have reported the use of the periwound technique with asymmetric biphasic pulsed current types[5,6,13] and the direct technique with low-intensity direct current[2] or monophasic pulsed current types.[7,9–11] Exceptions include the study by Wood et al.,[15] which used pulsed low-intensity direct current with application of electrodes at opposite sides of the wound on clinical normal skin. This study, however, did not report on the type of electrode that was used. Another exception is a study by Lundeberg et al.,[12] in which alternating current was used with application of stimulation outside the ulcer surface area.

Finally, another type of electrode arrangement that has been used includes the use of a Dacron silver mesh sock and sleeve electrode system to deliver high-voltage monophasic pulsed current as an adjunct to healing diabetic foot ulcers.[73] Researchers assessing the use of this system in providing eight hours of stimulation nightly found enhanced wound healing when study results were stratified according to patient compliance.

Of interest to clinicians is the decision memorandum by the CMS, in which electrical stimulation is defined as "the application of electrical current through electrodes applied directly to the skin in close proximity to the ulcer."[69]

Indications

Various categorizations have been provided for integument wounds by previous authors. Four main categories that have been reported to be treated with electrical stimulation are wounds as a result of pressure (decubitus), venous insufficiency, arterial insufficiency, or diabetes mellitus.[10,16,68,74] The present discussion will provide a brief review of potential pathophysiologies that may result in wounds from these categories.

Pressure wounds result from application of external force sufficient to exceed capillary filling pressure interrupting blood flow.[75] These individuals include patients with spinal injury, and patients immobilized in critical or extended care facilities, or following hip fracture. Wounds resulting from venous insufficiency are a hallmark of stasis dermatitis in the lower extremities.[75] These wounds are due to impaired venous outflow, venous insufficiency, and occur in patients with preexisting conditions such as venous thrombosis or valvular incompetence, that is, varicose veins. Wounds due to arterial insufficiency result from an interruption of blood flow into the tissues. The pathophysiologic etiologies responsible for these wounds are more diversified. These wounds may occur as a result of vasculitis in patients with polyarteritis nodosa or in peripheral vascular disorders such as atherosclerotic occlusive disease or thromboangiitis obliterans.[75] Alternatively, arterial insufficiency may be a manifestation of rheumatic disorders such as systemic lupus erythematosus or rheumatoid arthritis.[6] Integument wounds resulting from diabetes mellitus are complex in origin, resulting from peripheral neuropathy and/or dysfunction of both the large and small arteries.[77] These wounds occur commonly on the planter surface of the foot, but may also appear on the dorsal surface or at other locations, and result from loss of sensation due to peripheral neuropathy and decreased blood flow due to arterial damage. Finally, although not commonly classified in one of the four previous categories, integument wounds resulting from increased sympathetic activity also occur. Raynaud's disease/phenomenon results in intense vasoconstriction of the digits of the upper and occasionally lower extremities.[75] Multiple etiologies exist for this disorder, varying from idiopathic to previous mechanical or thermal injury at the site. Electric stimulation increases localized blood flow to the ischemic digits.[44,78] Thus, integument wounds may result from multiple pathophysiologies.

Contraindications and Precautions

Very few actual contraindications exist in regard to electric stimulation for tissue repair. The majority of situations result in precautions with regard to the electric stimulation due to the anatomic location of the wound. Several contraindications are based on empirical assessment. The federal Food and Drug Administration (FDA) has issued a statement of contraindication concerning application of TENS devices for both patients with synchronous (demand) cardiac pacemakers, and application of these devices over the carotid sinus.[79] Although the FDA statement concerns transcutaneous electrical stimulation for pain relief, any transcutaneous electrical stimulator with a varying electric field may fall under the ruling. The logic for the contraindication in patients with demand cardiac pacemakers is that a changing electric field of the transcutaneous electrical nerve stimulator may interfere with the performance of the cardiac pacemaker. Literature supporting TENS interference with demand cardiac pacemakers is contradictory. Several investigations have documented placement of TENS for pain relief in both the axial and appendicular regions of the body without interference of the cardiac pacemaker.[80,81] In contrast, a case report of two patients documented cardiac pacemaker dysfunction in patients receiving TENS for pain relief.[82] Stimulation of the carotid sinus may result in a vasovagal response, and stimulation of other structures in the anterior of the neck, such as the larynx may result in laryngeal spasm and asphyxiation.[16] Other areas considered to be contraindications to the use of electrical stimulation include those overlying vital organs or nerves, such as the heart.[83] Additionally, transcerebral application of electrical muscle stimulator (EMS) devices is contraindicated.[84]

Various types of skin lesions, such as basal cell carcinoma, squamous cell carcinoma, or melanoma at the application

Before You Begin

Remember to rule out contraindications to electrical stimulation.

site, may all be contraindications. This contraindication exists for both the presence of one of these neoplasia, or previous documentation of the neoplasia at the application site. Electrical stimulation of these neoplastic cells may result in further mitogenic activity,[16] or increased blood flow to the tissue may assist in the neoplastic metastasis. Other types of skin lesions may be considered to be contraindications for the application of electrical stimulation devices if the underlying etiology, such as thrombophlebitis, precludes the use of electrical stimulation.[84]

Various characteristics, such as osteomyelitis present in the bone beneath the integument wound, have also been described as a contraindication to electrical stimulation of the wound. The explanation for this contraindication is that premature closing of the integument may result in an abscess formation.[4,16] Additionally, increased blood flow to the tissue as a result of electrical stimulation may result in septicemia or bacteremia. Actively bleeding wounds are another example of described contraindications to the use of electrical stimulation.[17]

The presence of metal ions from antimicrobial medications[4] or metallic implants in the underlying tissue may pose a contraindication. Direct electrical currents may drive metal ions from antimicrobial medications into the tissues. Alternatively, electrical stimulation with biphasic or pulsed monophasic waveforms may result in inappropriate heating of metal ions or metallic implants damaging the surrounding tissue. Treatment of wounds in the lumbar or lower abdominal region in pregnant women should also be considered a contraindication. Although no documentation exists that transcutaneous currents at these energy levels are sufficient, the potential for mutagenic effects on the fetus in utero exist.

Several subpopulations of patients may be included in those in whom caution should be utilized when applying electrical stimulation for tissue repair. Treatment of wounds in the cranium or upper cervical area with electrical stimulation should be considered judiciously, and the treatment monitored closely. Additional precautions should be taken in these treatments if the patient has documented evidence of epilepsy, cerebrovascular accident, or reversible ischemic neurologic deficit. Electrical stimulation of this region in these patients may initiate an epileptic event or alter cerebral blood flow exacerbating cerebrovascular accident or reversible ischemic neurologic deficit. Finally, although a patient who is insensate at the wound site may be considered a contraindication to application of electrical stimulation for tissue repair, the application of electrical stimulation at this wound site is considered appropriate. Due to the insensate condition of the wound site, precaution should be used in establishing the initial electrical stimulation parameters. Several different types of patients may present insensate at the wound site, including patients with pressure ulcers resulting from spinal injury or diabetic wounds.

Adverse Site Responses

Several adverse responses may also occur at the application site. During application of the electric current the patient may complain of an unpleasant buzzing or tingling. This response is both amplitude dependent and frequency dependent. Additionally, if the electrode surface area is insufficient for the electrical amplitude or there is an uneven distribution of current density, a local hyperthermic reaction may occur resulting in a thermal burn. One study has reported a single instance of bleeding at the ulcer site associated with the use of pulsed current.[85] Finally, contact dermatitis may occur at the application site resulting from components of the electrode. Any of the components of the electrode may initiate this response. The contact dermatitis may be expressed by two distinctly different inflammatory processes: irritant and allergic dermatitis.[86] Irritant dermatitis is a non–immune-mediated response and is a result of the direct action of the irritant on the skin. In contrast, allergic dermatitis represents a type IV delayed cell-mediated immune hypersensitivity response. The clinician may differentiate these two responses. In irritant dermatitis, the cutaneous response is directly proportional to the amount of the irritant applied. In contrast, allergic dermatitis, only minute quantities are necessary to elicit an overt response. Repeated dermal exposures to compounds initiating irritant dermatitis may eventually result in allergic dermal responses.

Treatment Considerations

To date, electrical stimulation devices for wound healing have not been approved or received premarket approval by the FDA.[83] Safety and effectiveness of the devices must be demonstrated in order to obtain premarket approval.[83] At this time, the only FDA-approved indication for the use of electrical stimulation, as related to the previous discussion on potential mechanisms of action in wound care, is in the promotion of increased local blood flow.[4,87,88] Other FDA-approved indications may include pain suppression, maintaining or increasing joint range of motion, and prevention of muscle atrophy.[88] Electrical stimulation for patients with wounds is used as an off-label indication.[87] Clinicians are advised to consider this information when selecting a protocol with electrical stimulation and to review all appropriate guidelines as part of the decision-making process. Further sources of information on this topic may be found elsewhere.[4,87,89]

Application

The use of two application techniques will be considered in this chapter: the direct technique (as used with high-voltage monophasic pulsed current—active electrode placed on the wound bed, with dispersive electrode located 15 to 20 cm distant to the wound), and the periwound technique (as used with alternating or asymmetric biphasic pulsed current—electrodes placed adjacent to the wound bed on intact skin). In comparison to the direct technique, several additional considerations may apply to the use of the periwound technique. The periwound technique may result in less current density within the wound.[6] The periwound technique, as applied with both electrodes over skin with normal innervation, may be more advantageous when attempting to activate sensory nerves in the skin.[6] In addition, other advantages for the periwound technique include less potential for disturbance of the wound bed, and a reduced chance of cross-contamination between the wound and the electrode.[6] Finally, while indirect application methods of wound care (such as ultrasound to periulcer skin) may require minimal specialized training, the use of direct techniques with application of the modality directly to the wound bed are considered to require more advanced specialized training for the proper use of equipment and techniques.[89]

With each technique, clinicians should be aware that charge dosage, current density, and depth of penetration may vary when changes occur in stimulation parameters, electrode size, electrode arrangement, and specific wound characteristics. Since patients with wounds may have impaired sensation at the wound itself (depending on depth of the wound), and in the skin surrounding the wound, these factors should be among those considered when selecting treatment parameters and stimulation intensity.

Stimulation parameters have been proposed for the use of electrical stimulation in tissue healing for wound care. Kloth[16] has described formulas for calculating electrical charge dosages for low- and high-voltage pulsed current electrical simulation. A dosage range of 250 to 500 µC/sec has been found to be a shared quality among several studies.[16] Another stimulation parameter is that of charge density, or the amount of electrical charge per unit of a cross-sectional area of an electrode.[16] This value relates to electrode size; for example, the larger the size of the electrode, the smaller is the charge current density.[4] Absolute charge density transfer is obtained by multiplying the average spatial current density by the effective duty cycle and by the total duration of treatment.[90] Reich[90] suggested, based on an observed trend in several studies, that an absolute charge density transfer of 0.1 to 2.0 C/cm^2 may be effective in enhancing healing. Reich encouraged that further research be done in this area.

Many protocols call for the use of submotor stimulation intensity (amplitude) levels. For patients with impaired sensation, caution should be used to confirm the use of submotor intensities and to prevent the use of excessive current intensities.[17] Finally, while selecting stimulus intensity using the direct technique, clinicians should recall that the wound lacks skin and impedance is lower than the surrounding tissues.[91]

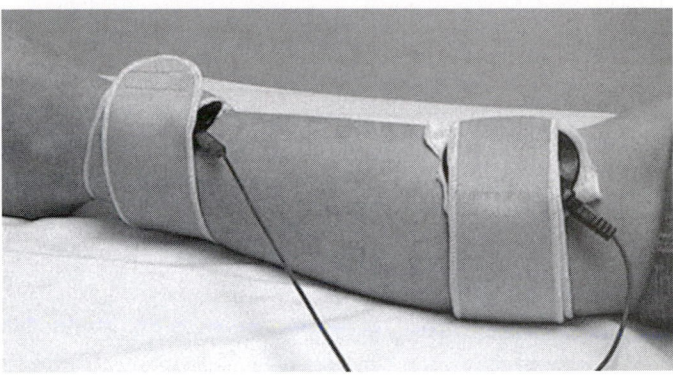

Figure 11-9 Model illustrating the use of the direct monopolar technique using carbon rubber electrodes. With this technique, one electrode is placed over the wound and a dispersive electrode is placed 15 to 20 cm away on intact skin.

Direct Technique (as used with high-voltage monophasic pulsed current research studies[9-11])

With this technique, the electrode may be placed directly on the wound, using saline-moistened sterile gauze. The moistened gauze is placed within the wound bed following wound irrigation or debridement as needed. Treatment electrode types have consisted of metalline gauze,[10] carbon electrode, or aluminum foil.[9] Metalline gauze electrodes, as used in the study by Houghton et al.,[10] are sterile, single-use electrodes. Carbon electrodes require a cleaning process with an approved disinfectant,[4,17] while aluminum foil electrodes are disposed of following a single application.[17] The treatment electrode is secured in place over the wound, while the dispersive electrode is placed on intact skin (see Figs. 11-9 and 11-10 for examples of the direct technique). Dispersive elec-

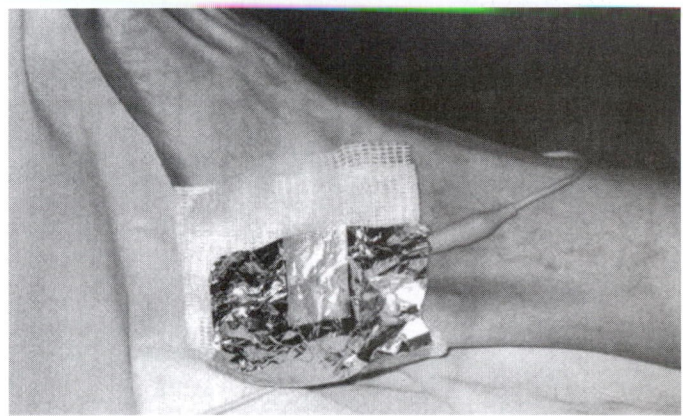

Figure 11-10 Illustration of the direct monopolar technique using an aluminum foil electrode over the wound. With this technique, one electrode is placed over the wound and a dispersive electrode is placed 15 to 20 cm away on intact skin. (Reprinted with permission from Sussman, C, and Byl, NN: Electrical stimulation for wound healing. In Sussman, C, and Bates-Jensen, BM [eds]: Wound Care, ed 2. Aspen Publishers, Gaithersburg, MD, 2001, pp 497–545.)

trode placement has been described as 15 cm cephalad to the wound,[16] 20 cm proximal to the wound,[10] or on the medial thigh as used in a study for healing of pressure ulcers in patients with spinal cord injury.[9] Dispersive electrode size has not always been reported; one study used a size of 20 × 25 cm,[9] whereas Kloth[16] recommends for dispersive electrode size to be similar to the wound surface area.

Periwound Technique (as used with asymmetrical biphasic pulsed current research studies[5,6,13])

With this technique, two electrodes are placed on intact skin adjacent to the wound. Electrode types have consisted of self-adhesive skin electrodes[13] or carbon rubber electrodes.[5,6] In studies that have specified electrode location, placement is generally proximal and distal to the wound (Fig. 11-11), although medial and lateral placement has been used for ulcers in region of the coccyx.[6]

Application Check List

- Determine if treatment with electrical stimulation is appropriate and decide upon the desired treatment parameters (equipment and current type, the type of technique to be used).

- Prior to each treatment, assess the wound, periwound, and wound drainage characteristics.

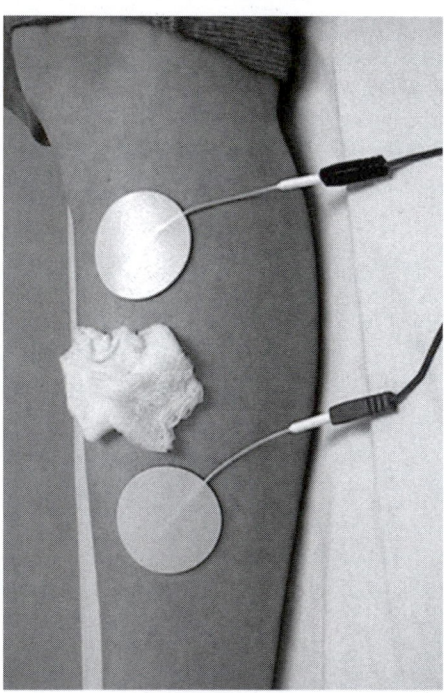

Figure 11–11   Model illustrating the use of the indirect bipolar technique with proximal/distal (6:00 and 12:00 o'clock) placement of self-adhesive electrodes. The gauze pad represents the location of the wound. With this technique, electrodes are placed on intact skin adjacent to the wound.

- Provide patient instructions: Explain the procedure/equipment to be used and describe the anticipated effects of treatment (see patient instruction section later in this chapter).

- Check electrical stimulation equipment to be sure it is intact and functioning properly.

- After checking to be sure the electrical stimulation unit is not turned on and the intensity control is in the off position, apply electrical stimulation electrodes (application techniques will differ depending upon whether the direct or periwound technique is used).

Direct Technique

- Prepare wound.

- Ensure that the wound is free of any metallic substances or petrolatum products.

- Determine the desired polarity of the treatment electrode.

- Apply saline-moistened sterile gauze to the wound, followed by application of the treatment electrode.

- Select dispersive electrode of size similar to wound surface area.

- Apply dispersive electrode 15 to 20 cm from the wound on intact skin.

Periwound Technique

- Prepare wound (maintain current wound dressing in place over the wound or irrigate wound and apply new dressing prior to electrical stimulation treatment).

- Ensure that the wound is free of any metallic substances or petrolatum products.

- Apply treatment electrodes on intact skin near the edges of the wound. See Box 11-1 for specific electrode application parameters.

- Set the electrical stimulation parameters (see Boxes 11-1 and 11-2).

- When ready, turn on the electrical stimulation unit and gradually increase intensity until the desired range is reached.

- For initial treatments, use lower dosage parameters in order to assess skin tolerance before full protocol dosage parameters are used.

- Ensure that the patient is comfortable, and provide the patient with a call light or bell.

- Recheck with the patient during the treatment session to determine the patient's continued comfort and tolerance to treatment.

- When treatment is concluded, decrease intensity to the off position, remove electrodes, and follow the appro-

BOX 11-1   Electrical Stimulation Parameters: Asymmetric Biphasic Pulsed Current or Alternating Current

This box summarizes research protocols for the use of asymmetric biphasic pulsed currents or alternating pulsed currents.

- *Asymmetric Biphasic Current*—Research protocol for pressure ulcers and diabetic ulcers.[5,6] *Pulse frequency and duration*—50 Hz, 100 μsec phase duration, 7:7 on/off time (sec). *Stimulus intensity*—below contraction level. *Treatment duration*—30 minute treatment sessions, totaling 30 to 90 minutes daily. *Electrode configuration*—carbon rubber electrodes of similar size placed on intact skin less than 1 cm from edge of the wound. Electrodes typically placed proximal and distal to the ulcer, but medial and lateral placement was used for ulcers in the region of the coccyx. The electrode whose polarity was negative during the leading phase of the waveform was placed proximal to the wound. *Electrode size*—dependent on wound size and location, sizes ranged from 2.5 × 2.5 cm to 5 × 10 cm.

- *Asymmetric Biphasic Current*—Research protocol for pressure ulcers.[80] *Pulse frequency and duration*—40 Hz, 0.25 milliseconds pulse duration, 4 second stimulation trains. *Stimulus intensity*—tetanic contractions produced, generally at 15 to 25 mA. *Treatment duration*— 2 hours daily. *Electrode configuration*—two self-adhesive skin electrodes placed on healthy skin at the edge of the wound. *Electrode size*—adjusted to wound size, average size was 30 ± 10 cm² each.

- *Alternating Constant Current Square Wave Pulses* (with inference of an asymmetrical unbalanced wave)—Research protocol for diabetic leg ulcers due to venous stasis.[12] *Pulse frequency and duration*—80 Hz, alternating constant current with pulse width 1 millisecond. *Stimulus intensity*—intensity-evoking paresthesia. *Treatment duration*—20 minutes twice daily. *Electrode configuration*—stimulation applied just outside the ulcer surface area. Polarity of treatment electrode was changed after each treatment. *Electrode size*—treatment electrode was 4 × 6 cm.

BOX 11-2   High-Voltage Monophasic Pulsed Current

The following description summarizes the electrical stimulation parameters described by Kloth[49] using a high-voltage electrical stimulation device as an example.

- *Voltage* 75 to 150 V
- *Pulse frequency* of 100 pps
- *Treatment duration* of 60 minutes, 7 days per week
- *Polarity* of the wound treatment electrode is varied according to the wound phase or the clinical needs of the wound.*

*Please see the reference source[16] for further information regarding polarity of the wound treatment electrode. While this protocol suggests varying the treatment electrode polarity during the episode of care, two studies using high-voltage pulsed current[9,10] have used protocols in which the treatment electrode was maintained at negative polarity throughout the duration of the study.

Patient Instructions

- Explain that research findings have supported the use of electrical stimulation as an effective adjunctive therapy for chronic wounds that have not shown signs of healing during the past 30 days.

- As indicated, relate that studies have shown that chronic wounds similar to the patient's wound have responded favorably to the use of electrical stimulation.

- Describe the anticipated effect of electrical stimulation on the healing of the patient's wound, including advantages/disadvantages and potential adverse effects.

- Discuss the equipment to be used and indications/contraindications for the use of the equipment. Explain the specific procedure. Include any directions or guidelines suitable to the patient's participation in the treatment.

- Explain the measures that will be used to help determine if the treatment is effective.

- Describe the duration of each treatment session and for the overall episode of care.

- Explain that treatment will be performed with the patient's consent. The treatment is not expected to produce any discomfort, but the patient may experience a tingling sensation under the electrodes in areas of intact sensation.

- Advise the patient not to disturb or remove the electrodes during the treatment session.

- Advise the patient to continue to follow other recommendations for the treatment of his or her wound.

- Ask the patient to use the call light or bell if any discomfort is experienced or if any questions arise during the treatment session.

priate disinfection or disposal procedures. Check the wound/periwound and the skin under the electrodes for any signs of allergic reaction or thermal injury. Clean electrode wires with an approved disinfectant.

- Document the treatment performed.

A recent study assessing the effect of high-voltage pulsed current applied to chronic vascular leg ulcers[10] used the following stimulation parameters: pulse frequency at 100 Hz, peak intensity 150 V, pulse duration of 100 microseconds, and treatment duration of 45 minutes for 3 days a week. Negative polarity of the treatment electrode was maintained throughout the 4-week study. Study results indicated that high-voltage pulsed current reduced wound surface area to approximately one half the initial wound size, and that this effect was over two times greater than that seen with wounds treated with sham electrical stimulation unit.

Discussion Questions

1. What is the "current of injury"?
2. How may the galvanotaxis theory be used in the treatment of wounds?
3. What are the types of ES current associated with increases in blood flow?
4. How can I find out what type of waveform an ES device supplies?
5. For an infected wound, what are two ways in which the use of ES may promote antimicrobial action?
6. What are the direct monopolar and indirect bipolar techniques for ES treatment of wounds?
7. What are the advantages of each technique?

CASE STUDY

The following case study is characteristic of a patient example for the use of electrical stimulation for a nonhealing ulcer.

Patient's age: 71

Initial Assessment

Reason for Referral

The patient came to physical therapy secondary to a left dorsal foot ulcer that would not heal. Patient reported undergoing orthopedic surgery on the left foot three months prior to initial physical therapy evaluation and development of a blood blister post surgery. Patient reported the wound continued to break down. The patient received home health nursing for several weeks with no significant progress. Patient stated previous ulcer care had consisted of cleaning the wound with Betadine at home and applying a topical antibiotic ointment with a gauze dressing.

Medical History

No history of diabetes, heart disease, or vascular insufficiency reported.

Wound Examination

The wound presented with irregular borders measuring 3.0 cm at the widest point and 4.5 cm in length. There was no undermining or tunneling of the wound. The wound had a partial thickness skin loss with a moderate amount of exudate. The wound bed consisted of approximately 30% red granulated tissue and approximately 70% yellow necrotic adherent tissue. Patient also presented with erythema surrounding the wound and moderate edema of left lower extremity.

Signs of Vascular Insufficiency

Signs of venous insufficiency included hair loss on the foot, erythema surrounding the wound, and edema of the left lower extremity.

Treatment

Each treatment consisted of saline cleansing and selective debridement prior to electrical stimulation.

Electrical stimulation using high voltage pulsed current was initiated on the third visit (1.5 weeks post start of care) with the following parameters: (−) polarity of the treatment electrode was primarily used throughout treatment episode with a few occasions of (+) polarity. Treatment duration was 25 to 30 minutes with frequency of 5 times a week for 3 weeks, then decreased to 3 times a week for 2 weeks, for a total of 20 treatments.

Electrical stimulation was discontinued after 5.5 weeks secondary to a fully granulated wound base with lack of necrotic tissue and signs of increased epithelialization. Wound size had decreased approximately 40% to 50%.

In addition to electrical stimulation, wound dressings consisted of a petrolatum impregnated gauze for 3 visits, enzymatic debridement ointment for 7 visits, then progressed to alginate dressing for 9 visits. Dressing change to alginate dressing was secondary to the presence of greater than 70% granulated tissue in the wound bed. Once granulation tissue exceeded 95%, dressing was changed to petrolatum impregnated gauze with a four layer bandaging system to promote edema control.

Wound Measurements

TIME	WIDTH (cm)	LENGTH (cm)
0 (Start of care)	3.0	4.5
4.5 Weeks	2.0	3.2
6 Weeks	1.6	2.7
8.5 Weeks	0.8	1.8
11 Weeks	0.3	0.5

Outcomes

In 4.5 weeks, the wound measured 2.0 cm in width, 3.2 cm in length, and had greater than 95% granulation tissue.

In 6 weeks, the wound decreased in wound size by 40% to 50%.

At 11 weeks, the patient was discharged secondary to presenting with a clean wound base and being independent with home dressing care. The patient was scheduled to follow up with the physician.

Acknowledgment

The authors appreciate the assistance of Amy Przybyszewski, student physical therapist, in the preparation of this chapter.

Additional Sources

Databases

American Physical Therapy Association. Available at http://www.apta.org/ (Guide to Physical Therapist Practice, ed 2. Phys Ther 81[1], 2001).

APTA Online Courses (text based) (No. 2: Wound Healing and Management; No. 8: Clinical Electrotherapy: Physiology and Basic Concepts). Available at http://www.apta.org/

Centers for Medicare and Medicaid Services. Available at http://www.cms.hhs.gov/

Centers for Medicare and Medicaid Services. Electrostimulation for wounds: Decision memorandum (CAG-00068N). Centers for Medicare and Medicaid Services, 2002. Available at http:// www.cms.hhs.gov/ncdr/memo.asp?id=27 Accessed November 25, 2003.

CINAHL–Cumulative Index of Nursing and Allied Health Literature. Available at http://www.cinahl.com/

The Cochrane Library. Available at http://www.update-software.com/cochrane/

MEDLINE/PubMed: reference source for biomedical journals. Available at http://www.ncbi.nlm.nih.gov/entrez/query.fcgi

References

1. Becker, RO: The electrical control of growth processes. Med Times 95:657–669, 1967.
2. Carley, PJ, and Wainapel, SF: Electrotherapy for acceleration of wound healing: low intensity direct current. Arch Phys Med Rehabil 66:443–446, 1985.
3. Weiss, DS, Kirsner, R, and Eaglstein, WH: Electrical stimulation and wound healing. Arch Dermatol 126:222–225, 1990.
4. Sussman, C, and Byl, NN: Electrical stimulation for wound healing. In Sussman, C, and Bates-Jensen, BM (eds): Wound Care, ed 2. Aspen Publishers, Gaithersburg, MD, 2001, pp 497–545.
5. Baker, LL, Chambers, R, DeMuth, SK, et al: Effects of electrical stimulation on wound healing in patients with diabetic ulcers. Diabetes Care 20:405–412, 1997.
6. Baker, LL, Rubayi, S, Villar, F, et al: Effect of electrical stimulation waveform on healing of ulcers in human beings with spinal cord injury. Wound Rep Regul 4:21–28, 1996.
7. Feedar, JA, Kloth, LC, and Gentzkow, GD: Chronic dermal ulcer healing enhanced with monophasic pulsed electrical stimulation. Phys Ther 71:639–649, 1991.
8. Gentzkow, GD, Pollack, SV, Kloth, LC, et al: Improved healing of pressure ulcers using Dermapulse, a new electrical stimulation device. Wounds 3:158–170, 1991.
9. Griffin, JW, Tooms, RE, Mendius, RA, et al: Efficacy of high voltage pulsed current for healing of pressure ulcers in patients with spinal cord injury. Phys Ther 71:433–442, 1991, discussion 442–444.
10. Houghton, PE, and Campbell, KE: Choosing an adjunctive therapy for the treatment of chronic wounds. Ostomy Wound Manage 45:43–52, 1999.
11. Kloth, LC, and Feedar, JA: Acceleration of wound healing with high voltage, monophasic, pulsed current. Phys Ther 68:503–508, 1988.
12. Lundeberg, TC, Eriksson, SV, and Malm, M: Electrical nerve stimulation improves healing of diabetic ulcers. Ann Plast Surg 29:328–331, 1992.
13. Stefanovska, A, Vodovnik, L, Benko, H, et al: Treatment of chronic wounds by means of electric and electromagnetic fields. Part 2. Value of FES parameters for pressure sore treatment. Med Biol Eng Comput 31:213–220, 1993.
14. Wolcott, LE, Wheeler, PC, Hardwicke, HM, et al: Accelerated healing of skin ulcer by electrotherapy: preliminary clinical results. South Med J 62:795–801, 1969.
15. Wood, JM, Evans, PE 3rd, Schallreuter, KU, et al: A multicenter study on the use of pulsed low-intensity direct current for healing chronic stage II and stage III decubitus ulcers. Arch Dermatol 129:999–1009, 1993.
16. Kloth, LC: Electrical stimulation for wound healing. In Kloth, LC, and McCulloch, JM (eds): Wound Healing Alternatives in Management, ed 3. FA Davis, Philadelphia, 2002, pp 271–315.
17. Myers, BA: Electrotherapeutic modalitites, physical agents, and mechanical modalities. In Myers, BA (ed): Wound Management: Principles and Practice. Prentice-Hall, Upper Saddle River, NJ, 2004, pp 152–183.
18. Sommer, C: Immunity and inflammation. In Porth, CM (ed): Pathophysiology: Concepts of Altered Health States, ed 6. Lippincott Williams & Wilkins, Philadelphia, 2002, pp 331–355.
19. Porth, CM: Cellular adaptation, injury, and death and wound healing. In Porth, CM (ed): Pathophysiology: Concepts of Altered Health States, ed 6. Lippincott Williams & Wilkins, Philadelphia, 2002, pp 95–113.
20. Gogia, PP: Physiology of wound healing. In Gogia, PP (ed): Clinical Wound Management. SLACK Incorporated, Thorofare, NJ, 1995, pp 1–12.
21. Burr, HS, Harvey, SC, and Taffel, M: Bio-electric correlates of wound healing. Yale J Biol Med 103–107, 1938.
22. Cunliffe-Barnes, TC: Healing rate of human skin determined by measurement of the electrical potential of experimental abrasions: a study of treatment with petrolatum and with petrolatum containing yeast and liver extracts. Am J Surg 69:82–88, 1945.
23. Jaffe, LF, and Vanable, JW Jr: Electric fields and wound healing. Clin Dermatol 2:34–44, 1984.
24. Foulds, IS, and Barker, AT: Human skin battery potentials and their possible role in wound healing. Br J Dermatol 109: 515–522, 1983.
25. Borgens, RB, Vanable, JW Jr, and Jaffe, LF: Bioelectricity and regeneration: large currents leave the stumps of regenerating newt limbs. Proc Natl Acad Sci U S A 74:4528–4532, 1977.
26. Lee, RC, Canaday, DJ, and Doong, H: A review of the biophysical basis for the clinical application of electric fields in soft-tissue repair. J Burn Care Rehabil 14:319–335, 1993.
27. Kerstein, MD: Moist wound healing: the clinical perspective. Ostomy Wound Manage 41:37S–44S, 1995, discussion 45S.
28. Ovington, LG: Dressings and ajunctive therapies: AHCPR guidelines revisited. Ostomy Wound Manage 45:94S–106S, 1999, quiz 107S–108S.
29. Rajnicek, AM, Stump, RF, and Robinson, KR: An endogenous sodium current may mediate wound healing in Xenopus neurulae. Dev Biol 128:290–299, 1988.
30. Kloth, LC, and McCulloch, JM: Promotion of wound healing with electrical stimulation. Adv Wound Care 9:42–45, 1996.

31. Gault, WR, and Gatens, PF Jr: Use of low intensity direct current in management of ischemic skin ulcers. Phys Ther 56:265–269, 1976.

32. Fukushima, K, Senda, N, Inui, H, et al: Studies on galvanotaxis of leukocytes. Med J Osaka Univ 4:195–208, 1953.

33. Orida, N, and Feldman, JD: Directional protrusive pseudopodial activity and motility in macrophages induced by extracellular electric fields. Cell Motil 2:243–255, 1982.

34. Bourguignon, GJ, and Bourguignon, LY: Electric stimulation of protein and DNA synthesis in human fibroblasts. FASEB J 1: 398–402, 1987.

35. Cooper, MS, and Schliwa, M: Electrical and ionic controls of tissue cell locomotion in DC electric fields. J Neurosci Res 13: 223–244, 1985.

36. Mertz, PM, Davis, SC, Cazzaniga, AL, et al: Electrical stimulation: acceleration of soft tissue repair by varying the polarity. Wounds 5:153–159, 1993.

37. Brown, M, McDonnell, M, and Menton, DN: Polarity effects on wound healing using electrical stimulation in rabbits. Arch Phys Med Rehabil 70:624–627, 1989;

38. Barranco, SD, Spadaro, JA, Berger, TJ, et al: In vitro effect of weak direct current on Staphylococcus aureus. Clin Orthop 100: 250–255, 1974.

39. Guffey, JS, and Asmussen, MD: In vitro bactericidal effects of high voltage pulsed current versus direct current against Staphylococcus aureus. J Clin Electrophysiol 1:5–9, 1989.

40. Kincaid, CB, and Lavoie, KH: Inhibition of bacterial growth in vitro following stimulation with high voltage, monophasic, pulsed current. Phys Ther 69:651–655, 1989.

41. Laatsch, LJ, Ong, PC, and Kloth, LC: In vitro effects of two silver electrodes on select wound pathogens. J Clin Electrophysiol 7:10–15, 1995.

42. Rowley, BA, McKenna, JM, Chase, GR, et al: The influence of electrical current on an infecting microorganism in wounds. Ann N Y Acad Sci 238:543–551, 1974.

43. Szuminsky, NJ, Albers, AC, Unger, P, et al: Effect of narrow, pulsed high voltages on bacterial viability. Phys Ther 74: 660–667, 1994.

44. Kaada, B: Vasodilation induced by transcutaneous nerve stimulation in peripheral ischemia (Raynaud's phenomenon and diabetic polyneuropathy). Eur Heart J 3:303–314, 1982.

45. Scudds, RJ, Helewa, A, and Scudds, RA: The effects of transcutaneous electrical nerve stimulation on skin temperature in asymptomatic subjects. Phys Ther 75:621–628, 1995.

46. Wong, RA, and Jette, DU: Changes in sympathetic tone associated with different forms of transcutaneous electrical nerve stimulation in healthy subjects. Phys Ther 64:478–482, 1984.

47. Baker, LL, Chambers, R, Merchant, L, et al: The effects of electrical stimulation on cutaneous oxygen supply in normal older adults and diabetic patients. Abstract. Phys Ther 66:749, 1986.

48. Dodgen, PW, Johnson, BW, Baker, LL, et al: The effects of electrical stimulation on cutaneous oxygen supply in diabetic older adults. Abstract. Phys Ther 67:793, 1987.

49. Gilcreast, DM, Stotts, NA, Froelicher, ES, et al: Effect of electrical stimulation on foot skin perfusion in persons with or at risk for diabetic foot ulcers. Wound Repair Regen 6:434–441, 1998.

50. Mawson, AR, Siddiqui, FH, Connolly, BJ, et al: Effect of high voltage pulsed galvanic stimulation on sacral transcutaneous oxygen tension levels in the spinal cord injured. Paraplegia 31:311–319, 1993.

51. Peters, EJ, Armstrong, DG, Wunderlich, RP, et al: The benefit of electrical stimulation to enhance perfusion in persons with diabetes mellitus. J Foot Ankle Surg 37:396–400, 1998, discussion 447–448.

52. Heath, ME, and Gibbs, SB: High-voltage pulsed galvanic stimulation: effects of frequency of current on blood flow in the human calf muscle. Clin Sci (Lond) 82:607–613, 1992.

53. Miller, BF, Gruben, KG, and Morgan, BJ: Circulatory responses to voluntary and electrically induced muscle contractions in humans. Phys Ther 80:53–60, 2000.

54. Hecker, B, Carron, H, and Schwartz, DP: Pulsed galvanic stimulation: effects of current frequency and polarity on blood flow in healthy subjects. Arch Phys Med Rehabil 66:369–371, 1985.

55. Tracy, JE, Currier, DP, and Threlkeld, AJ: Comparison of selected pulse frequencies from two different electrical stimulators on blood flow in healthy subjects. Phys Ther 68:1526–1532, 1988.

56. Walker, DC, Currier, DP, and Threlkeld, AJ: Effects of high voltage pulsed electrical stimulation on blood flow. Phys Ther 68: 481–485, 1988.

57. Cosmo, P, Svensson, H, Bornmyr, S, et al: Effects of transcutaneous nerve stimulation on the microcirculation in chronic leg ulcers. Scand J Plast Reconstr Surg Hand Surg 34:61–64, 2000.

58. Cramp, AF, Gilsenan, C, Lowe, AS, et al: The effect of high- and low-frequency transcutaneous electrical nerve stimulation upon cutaneous blood flow and skin temperature in healthy subjects. Clin Physiol 20:150–157, 2000.

59. Lundeberg, T, Kjartansson, J, and Samuelsson, U: Effect of electrical nerve stimulation on healing of ischaemic skin flaps. Lancet 2:712–714, 1988.

60. Wikstrom, SO, Svedman, P, Svensson, H, et al: Effect of transcutaneous nerve stimulation on microcirculation in intact skin and blister wounds in healthy volunteers. Scand J Plast Reconstr Surg Hand Surg 33:195–201, 1999.

61. Porth, CM: Control of the circulation. In Porth, CM (ed): Pathophysiology: Concepts of Altered Health States, ed 6. Lippincott Williams & Wilkins, Philadelphia, 2002, pp 399–428.

62. Mawson, AR, Siddiqui, FH, Connolly, BJ, et al: Sacral transcutaneous oxygen tension levels in the spinal cord injured: risk factors for pressure ulcers? Arch Phys Med Rehabil 74:745–751, 1993.

63. Cramp, AF, Noble, JG, Lowe, AS, et al: Transcutaneous electrical nerve stimulation (TENS): the effect of electrode placement upon cutaneous blood flow and skin temperature. Acupunct Electrother Res 26:25–37, 2001.

64. U.S. Department of Health and Human Services: Clinical Practice Guideline No. 15. Treatment of Pressure Ulcers. U.S. Department of Health and Human Services, Rockville, MD, 1994.

65. Sheffet, A, Cytryn, AS, and Louria, DB: Applying electric and electromagnetic energy as adjuvant treatment for pressure ulcers: A critical review. Ostomy Wound Manage 46:28–33, 36–40, 42–44, 2000.

66. Collum, N, Nelson, EA, Flemming, K, et al: Systematic reviews of wound care management: (5) beds; (6) compression; (7) laser

therapy, therapeutic ultrasound, electrotherapy and electromagnetic therapy. Health Technol Assess 5, 2001.

67. Akai, M, and Hayashi, K: Effect of electrical stimulation on musculoskeletal systems: A meta-analysis of controlled clinical trials. Bioelectromagnetics 23:132–143, 2002.

68. Gardner, SE, Frantz, RA, and Schmidt, FL: Effect of electrical stimulation on chronic wound healing: A meta-analysis. Wound Repair Regen 7:495–503, 1999.

69. Centers for Medicare and Medicaid Services: Electrostimulation for Wounds: Decision Memorandum (#CAG-00068N). 2002; accessed December 6, 2003. Web Page. Available at: http://www.cms.hhs.gov/mcd/index

70. Assimacopoulos, D: Low intensity negative electric current in the treatment of ulcers of the leg due to chronic venous insufficiency. Preliminary report of three cases. Am J Surg 115:683–687, 1968.

71. American Physical Therapy Association: Electrotherapeutic Terminology in Physical Therapy: Section on Clinical Electrophysiology, Alexandria, VA, 1990.

72. Stromberg, BV: Effects of electrical currents on wound contraction. Ann Plast Surg 21:121–123, 1988.

73. Peters, EJ, Lavery, LA, Armstrong, DG, et al: Electric stimulation as an adjunct to heal diabetic foot ulcers: A randomized clinical trial. Arch Phys Med Rehabil 82:721–725, 2001.

74. Tunis, S, Shuren, J, Ballantine, L, et al: Medicare Coverage Policy—NCDS: Electrostimulation for Wounds. July 23, 2002. Web Page.

75. Porth, CM: Alterations in blood flow in the systemic circulation. In Porth, CM (ed): Pathophysiology: Concepts of Altered Health States, ed 6. Lippincott Williams & Wilkins, Philadelphia, 2002, pp 429–458.

76. Bancroft, DA, and Pigg, JS: Alterations in skeletal function: Rheumatic disorders. In Porth, CM (ed): Pathophysiology: Concepts of Altered Health States, ed 6. Lippincott Williams & Wilkins, Philadelphia, 2002, pp 1367–1390.

77. Guven, S, Kuenzi, JA, and Matfin, G: Diabetes mellitus. In Porth, CM (ed): Pathophysiology: Concepts of Altered Health States, ed 6. Lippincott Williams & Wilkins, Philadelphia, 2002, pp 925–952.

78. Kaada, B: Systemic sclerosis: successful treatment of ulcerations, pain, Raynaud's phenomenon, calcinosis, and dysphagia by transcutaneous nerve stimulation. A case report. Acupunct Electrother Res 9:31–44, 1984.

79. Food and Drug Administration Guidelines for Electromedical Devices. 1975.

80. Rasmussen, MJ, Hayes, DL, Vlietstra, RE, et al: Can transcutaneous electrical nerve stimulation be safely used in patients with permanent cardiac pacemakers? Mayo Clin Proc 63:443–445, 1988.

81. Shade, SK: Use of transcutaneous electrical nerve stimulation for a patient with a cardiac pacemaker. A case report. Phys Ther 65:206–208, 1985.

82. Chen, D, Philip, M, Philip, PA, et al: Cardiac pacemaker inhibition by transcutaneous electrical nerve stimulation. Arch Phys Med Rehabil 71:27–30, 1990.

83. Ojingwa, JC, and Isseroff, RR: Electrical stimulation of wound healing. J Investig Dermatol 36:1–12, 2002.

84. American Physical Therapy Association: Clinical Electrotherapy: Physiology and Basic Concepts, APTA Continuing Ed Series No. 8. 2003; accessed November 25, 2003. Available at http://www.apta.org

85. Mulder, GD: Treatment of open-skin wounds with electric stimulation. Arch Phys Med Rehabil 72:375–377, 1991.

86. Cohen, DE, and Rice, RH: Toxic responses of the skin. In Klasssen, CD (ed): Casarett and Doull's Toxicology: The Basic Science of Poisons, ed 6. McGraw-Hill, Medical Publishing Division, New York, 2001, pp 653–672.

87. Kloth, LC: The APTA electrical stimulation lawsuit and its aftermath. American Physical Therapy Association. Adv Wound Care 12:472–475, 1999.

88. Unger, PG: Update on high-voltage pulsed current research and application. Top Geriatr Rehabil 16:35–46, 2000.

89. Houghton, PE, Kincaid, CB, Lovell, M, et al: Effect of electrical stimulation on chronic leg ulcer size and appearance. Phys Ther 83:17–28, 2003.

90. Reich, JD, and Tarjan, PP: Electrical stimulation of skin. Int J Dermatol 29:395–400, 1990.

91. Mehreteab, TA: Clinical Uses of Electrical Stimulation. Appleton & Lange, Norwalk, CT, 1994, pp 283–293.

92. Kirsner, RS, and Bogensberger, G: The normal process of healing. In Kloth, LC, and McCulloch, JM (eds): Wound Healing Alternatives in Management, ed 3. FA Davis, Philadelphia, 2002, pp 3–34.

93. Nelson, RM, and Currier, DP (eds): Clinical Electrotherapy. Norwalk, CT, Appleton & Lange, 1987.

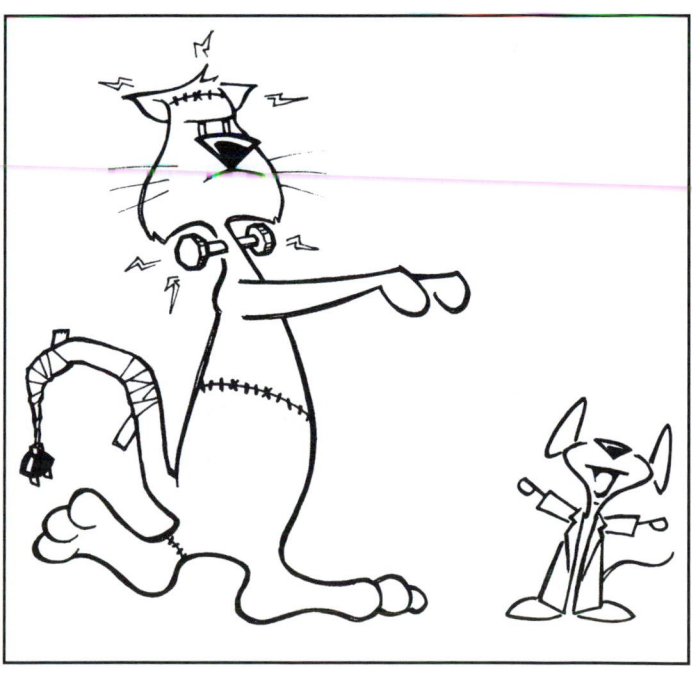

Objectives

- Discuss the concepts of pain management as opposed to pain relief.
- Outline the procedures for the utilization of electrical stimulation to promote analgesia.
- Review the concepts of endogenous mechanisms for pain management.
- Discuss the clinical decision making involved for determining the appropriate parameters for electrical stimulation.
- Discuss appropriate documentation for the use of electrical stimulation to promote analgesia.
- Compare clinical and patient options for pain management with electrical stimulation.

Key Terms

Endogenous	Opiate	Sensory analgesia
Noxious	Pain management	

Barbara J. Behrens PTA, MS   *Kathleen M. Kenna, PT*

Pain Management with Electrical Stimulation

Outline

> *"So are you making my hand hurt so that I forget about my back?"*
>
> *"Is that really supposed to do something? All I feel is tingling, no pain."*

Pain is a sensation that has both physical and psychological components to it. As discussed in Chapter 1, it has been studied, and numerous instruments have been developed in an attempt to capture its extent. The capturing of this type of data has been a perpetual battle due in part to the simple fact that the individual experiencing the discomfort is really the only one who knows how much discomfort he or she is experiencing. The individual is also the only one to know how this level of discomfort is affecting his or her life. Numerous physical agents have had a positive impact on decreasing the level of discomfort perceived by the patient. Electrical stimulation is one of those physical agents that has been used successfully for more than 40 years to provide sensory stimulation and to "gate" the painful stimulation from reaching the brain. This served as the foundation for Melzack and Wall's Gate Control Theory for pain relief and subsequent work.[1]

Pain commonly brings people to seek therapeutic intervention. The clinician has many types of physical agents to choose from to effectively manage the patient's underlying pathology, symptoms, and associated dysfunctions. Thermal and mechanical agents have been presented in this text as tools to address a variety of patient problems. In this chapter, the use of electrical stimulation as a therapeutic intervention for pain management is presented. The following areas are addressed:

- General principles of pain management with the use of electrical stimulation

- Treatment rationale and method
- Treatment expectations and progression
- Appropriate documentation

Remember, pain management is only one aspect of the complete care of the patient. Depending upon the additional rehabilitation needs of the individual, other therapeutic interventions will be used.[2–5] Electrical stimulation, as with any other treatment intervention, is to be implemented to help achieve functional goals for a patient. For example, to facilitate greater force gains in a shorter period of time enabling a patient to perform recreational and activities of daily living, a patient may use electrical stimulation for postoperative physical therapy interventions.[5]

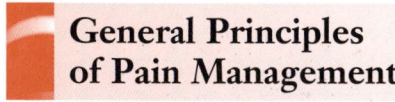

General Principles of Pain Management

Therapeutic intervention with the use of electrical stimulation can provide an analgesic effect. This occurs through a number of postulated neurophysiologic mechanisms (see Chapter 1 for this information). Box 12-1 summarizes the terminology for pain management.

Pain management involves controlling the perception and/or sensation of pain. Management of pain allows the patient to better control his or her discomfort. This can lead to improved function. Electrical stimulation is a physical agent that can be used as one tool for pain management.[6]

Electrical stimulation is believed to produce analgesic effects through the stimulation of the peripheral and central

nervous system. Electrical stimulation devices are available as both clinical and portable models that the patient can use at appropriate times during the day as needed. The portable units are generally the size of a "beeper" and run on rechargeable batteries. The portability of the electrical stimulators allows the patient greater autonomy in his or her own care as well as the option for use of extended periods of stimulation. When the unit and electrodes are used appropriately, side effects are minimal. There is a chance for a chemical burn at the stimulation site, hypersensitivity reactions to the stimulation, or allergic reactions to the self-adhering electrodes.

Physiology Review

Pain sensation occurs as a result of damage to sensory receptors in the skin and internal structures. This damage may be of several different forms, and thus cause the excitation of different sensory receptors. One type of sensory receptor includes the nerve fiber types that are the mediators of pain impulses or noxious sensation in the central nervous system—the A-delta and C fibers. Both of these fiber types are responsible for noxious (painful) sensations. A-delta fibers provide fast pain sensation, and C fibers provide a deeper, dull or achy pain sensation. A-beta fibers transmit discriminative touch stimuli from the skin.

According to the original work of Melzack and Wall,[1] the sensory pain fibers also have the property of being able to be blocked and to stop their ability to transmit their input to the brain, thus temporarily altering pain perception. This original work sparked the development of a tremendous market for electrical stimulation devices that could be used for this purpose. The devices were termed transcutaneous electrical nerve stimulation (TENS) units. TENS has since been used to accomplish pain relief for a multitude of conditions.[7–10]

TENS actually refers to the application of electrical stimulation across the skin, which really applies to most of the electrical stimulation that is applied in physical therapy clinical settings, except for needle insertion for electromyographic (EMG) studies. (For more information, refer to Chapter 1.)

Pain Fiber Types, Central Pathways, and TENS

Once a pain receptor is stimulated, the nerve fiber transmits a signal to the dorsal horn of the spinal cord. A few ascending and descending fibers branch off to form Lissauer's tract and communicate with neighboring spinal segments. The main fiber continues in the dorsal horn to make connections with neurons of the lamina I, II, III, IV, and V. Lamina II is also known as the substantia gelatinosa. Synaptic connections are then made with neurons, giving rise to the lateral spinothalamic tract. These neurons cross over to the opposite side of the spinal cord at the ventral white commissure. The fibers of the lateral spinothalamic tract ascend the spinal cord and enter the brainstem.

Because TENS has the ability to block ascending transmission of nerve fibers, it has the ability to gate pain perception. There is a crossing over of information to the opposite side of the spinal cord, so it is also possible in theory to gate pain perception on the right with stimulation on the left at the same spinal level. Pain has both physical and psychological factors associated with it. Research, however, has indicated that there is a more complex mechanism than just the specificity theory that clinicians have been relying on to explain their successes with TENS.[11]

Sensory Analgesia

Sensory analgesia can be produced by causing a "tingling" sensation. The stimulation may be activity of A-beta nerve fibers. The sensation produced may affect the "gating" mechanism at the spinal cord level, so pain impulses are not transmitted to the higher centers.[1] In effect, the patient experiences a tolerable stimulus that blocks pain impulses. Electrode placements can be directly over the painful site, along the corresponding dermatome, along the cutaneous nerve distribution of the painful area, or along the area superficial to the nerve trunk supplying the painful site. Parameters of stimulation are a rate of greater than 50 pulses per second (pps) to 125 pps, a pulse duration of 60 to 100 milliseconds, and an amplitude to produce a strong tingling sensation without a muscle contrraction.[6] Duration of treatment initially can be up to an hour to assess the therapeutic effect. Depending upon its effectiveness, this form of stimulation can be used up to 24 hours per day. Pain relief usually occurs during the time the stimulus is applied. This relief then may enable the patient to perform functional activities much sooner than if the TENS had not been used.[4,6,7,12]

Endogenous Opiate Liberation

Theoretically, stimulation of the endogenous opiate system can also lead to pain relief. Electrical stimulators capable of rates of 1 to 5 pps, a pulse duration greater than 200 milliseconds, and an intensity to create a muscle twitch may generate pain relief through this mechanism. The duration of treatment is 30 to 45 minutes. Electrode placement sites may include motor points that may also be acupuncture points or trigger points. (See the Appendix at the end of this chapter for more information regarding electrode placement.)

Stimulation of the A-delta and C fibers by the parameters described may affect the production of endorphins and enkephalin release that mimic the action of narcotic drugs to promote decreased perception of pain. Pain reduction usually lasts longer with this form of electrical stimulation than the application to produce sensory analgesia. This form of electrical stimulation may used for the treatment of intense or chronic pain.[13,14]

Other Considerations

When using electrical stimulation for promoting pain reduction, other factors need to be considered. The patient's attitude toward the use of electrical stimulation is important in the successful use of the modality. Explanations of the intended purpose and mechanism of affecting the pain experience need to be presented to the patient in appropriate, understandable terminology. Also, the expected results of treatment need to be discussed. Do not set the patient up for failure by trying to attain unrealistic goals. If a patient has heard of a form of electrical stimulation or has been treated with this modality in the past, find out more details about what the modality was, how it was used, and how effective it was for that patient. If the patient is biased toward the success of the treatment, build upon the experience and how the treatment has effectively been used on other patients with similar conditions. If electrical stimulation is used, the patient should be informed that there are a great variety of treatment parameters and electrode placements that can lead to a successful treatment outcome. If the stimulation was used in the past for sensory analgesia, emphasize the effectiveness of endogenous opiate stimulation or vice versa. If the patient indicates a certain type of electrode placement, discuss other options that can be used.

Most important, the practitioner needs to discuss expected results of the use of electrical stimulation by developing realistic goals. If a patient is of the attitude that electrical stimulation does not help or if he or she has had a bad experience with the modality, the practitioner may choose another technique for pain control (see Treatment Expectations, p. 218).

Narcotic pain medications produce analgesia by decreasing the perception of pain. The release of endogenous opiates by electrical stimulation produces pain relief through the same mechanism. If electrical stimulation is effective in alleviating pain, a decrease in the amount of prescribed medication may be indicated. This must be discussed with the physician who prescribed the medication prior to making a comment to a patient about changing the dosage level.

Before You Begin

Ask yourself the following questions:

- Has the patient already had a bad experience with electrical stimulation that you will have to overcome?
- Does the patient have a fear of electricity?
- Have you thoroughly explained what you are going to do and what the patient should expect?

Alcohol consumption by the patient needs to be considered by the clinician. Alcohol is considered a sedative-hypnotic agent. The effects of dose-dependent central nervous system depression from alcohol produce analgesia. Judgment is also impaired with alcohol consumption; therefore, home use of an electrical stimulator may not be recommended for patients who have a tendency to abuse alcohol by consuming large quantities on a regular basis. Intensity may have to be significantly increased in order to be perceived by the patient. In either case, safety of the patient becomes an issue. The clinician is to be prudent in informing the patient of this information.

The use of exercise is also a consideration when using electrical stimulation for pain relief. Patients will be able to detect sharp A-delta pain if an exercise is being done beyond the recommended range of motion or at an excessive level that could be causing tissue damage. Protective pain mechanisms remain intact when sensory analgesia is produced via electrical stimulation. Depending on the diagnosis of the patient, the desired response to treatment, and the perception of pain, electrical stimulation can be used to facilitate exercise by decreasing pain perception. Specific guidelines need to be reinforced for a home exercise program that is also being done by a patient who is using a portable electrical stimulation device.

Potential Treatments and How to Achieve Success

Clinical Decision Making

Many electrical stimulation devices exist that allow several treatment options. These include, but are not limited to, interferential current stimulators, high-voltage pulsed current muscle stimulators, and low-voltage units. The details of the various types of devices are presented in Chapter 14. Look at the parameters a given machine is capable of producing in order to determine if its use is appropriate for the type of treatment for which you want to use it.

The purpose of this section is to develop a process by which the clinician can determine the most appropriate forms of electrical stimulation treatments for a patient. In order to provide effective treatment, the clinician goes through a decision-making process that concludes in treatment alternatives for the patient. Through thorough examination and assessment, the clinician may identify the source of a patient's painful symptoms. Past medical history and the history of the present condition assist the clinician in identifying contraindications and precautions relevant to the use of electrical stimulation. A summary of contraindications and precautions is presented in Box 12-2. In the presence of contraindications, a different pain-reducing modality that presents fewer risks to the patient should be selected. If precautions are present, the patient should be monitored closely for signs of adverse reactions to treatment. If electrical stimulation is the chosen treatment, parameters are further delineated by identifying the type of pain present, the location of the pain, the characteristics of the pain, and the other rehabilitative needs of the patient. The findings influence treatment parameters, options for electrode placement, and goal setting. A decision-making paradigm is presented in Figure 12-1.

The portability of some electrical stimulation units allows for home use of the device, thus providing the patient treatment opportunities as needed for pain relief. The patient needs sufficient joint range of motion and dexterity to apply electrodes, to plug in wires, and to operate the controls. If the patient is not physically capable of using the machine, the individual may have another person at home that can apply the electrodes and adjust the controls as needed. The patient should also have the ability to understand the appropriate use of the machine. Clinicians should be able to explain the purpose and use of the device in understandable terms. The

---

BOX 12-2   Contraindications and Precautions with the Use of Electrical Stimulation for Pain Management

Contraindications

Demand type cardiac pacemaker
Carotid sinus, stimulation over the area may result in a hypotensive incident
Directly over the eye
Epilepsy
Malignancies (see below)
Loss of or decreased sensation

Precautions

Patients with known cardiac disease or arrhythmias should be closely monitored for signs of adverse effects.
Directly over an open wound.
Directly over the lumbar paraspinals and abdominal area during pregnancy, except during labor and delivery in uncomplicated pregnancies.
For patients with diagnosed malignancies that have been diagnosed as terminal, it may be utilized for pain control with informed consent of the patient.
In addition the electrical stimulator is for external use only and should be kept out of the reach of children.

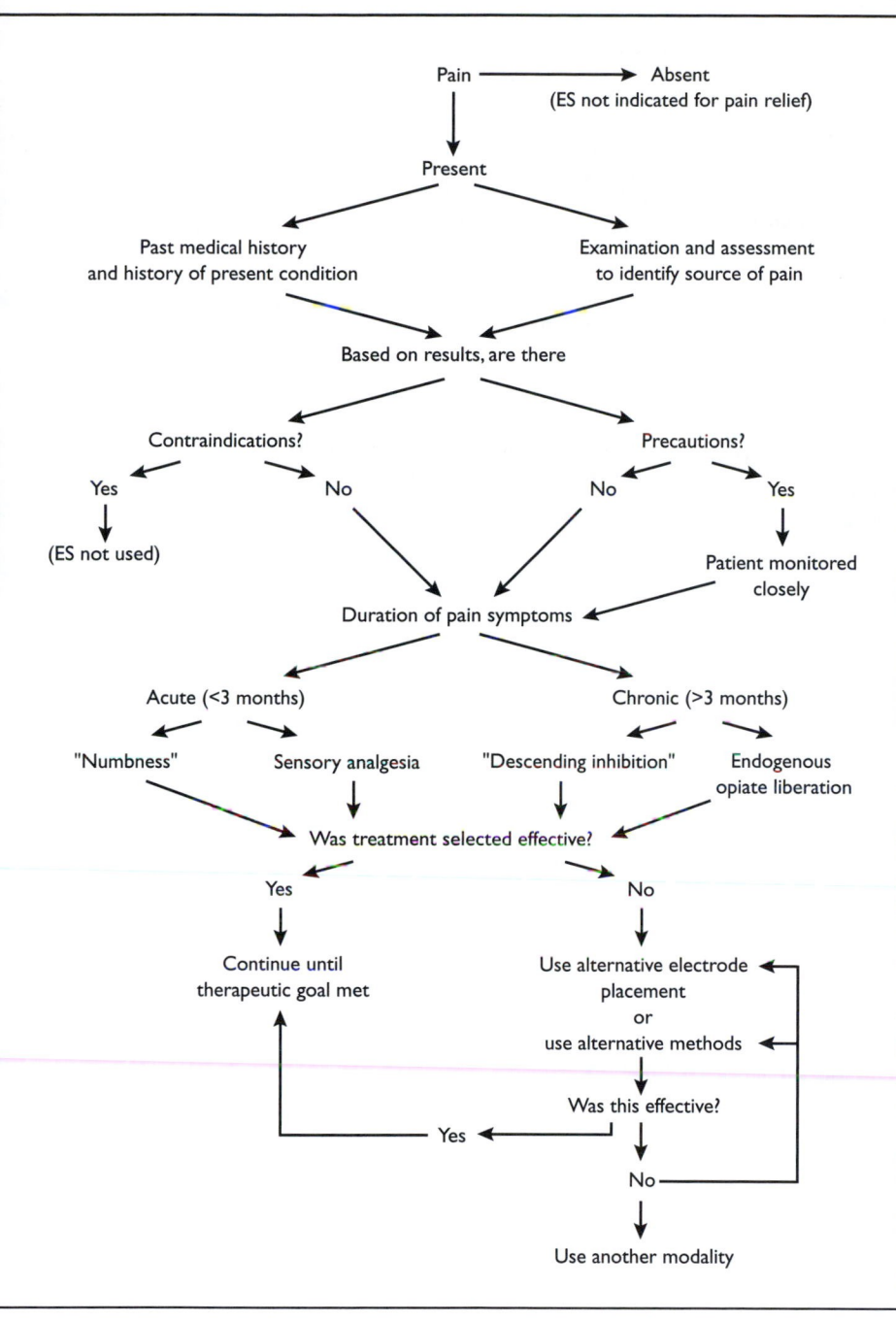

Figure 12-1 Clinical decision-making paradigm.

patient should also be instructed to monitor skin condition and respond accordingly.

Some form of written and/or pictorial home instruction material outlining the safe use of the unit should be provided. All important information concerning the safe and appropriate use of the unit should be included. This form should include, but is not limited to, the following information:

- Purpose of the unit
- Settings of the controls (pulse duration, pulse rate)
- Some form of pain assessment chart to monitor results

- Electrode placement site charts
- Battery insertion instructions
- Electrode care and instructions for use
- The name and telephone number of the clinician or another resource person to answer questions
- A list of "do's and don'ts" regarding the use of the device
- Potential trouble shooting tips for the unit
- Instructions on appropriate skin care

A sample form is given in Figure 12-2.

TENS
Home Instruction Form

Your clinician will determine the electrode placement sites and method of stimulation that will provide the most effective degree of pain control with the shortest treatment time. Your cooperation is essential to this process.

Complete the chart below recording your pain ratings as requested. If you have any questions call your clinician.

| 1   2   3   4   5   6   7   8   9   10 |
| No   Maximal |
| pain   pain |

pre-TENS rating	Treatment time	post-TENS rating	Relief time	Comments
_____	_____	_____	_____	_____
_____	_____	_____	_____	_____
_____	_____	_____	_____	_____
_____	_____	_____	_____	_____
_____	_____	_____	_____	_____
_____	_____	_____	_____	_____
_____	_____	_____	_____	_____
_____	_____	_____	_____	_____
_____	_____	_____	_____	_____
_____	_____	_____	_____	_____
_____	_____	_____	_____	_____

Setting up the TENS unit . . .

The following descriptions will assist you in setting the controls on the TENS unit. Do not experiment with the settings unless instructed to do so by the clinician.

I Conventional

Pulse Duration: (PD, width)	Preset to the lowest setting
Frequency: (Hz, PPS, rate)	Preset to the highest setting
Amplitude: (intensity)	Increase to a comfortable level of tingling. Increase if it "fades."
Treatment time:	Leave it ON until you do not feel pain. Do not leave it turned ON for more than 60 minutes without turning if OFF to see how it feels.

II Acupuncturelike

Pulse Duration: (PD, width)	Preset to the highest setting
Frequency: (Hz, PPS, rate)	Preset to the lowest setting
Amplitude: (intensity)	Increase until muscle "thumping" occurs
Treatment time:	25 to 30 minutes while resting.

III Brief Intense

Pulse Duration: (width)	Preset to the highest setting
Frequency: (Hz, PPS, rate)	Preset to the highest setting
Amplitude: (intensity)	Increase to the strongest level tolerable.
Treatment time:	5 to 30 minutes as instructed

Electrode Placement Sites

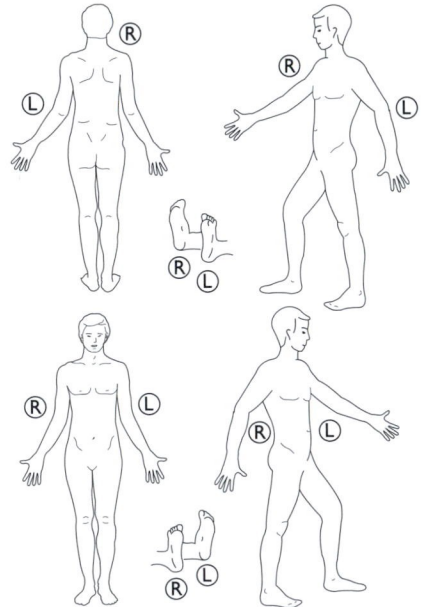

These electrode placement sites should be used. "X's" are one channel, and "O's" are the other channel.

TENS Reminders . . .

1. Do not wear the TENS unit while bathing, showering, or sleeping. Remove the electrodes and replace them after the activity.
2. The TENS unit may be worn at all other times, and turned ON whenever you are experiencing pain. There is no limit to the number of times (treatments) per day.
3. The TENS unit should be turned OFF when not in use, to insure a longer battery life.
4. If your TENS unit has rechargeable batteries, the extra set should be plugged into the recharger to ensure the availability of charged batteries at all times.
5. Carefully inspect the electrodes before applying them. Make sure that there is no metal or bare rubber showing through the side of the electrode that touches your skin. If the electrodes do break down, replace them.
6. If you need more electrodes, or new lead wires, call the TENS distributor.

Notes:

Important #'s:

Date: _____   Model: _____   Serial # _____

Clinician: _____

TENS Distributor: _____

Figure 12-2 Sample written and pictorial home instruction material. (Diagram courtesy of Barbara J. Behrens, PTA, MS.)

Treatment Methods

Rationale for Electrode Placement

Chapters 10 and 11 discuss electrode placement sites for a number of treatment applications. This section will deal specifically with electrode placement site selection for analgesia.

Optimal stimulation sites for electrodes are those that will facilitate goal accomplishment through the delivery of current. If the skin resistance is too high, the target tissue may not be reached at a comfortable level of current. Motor points, trigger points, and acupuncture points all represent electrically active and identifiable points that enhance the potential flow of current into the target tissue.

Motor points are the anatomic location where the peripheral nerve enters the muscle. The amount of electrical current necessary to elicit a motor response from a muscle will be less over the motor point than other areas of the muscle. Placement of an electrode over this area facilitates a motor response of the underlying muscle belly with a lower intensity setting than other nonspecific sites. Whenever the desired response involves a motor response or muscle contraction, motor points should be selected for use.[15–17]

Trigger points are those areas that exhibit hypersensitivity to both pressure and electrical stimulation. Palpation of these sites causes pain to radiate away from the site.[15–18] Trigger points have a decreased resistance to electrical energy. There is a direct correlation between the location of trigger points and motor points.[17] Selection of a trigger point for electrical stimulation would tend to yield better results than not selecting one, because these points represent an area of decreased resistance.

Acupuncture points represent another type of point that has been described for use with electrical stimulation devices. These points are located over the entire surface of the body and have been mapped out for centuries. Acupuncture points may lie over muscle or connective tissue. They are also electrically active, exhibiting a decreased resistance to the flow of electrical current.[17] If the desired response to the electrical stimulation is a diffuse sensory analgesia, then acupuncture points may afford the greatest availability of sites for electrode placements.

Diffuse sensory analgesia can be readily accomplished through the use of two channels of electrodes for a total of four electrodes. These two channels can be set up in a crisscrossed pattern. This pattern will promote an increase in sensation throughout the area with less discrimination of actual location of individual electrodes, as long as the electrodes surround the painful region. This setup will be enhanced with the use of acupuncture points. (Refer to Appendix at the end of this chapter.)

The rationale for electrode placement is based on the type of response the clinician is trying to elicit through electrical stimulation. If a muscle twitch is desired, motor points are the placement of choice. If sensory analgesia is desired, the use of acupuncture points is warranted. The utilization of optimal stimulation points does not guarantee the desired amount of sensation. The appropriate parameters must be used to create the desired analgesic effect.

Treatment methods for pain relief to be produced by electrical stimulation fall into four categories. Each method theoretically produces pain relief by a different neurophysiologic effect generated by the use of different parameters of the electrical stimulation device. All methods have been demonstrated to be effective forms of treatment when used appropriately.[1,2,4–7,9,10]

Producing Analgesia for a Painful Procedure

Some manual techniques may be painful for a patient when the technique is being performed. It is possible to produce analgesia via "a strong tingling sensation" to ease the discomfort of the procedure through the use of electrical stimulation. Parameters for this technique are summarized in Box 12-3. Effective carryover of pain relief is brief, because once the stimulation is turned off, normal sensation returns very rapidly.

Producing Sensory-Level Analgesia

Sensory analgesia is suggested to activate the "gating" mechanism in the spinal cord. This reduces pain impulses from reaching the brain to be processed.[1] Appropriate parameters and treatment indications are described in Box 12-4. Effective

---

BOX 12-3   Parameters for Producing Analgesia During a Painful Procedure[34]

Frequency:	150 + pulses per second
Pulse Duration:	Greater than 150 μsec
Intensity:	A strong tingling sensation to tolerance. *Note:* a nonrhythmical muscle contraction may be produced at this intensity
Electrode Placement Sites:	Along involved dermatome, two points where the nerve is superficial
Treatment Time:	5 minutes prior to initiation of the painful technique, 15–30 minutes total time.
Indications:[2,34]	Acute pain, pain associated with wound debridement, pain associated with transverse friction massage, pain associated with aggressive stretching techniques, pain associated with aggressive joint mobilization techniques

<table>
<tr><td colspan="2">BOX 12-4   **Parameters for Producing Sensory - Level Analgesia**</td></tr>
<tr><td>Frequency:</td><td>75–150 pulses per second</td></tr>
<tr><td>Pulse duration:</td><td>Less than 200 µsec</td></tr>
<tr><td>Intensity:</td><td>Strong, but comfortable tingling sensation</td></tr>
<tr><td>Electrode Placement Sites:</td><td>Surrounding the site of pain</td></tr>
<tr><td>Indications:</td><td>Acute pain conditions, chronic pain conditions</td></tr>
</table>

<table>
<tr><td colspan="2">BOX 12-6   **Parameters for Endogenous Opiate Liberation[36]**</td></tr>
<tr><td>Frequency:</td><td>1–5 pulses per second</td></tr>
<tr><td>Pulse Duration:</td><td>200–300 µsec</td></tr>
<tr><td>Intensity:</td><td>Muscle twitch</td></tr>
<tr><td>Electrode Placement Sites:</td><td>Motor points</td></tr>
<tr><td>Treatment Time:</td><td>30–45 minutes</td></tr>
<tr><td>Indications:</td><td>Chronic pains syndromes</td></tr>
</table>

carryover is pain relief that persists after the stimulation is no longer present.

Noxious Stimulation to Produce Analgesia

Electrical stimulation, which is theorized to induce "descending inhibition," uses a noxious form of stimulation to help control pain. The painful stimulus activates the smaller pain fibers, which then make connections in the brainstem reticular formation. Information is then conducted to the midbrain to an area called the periaqueductal gray matter. This area of the brain activates a descending pathway that inhibits pain at the spinal cord level.[1] Analgesia occurs quickly with this form of stimulation and effective carryover can last a few minutes to a few hours. Treatment parameters and indications are presented in Box 12-5. A disadvantage of this form of stimulation is that the patient must experience noxious stimuli to produce the desired effect.

Endogenous Opiate Liberation

Low-rate electrical stimulation can potentially produce analgesia through the liberation of endogenous opiates. Parameters for pain relief by this method and indications are summarized in Box 12-6. The onset of pain relief may occur

<table>
<tr><td colspan="2">BOX 12-5   **Parameters for Producing "Hyperstimulation Analgesia"**</td></tr>
<tr><td>Frequency:</td><td>1–4 pulses per second</td></tr>
<tr><td>Pulse Duration:</td><td>≥ 1 msec</td></tr>
<tr><td>Intensity:</td><td>Highest tolerable level of noxious stimulation</td></tr>
<tr><td>Electrode Placement Sites:</td><td>Active electrode is a small diameter probe that is placed over a point with decreased resistance to the flow of current. It may be an acupuncture point, trigger point, or motor point. The dispersive electrode can be held by the patient or placed on the skin at a point distal to the site of stimulation.</td></tr>
<tr><td>Treatement Time:</td><td>30 seconds per point</td></tr>
<tr><td>Indications:</td><td>Acute or chronic pain syndromes</td></tr>
</table>

by the end of a treatment session or several hours later with potentially long-term carryover of pain relief.

Treatment Expectations

When utilizing electrical stimulation as a tool in a pain management program, realistic goals must be considered. Goal determination is based upon evaluative findings, the nature of the disabling condition, the previous activity level of the patient, the patient's psychosocial condition, and the prognosis of recovery. The goals established will also vary depending on the stage of the healing process and the nature of the pain acute versus chronic. If a patient is not "invested in" or motivated toward his or her own recovery, the efforts of a clinician may have limited success.

A patient who is experiencing acute pain experiences decreased pain intensity and pain patterns as a result of the resolution of the inflammatory response and the healing process. During the acute phase, patients may experience pain at rest as well as with any movement.[12] The use of electrical stimulation can facilitate the healing process because of physiologic responses to the modality. Once pain decreases, the patient may also experience a decrease in the intensity of muscle guarding. The use of electrical stimulation can be used to help break up the pain-spasm-pain cycle. Goals for a patient during the acute phase of the inflammatory response and the healing process include decreasing the intensity of pain at rest and with movement. This response, if elicited by the use of electrical stimulation, may occur within the treatment time of 20 to 30 minutes. The desired response with other patients may be elicited only while the patient is using an electrical stimulation device. In that case, the patient may be a good candidate for a portable device to be used at times outside the clinical setting.

As the healing process enters the subacute phase, pain may be experienced at the end range of motion.[12] Pain at rest has usually resolved by this time. This process tends to occur from 7 to 21 days after the onset of injury, but may last up to 6 weeks. Tendons and ligaments may take several weeks to go through this initial healing phase. The severity of injury will also determine the duration of the subacute phase. The use of electrical stimulation may continue to be a treatment option for the patient; however, the underlying purpose for its use will change. The purpose now becomes directed toward controlling the pain that is created as a result of other therapeutic interventions that stress the tissue at end range of motion. The patient may have little discomfort prior to treatment, but the gentle therapeutic techniques used to enhance range of motion may cause an increase in pain perception. Electrical stimulation may then be used as a post-treatment modality. In this situation, the goal would be to bring the pain level back to a pretreatment level.

When the healing process has reached the maturation and remodeling phase, therapeutic interventions tend to become more aggressive to promote the patient's functional abilities. Progressive stretching, strengthening, and functional activities are commonly the emphasis of treatment. Therapeutic techniques at this phase are intended to stress the immature collagen fibrils laid down in the subacute phase to develop stronger chemical bonds and to orient fibers in a direction that is conducive to function. This process lasts for an additional 8 to 14 weeks after the initial injury. The denser the connective tissue, the longer is the process. During this phase of healing, pain may be experienced at the end range of motion when overpressure is applied to shortened or weakened structures. Electrical stimulation can be used for the purpose of treating pain created by the therapeutic intervention with the intent to bring pain levels back to pretreatment levels.

The purpose of the use of electrical stimulation during the normal course of the healing of an acute injury is a transition from managing pain at rest, to post-treatment pain reduction. Each patient's response will vary; therefore, the goals formulated are to be individualized for the patient and adjusted accordingly. If pain is at a tolerable level, not interfering with recovery, or can be controlled by other physical agents effectively, the use of electrical stimulation may be discontinued.

Individuals with chronic pain conditions may also benefit from the use of electrical stimulation. The expectation of eliminating pain symptoms may be unrealistic for the majority of patients; thus, the goal of electrical stimulation is to control pain to allow for better function.

Electrical stimulation may be effective for at least three different purposes in treating a chronic pain patient. Electrical stimulation can be used to decrease the intensity of the pain the patient is experiencing at rest. It can decrease the pain associated with the therapeutic techniques utilized to enhance muscle flexibility and functional activity during and after treatment. Finally, it can also help treat acute "flare-ups" or exacerbations in pain symptoms.

Treatment goals for the use of electrical stimulation with patients who have chronic pain may emphasize functional ability while keeping pain symptoms at a manageable level. The goal may be an effective reduction in pain that allows the patient to walk for longer periods of time or that provides greater comfort for a person to do work-related tasks. The patient should also be able to use a home electrical stimulation unit effectively to manage his or her pain symptoms.

The complete treatment of a patient with chronic pain is a multifaceted approach involving many medical disciplines and is beyond the scope of this text. Developing relaxation skills; improving coping skills; and increasing flexibility, strength, and endurance will further enhance patient recovery. The use of electrical stimulation is only one tool used to help these patients.

Although TENS will not provide success for pain relief for all patients, clinicians have successfully used this modality to help in pain management with many patients who seek relief of their symptoms. Combining the appropriate parameters and electrode placements with the principles of the healing process and the appropriate communication approach to the patient provides the treatment that has a high potential for success. Pain may not be eliminated, but it may be controlled sufficiently to facilitate a more comfortable recovery, facilitate other goals of treatment, and restore functional ability as a result of pain control.

Documentation of Treatments with Electrical Stimulation

The documentation of treatment parameters and patient responses are essential to the practice of determining the efficacy of any treatment. The treatment parameters that one clinician uses should be reproducible by another. Documentation is the key for accomplishing consistency in treatment between practitioners. When using the Subjective, Objective, Assessment, Plan (SOAP) note format for documentation, different aspects of the pain management should be noted throughout different headings of documentation.

Objective (O in SOAP) information for the documentation of pain management includes the measurable aspects of the patient's condition and the treatment rendered. Parameters used with electrical stimulation must be indicated. Documentation should include the type of electrical stimulation used, the mode of delivery, pulse duration (PD), frequency (F), rise and fall time (if used), treatment area, electrode placement sites, duration of treatment, and goal of or response to the intensity.

Summary

The use of electrical stimulation as a physical agent for the treatment of pain symptoms is multifaceted. The clinician should have a thorough understanding of the neurophysiologic basis of pain modulation and the variety of methods to achieve pain reduction with electrical stimulation. Treatment applications are based on this knowledge as well as the results of a thorough evaluation of the patient. Any modification of parameters is based on treatment outcome. This chapter presented a review of the underlying tenets of pain modulation and a variety of methods to achieve pain reduction. The paradigm of clinical decision making provides the practitioner with a framework of the process for treatment selection or modification to achieve the desired goals of electrical stimulation as an instrument for pain reduction.

Discussion Questions

1. What forms of electrical stimulation can be used to treat the pain associated with the performance of a painful manual technique such as a deep tissue massage? What parameters would you use and why?

2. Explain the neurophysiologic mechanisms of the effects of electrical stimulation in terms that a patient would understand.

3. A patient is diagnosed with phantom limb pain. What information would you need to know about this patient in order to recommend a form of electrical stimulation for treatment of this syndrome?

4. What are the advantages and disadvantages of electrical stimulation for analgesia compared with others that reduce pain perception?

5. Describe three possible forms of electrical stimulation treatments for an individual with a chronic pain syndrome.

CASE STUDY

Carol is cartoonist who has been referred to physical therapy for pain management techniques subsequent to a cervical strain injury. She was involved in a motor vehicle accident where she was hit from behind. She now has muscle guarding and marked decreases in her cervical range of motion in all directions. Her primary complaint is of occipital headaches. She lives alone and works from a home office. Most of her day is spent at an artist's table that is angled at 45 degrees. Medications to reduce muscle guarding and inflammation caused other complications in interaction with medications that she was taking.

References

1. Melzack, R: Pain: Past, present and future. Can J Exp Psych 47:615–629, 1993.
2. Hurley, DA, Minder, PM, McDonough, SM, et al: Interferential therapy electrode placement technique in acute low back pain: A preliminary investigation. Arch Phys Med Rehabil 82:485–493, 2001.
3. Draper, V, and Ballard, L: Electrical stimulation versus electromyographic biofeedback in the recovery of quadriceps femoris function following anterior cruciate ligament surgery. Phys Ther 71:455–465, 1991.
4. Gotlin, RS, Hershkowitz, S, Juris, PM, et al: Electrical stimulation effect on extensor lag and length of hospital stay after total knee arthroplasty. Arch Phys Med Rehabil. 75:957–959, 1994.
5. Lewek, M, Steven, J, and Snyder-Mackler, L: The use of electrical stimulation to increase quadriceps femoris muscle force in an elderly patient following total knee arthroplasty. Phys Ther 81:1565–1571, 2001.
6. Jarit, GJ, Mohr, KJ, Waller, R, et al: The effects of home interferential therapy on post-operative pain, edema, and range of motion of the knee. Clin J Sport Med 13:16–20, 2003.
7. Rakel, B, and Frantz, R: Effectiveness of transcutaneous electrical nerve stimulation on postoperative pain with movement. J Pain 4:455–464, 2003.
8. Sluka, KA, and Walsh, D: Transcutaneous electrical nerve stimulation: Basic science mechanisms and clinical effectiveness. J Pain 4:109–121, 2003.
9. Chesterton, LS, Foster, NE, Wright, CC, et al: Effects of TENS frequency, intensity and stimulation site parameter manipulation of pressure pain threshold in healthy human subjects. Pain 106:73–80, 2003.
10. Moore, SR, and Shurman, J: Combined neuromuscular electrical stimulation and transcutaneous electrical nerve stimulation for treatment of chronic back pain: A double-blind, repeated measures comparison. Arch Phys Med Rehabil 78:55–60, 1997.
11. Melzack, R, Coderre, TJ, Katz, J, et al: Central neuroplasticity and pathological pain. Ann N Y Acad Sci 933:157–174, 2001.
12. Zizic, TM, Hoffman, KC, Holt, PA, et al: The treatment of osteoarthritis of the knee with pulsed electrical stimulation. J Rheumatol 22:1757–1761, 1995.
13. Wells, PE, Frampton, V, and Bowsher, D: Pain Management by Physical Therapy. Appleton & Lange, Norwalk, CT, 1988.
14. Tollison, CD, Satterthwaite, JR, and Tollison, JW: Handbook of Pain Management, ed 2. Williams & Wilkins, Baltimore, 1994.
15. Travell, J, and Rinzler, SH: The myofascial genesis of pain. Postgrad Med 11:425–435, 1952.
16. Melzack, R: Myofascial trigger points: Relation to acupuncture and mechanisms of pain. Arch Phys Med Rehabil 62:114, 1981.
17. Melzack, R, Stilwell, DM, and Fox, EJ: Trigger points and acupuncture points for pain: Correlations and implications. Pain 3:3, 1977.
18. Baldry, P: Management of myofascial trigger point pain. Acupoint Med 20:2–10, 2002.

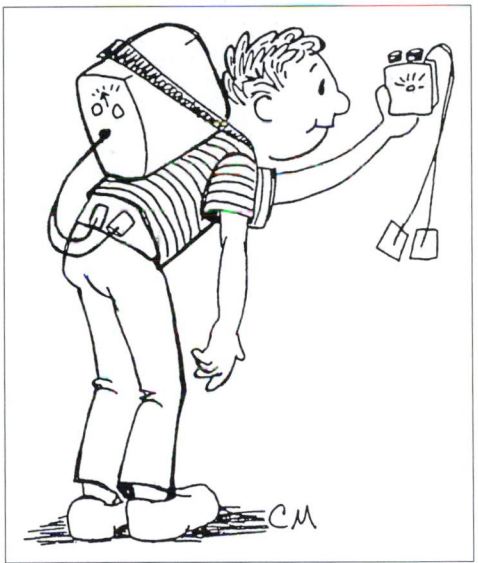

Appendix:
Optimal Stimulation Sites for TENS Electrodes

Key to Illustrations and Tables on Following Pages

▼	Acupuncture point	K. or K....	kidney meridian
○	Motor point	LI. or li....	large intestine
□	Trigger point	LU. r lu....	lung
● (gray)	Cutaneous nerve	LV. or lv....	liver
●	Peripheral nerve	P. or p....	pericardium
		SI. or si....	small intestine
BL. or bl....	bladder meridian	SP. or sp....	spleen
GB. or gb....	gallbladder meridian	ST. or st....	stomach
H. or h....	heart meridian	TW. or tw....	triple warmer

Researched and developed by Jeffrey S. Mannheimer, M.A., R.P.T., and Barbara J. Behrens, A.A.S.P.T.A. © 1980.

*From Mannheimer, JS and Lampe GN: Clinical Transcutaneous Electrical Nerve Stimulation. FA Davis, Philadelphia, 1984, pp 301, 306–307, 309–319, 324–325, with permission.

Spine and Occiput

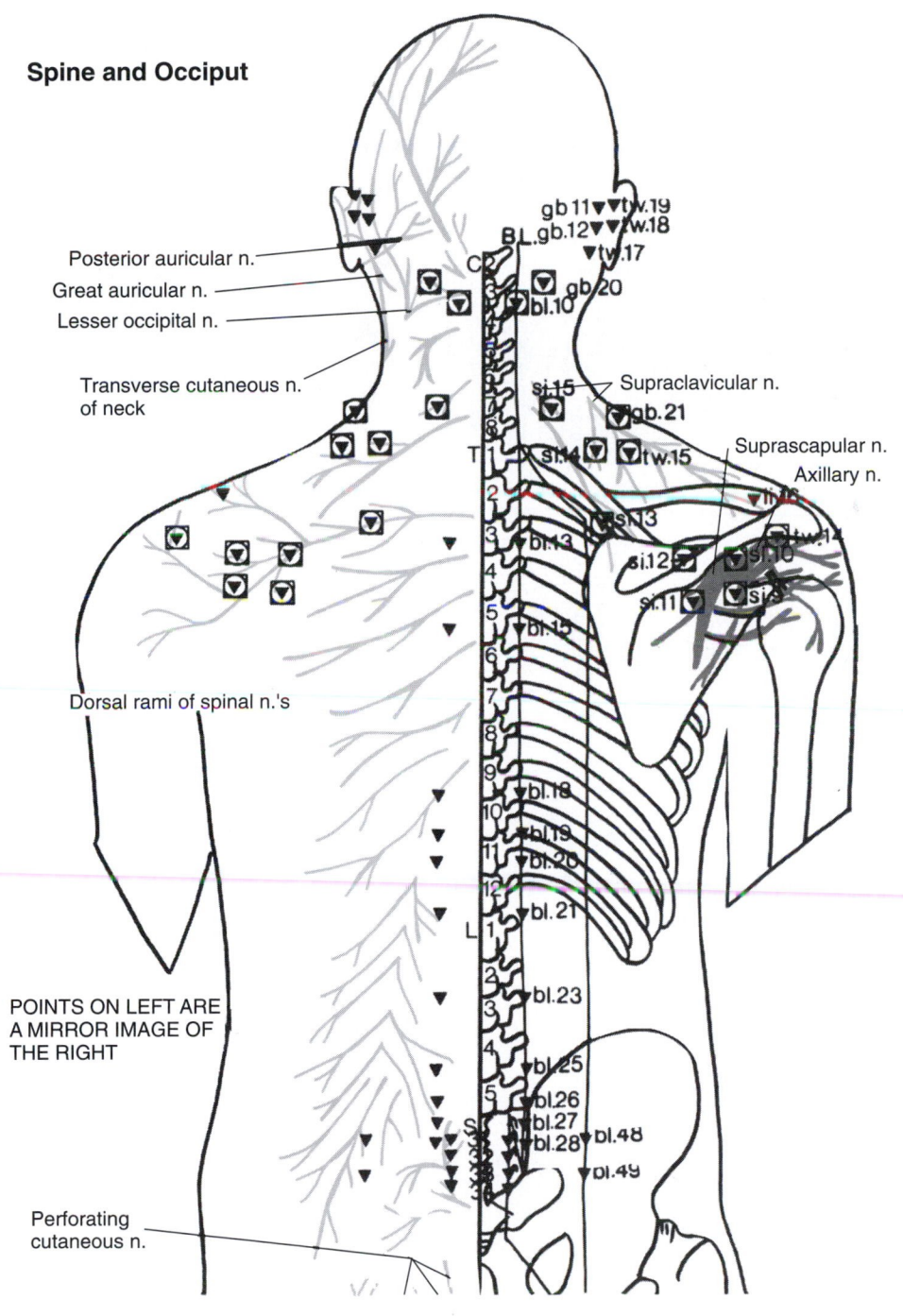

Posterior auricular n.

Great auricular n.

Lesser occipital n.

Transverse cutaneous n.
of neck

Dorsal rami of spinal n.'s

POINTS ON LEFT ARE
A MIRROR IMAGE OF
THE RIGHT

Perforating
cutaneous n.

gb 11   tw.19
gb.12   tw.18
B.L.   tw.17
C   gb.20
       bl.10
si.15   Supraclavicular n.
       gb.21
T   si.14   tw.15   Suprascapular n.
       si.13   Axillary n.
       bl.13   tw.14
       si.12   si.10
       si.11   si.9
L   bl.15
       bl.18
       bl.19
       bl.20
       bl.21
       bl.23
S   bl.25
       bl.26
       bl.27   bl.48
       bl.28
       bl.49

Table 12-1 Optimal Stimulation Sites for TENS Electrodes

OCCIPUT

LOCATION	SUPERFICIAL NERVE BRANCH	ACUPUNCTURE POINT	MOTOR POINT	TRIGGER POINT	SEGMENTAL LEVEL
Posterior ear upper third (TW 19) same level but slightly more medial on occiput (GB 11)	Great auricular, posterior branch communicates with lesser occipital, auricular branch of vagus, posterior auricular branch of facial. Transverse cutaneous nerve of neck	TW 19 GB 11 is just medial			Cranial C2–4
Posterior ear middle third (TW 18) same level but slightly more medial on occiput (GB 12)	Same as above	TW 18 GB 12 is just medial			Cranial C2–4
Behind ear in depression between angle of mandible and mastoid process	Great auricular, posterior branch and lesser occipital	TW 17			C2–4
Suboccipital depression, between sternocleidomastoid (SCM) and upper trapezius	Greater and lesser occipital nerves	GB 20 B 10 is nearby, slightly medial and inferior	Splenius capitis (branches from C2–4) semispinalis capitis	Splenius capitis Semispinalis capitis	C2–3

The explanation of optimal stimulation sites for the shoulder girdle as seen on this view can be found on the view of posterolateral shoulder and dorsal region of the upper extremity.

THE SPINE

LOCATION	SUPERFICIAL NERVE BRANCH	ACUPUNCTURE POINT	MOTOR POINT	TRIGGER POINT	SEGMENTAL LEVEL
In depression between medial border of posterior superior iliac spine (PSIS) and 1st sacral spinous process	Dorsal ramus of L2	B 27			L2
2" lateral to spinous process of S2	Dorsal ramus of L2	B 48	Gluteus maximus (upper motor pt) (inferior gluteal L5–S2)	Gluteus maximus	L2 L5–S2
2" lateral to spinous process of S4	Dorsal rami of L2–3	B 49	Gluteus maximus (lower motor pt) (piriformis directly below) (inferior gluteal) (L5–S2)	Gluteus maximus (piriformis directly below)	L2–3 L5–S2
Directly over 1st sacral foramen	Dorsal ramus of S1	B 31			S1

Directly over 2nd sacral foramen	Dorsal ramus of S2	B 32			S2
Directly over 3rd sacral foramen	Dorsal ramus of S3	B 33			S3
Directly over 4th sacral foramen	Dorsal ramus of S4	B 34			S4

The twelve cutaneous branches of thoracic posterior primary rami become superficial adjacent to the spinous processes. They each have multiple cutaneous twigs. Havelacque considers the dorsal ramus of T2 to be the largest and most diffuse.[265]

The cutaneous disbribution of the dorsal ramus of T2 reaches up to the posterior aspect of the acromion, covering the mid-back (to the region of T5–6) and laterally to the superior region of the posterior axillary fold. A number of optimal stimulation sites are depicted as overlying this nerve.

Cutaneous branches of the dorsal rami of L1–3 descend as far as the posterior part of the iliac crest, skin of the buttock and almost to the greater trochanter of the femur (see lower extremity, lateral and posterior views).[1(p1033), 93]

ANTEROMEDIAL SHOULDER AND VOLAR REGION OF UPPER EXTREMITY

LOCATION	SUPERFICIAL NERVE BRANCH	ACUPUNCTURE POINT	MOTOR POINT	TRIGGER POINT	SEGMENTAL LEVEL
Between first and second ribs, about 4" lateral to sternum, medial to coracoid process	Musculocutaneous nerve	LU 1	Coracobrachialis is nearby (musculocutaneous) (C6)		C5–7
Radial side of biceps brachii 2" below anterior axillary fold. 3" below anterior axillary fold	Musculocutaneous nerve and its lower lateral cutaneous branch	LU 3 LU 4	Biceps brachii (musculocutaneous) (C5–6)		C5–7
In antecubital fossa on crease at radial side of biceps tendon	Lateral cutaneous nerve of arm	LU 5	Brachialis (musculocutaneous) (C5–6)		C5–7
Just lateral to radial artery from 1st volar crease to just above radial styloid	Lateral cutaneous nerve of forearm communicating with superficial radial nerve	LU 7–9			C5–7 C6–8
Volar surface of hand at midpoint of 1st metacarpal	Superficial branch of radial nerve and palmar cutaneous of median	LU 10	Abductor pollicis brevis (median) (C8–T1)		C6–8 C5–T1 C5–7
Between heads of biceps brachii 2" below anterior axillary fold with medial cutaneous	Musculocutaneous and intercostal brachial nerves, may communicate nerve of forearm	P 2			T2 C8–T1
Just medial to biceps tendon in antecubital fossa	Median nerve and anterior branch of medial cutaneous nerve of forearm	P 3	Pronator teres (median) (C 6)		C5–T1 C8–T1
Between tendons of flexor carpi radialis (FCR) and palmaris longus (PL) 2" and 1½" above volar crease respectively	Median and anterior branch of medial cutaneous nerve of forearm	P 5 P 6 is 1" below			C5–T1 C8–T1

Anteromedial Shoulder and Volar Region of Upper Extremity

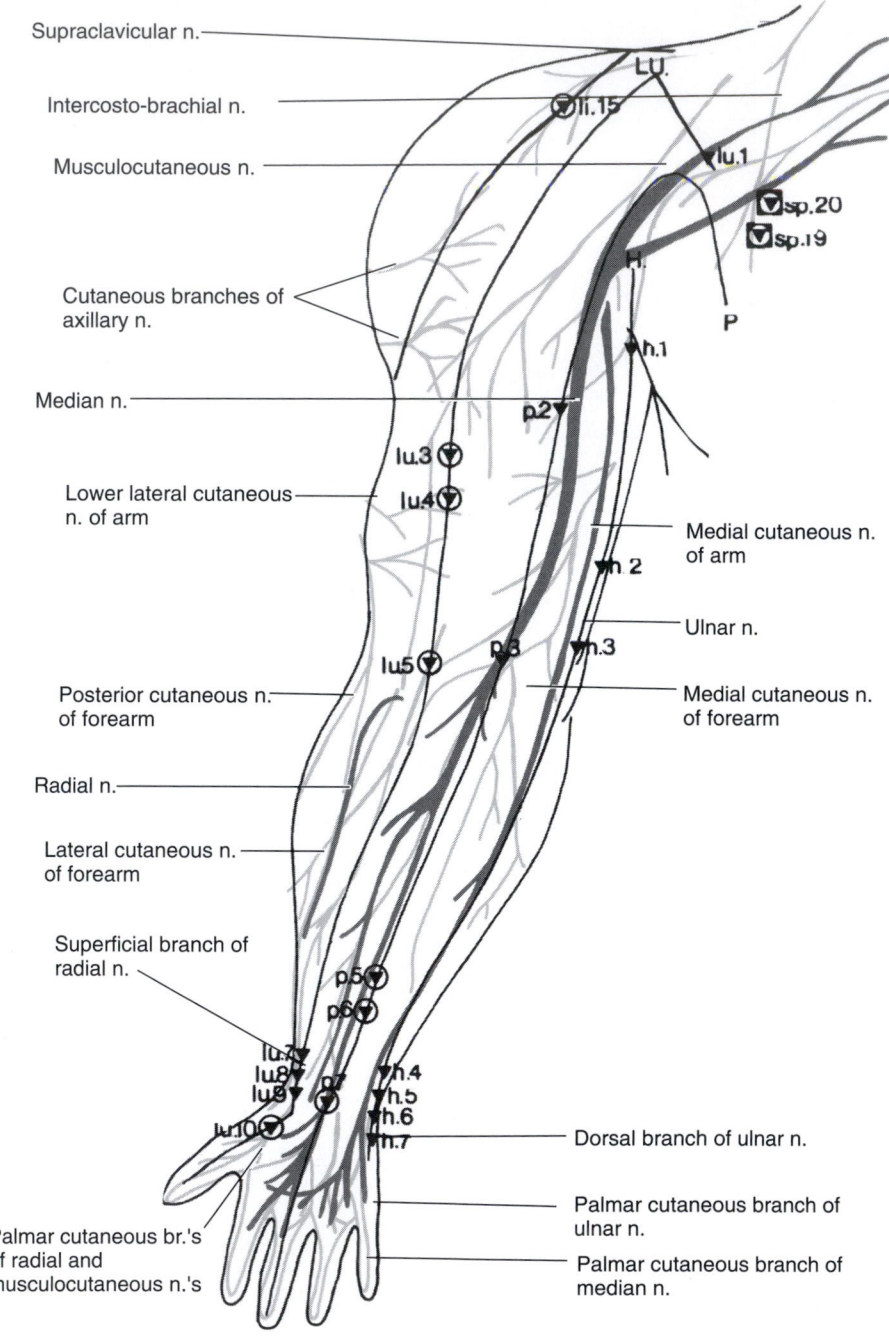

Table 12-1   Optimal Stimulation Sites for TENS Electrodes *(continued)*

ANTEROMEDIAL SHOULDER AND VOLAR REGION OF UPPER EXTREMITY

LOCATION	SUPERFICIAL NERVE BRANCH	ACUPUNCTURE POINT	MOTOR POINT	TRIGGER POINT	SEGMENTAL LEVEL
Between tendons of FCR and PL at midpoint transverse volar wrist crease	Median and anterior branch of medial cutaneous nerve of forearm and palmar cutaneous branch of median	P 7			C5–T1 C8–T1
Between ribs 2-3 and 3-4, midway between anterior axillary fold and sternum	Medial and intermedial supraclavicular nerves to 2nd rib, lateral cutaneous nerves of thorax (2-4), the 2nd nerve is the intercostal brachial nerve	SP 19-20	Pectoralis major (medial) and lateral anterior thoracic nerves)	Pectoralis major	C3–4 T2–4
Medial to brachial artery in axilla	Ulnar nerve, intercostobrachial, medial cutaneous nerve of arm and median nerve which is just lateral to artery	H 1			C7–T1 T2 C9–T1 C5–T1
In groove medial to lower 1/3 of biceps brachii medial to brachial artery	Median and medial cutaneous nerve of arm	H 2			C5–T1 C8–T1
Just superior to cubital tunnel by medial epicondyle	Medial cutaneous nerve of forearm	H 3			C8–T1
Ulnar aspect of wrist lateral to flexor carpi ulnaris (FCU) tendon from 1 1/2" above 1st volar wrist crease to pisiform bone	Ulnar nerve and its palmar cutaneous branch	H4-7			C7–T1
In depression anterior and inferior to acromion	Upper lateral cutaneous nerve branch of axillary	LI 15	Anterior deltoid (axillary) (C5-6)		C5–6

POSTEROLATERAL SHOULDER AND DORSAL REGION OF UPPER EXTREMITY

LOCATION	SUPERFICIAL NERVE BRANCH	ACUPUNCTURE POINT	MOTOR POINT	TRIGGER POINT	SEGMENTAL LEVEL
1 1/2" lateral to spinous process of C7	Medial branch of supraclavicular	SI 15	Levator scapulae (spinal accessory and dorsal scapular (C3-4)	Levator scapulae	Cranial C3–4
1 1/2" above superior angle of scapula at the level of the spinous process of T1	Lateral (posterior) branch of supraclavicular	SI 14 TW 15 is just lateral	Middle trapezius (spinal accessory (C3-4)	Middle trapezius	Cranial C3–4
Suprascapular fossa (medial end) 3" lateral to spinous process of T2	Lateral (posterior) branch of supraclavicular and dorsal ramus of T2	SI 13	Middle trapezius (spinal accessory) (C3-4)	Middle trapezius	Cranial C3–4 T2
At midpoint of suprascapular fossa	Dorsal ramus of T2	SI 12	Supraspinatus (suprascapular) (C5-6)	Supraspinatus	C5–6 T2

Posterolateral Shoulder and Dorsal Region of Upper Extremity

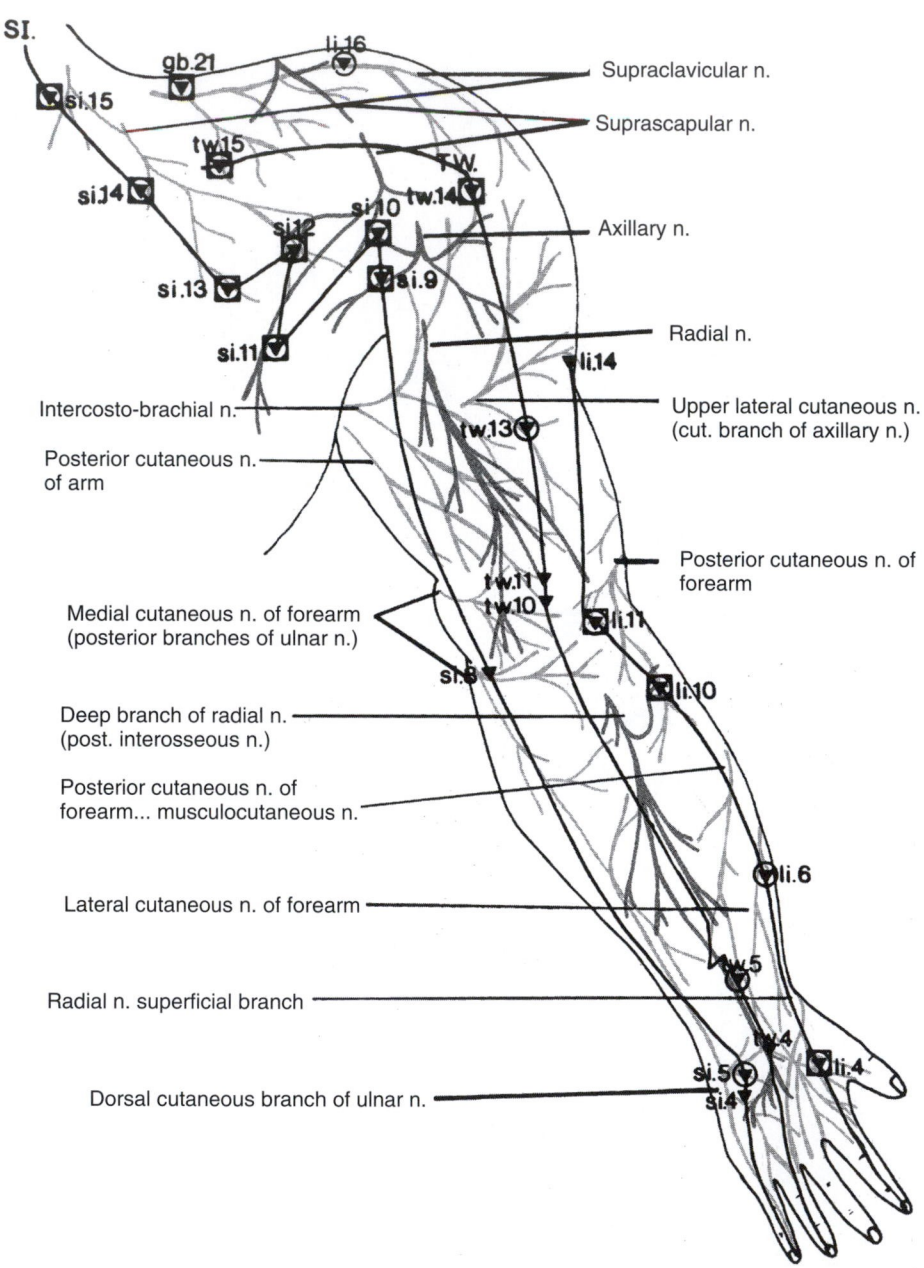

Table 12-1 Optimal Stimulation Sites for TENS Electrodes (continued)

POSTEROLATERAL SHOULDER AND DORSAL REGION OF UPPER EXTREMITY

LOCATION	SUPERFICIAL NERVE BRANCH	ACUPUNCTURE POINT	MOTOR POINT	TRIGGER POINT	SEGMENTAL LEVEL
At midpoint of infrascapular fossa	Dorsal ramus of T2	SI 11	Infraspinatus (suprascapular) (C5–6)	Infraspinatus	C5-6 T2
Directly above posterior axillary fold. Just below spine of scapula	Dorsal ramus of T2 and axillary (posterior branch), which continues as the upper lateral cutaneous nerve of the arm	SI 10 (axillary)	Posterior deltoid (C5–6)	Posterior deltoid T2	C5-6
Directly below SI 10. Just superior to posterior axillary fold	Axillary and dorsal ramus of T2	SI 9	Teres major (subscapular) (C5–6)	Teres major	C5-6 T2
In groove between olecranon and medial epicondyle of humerus	Ulnar nerve and its medial cutaneous branches	SI 8			C7–T1
In depression between pisiform bone and ulnar styloid	Dorsal and palmar cutaneous branches of ulnar nerve	SI 5			C7–T1
In depression between fifth metacarpal and triquetral	Dorsal and palmar cutaneous branches of ulnar nerve	SI 4	Palmaris brevis (median) (C8–T1)		C7–T1
On cephalad surface of upper trapezius directly above superior angle of scapula	Supraclavicular	GB 21	Upper trapezius (spinalaccessory)	Upper trapezius	Cranial C3–4
In depression posterior and inferior to acromion and above greater tubercle of humerus with arm in anatomical position	Intercostal brachial, upper lateral cutaneous nerve–branch of axillary, and dorsal ramus of T2	TW 14	Posterior deltoid (axillary) (C5–6)		C5–6 T2
Just below deltoid insertion by lateral head of triceps	Upper lateral cutaneous nerve branch of axillary	TW 13	Lateral head of tricps (radial) (C7–8)		C5–6
In depression I" above olecranon with the elbow flexed to 90°	Posterior cutaneous of arm (radial) medial cutaneous of forearm (ulnar posterior branches) posterior cutaneous nerve of forearm	TW 10, TW 11 is just above			C5–8 C8–T1 C5–8
Between radius and ulna on dorsal surface about 2" proximal to transverse wrist crease	Posterior cutaneous nerve of forearm, branch of radial communications with lateral cutaneous nerve of forearm, branch of musculocutaneous	TW 5	Extensor indicis proprius (radial) (C7)		C5–8 C5–6

Table 12-1   Optimal Stimulation Sites for TENS Electrodes *(continued)*

LOWER EXTREMITY, POSTERIOR VIEW

LOCATION	SUPERFICIAL NERVE BRANCH	ACUPUNCTURE POINT	MOTOR POINT	TRIGGER POINT	SEGMENTAL LEVEL
2" lateral to superior border of symphysis pubis	Anterior cutaneous branches of iliohypogastric, ilioinguinal and genitofemoral	LIV 10–12	Pectineus (femoral) (L2–4)		L1 L1 L1–2
Between 1st and 2nd metatarsals just above web space junction on dorsum of foot	Deep peroneal nerve via its medial terminal and interosseous branches	LIV 2–3	1st dorsal interosseus (lateral plantar) (S1–2)		L4–5 S1–2
From inguinal ligament to femoral triangle lateral to femoral artery	Anterior branch of obturator communicating with medial cutaneous. Forms subsartorial plexus.	SP 12 SP 13	Iliopsoas (femoral) (L2–4)		L2–4 L2–4
2" above medial aspect of patellar base	Medial cutaneous nerve of thigh and saphenous nerve (infrapatellar)	SP 10	Vastus medialis (femoral) (L2–4)	Vastus medialis	L2–4 L2–3
Just below medial condyle of tibia, level with tibial tuberosity between sartorius and gracilis	Saphenous nerve	SP 9			L3–4
Just superior to midpoint of patellar base	Intermediate cutaneous nerve of the thigh	Extra 31			L2–3
Medial to patellar tendon	Medial cutaneous nerve of thigh	Extra 32 (medial)			L2–3
In depression just below patella, lateral to tendon with knee flexed 2-3" above lateral aspect of patellar base	Medial and lateral cutaneous nerve of thigh and infrapatellar branch of saphenous which forms a patellar plexus	ST 35 Extra 32 (lateral)			L2–3 L3–4
	Intermediate and lateral cutaneous nerve of thigh	ST 33–34	Vastus lateralis (femoral) (L2–4)		L2–4
In depression just below patella, lateral to tendon with knee flexed	Medial and lateral cutaneous nerve of thigh and infrapatellar branch of saphenous which form a patellar plexus	ST 35 Extra 32 (lateral)			L2–3 L3–4
2" below inferior angle of patella, lateral to tibial crest	Infrapatellar branch of saphenous	ST 36	Superior motor point of anterior tibialis (deep peroneal) (L4–5,)	Anterior tibialis	L3–4
Below malleoli at center of dorsum of foot, lateral to anterior tibialis tendon	Superficial peroneal	ST 42			L4–S2

Lower Extremity, Anterior View

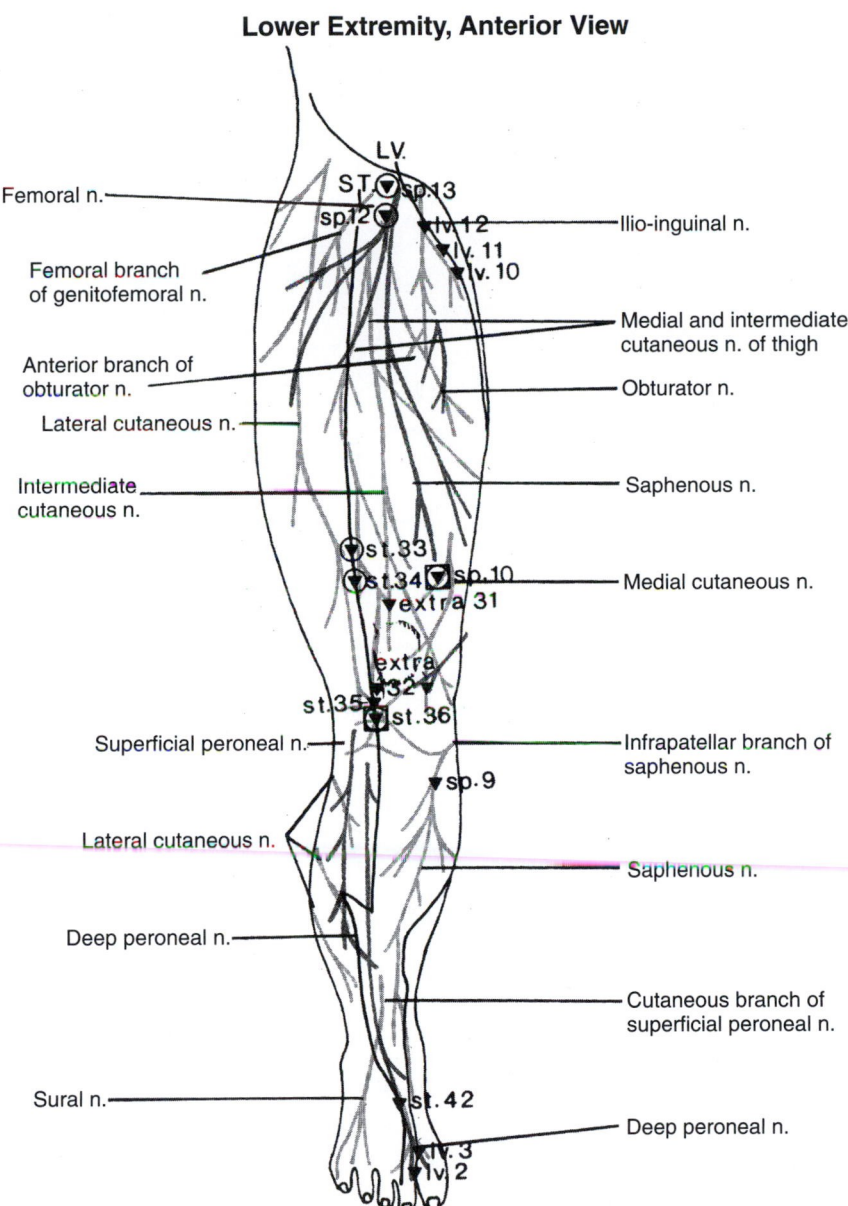

Femoral n.

Femoral branch
of genitofemoral n.

Anterior branch of
obturator n.

Lateral cutaneous n.

Intermediate
cutaneous n.

Superficial peroneal n.

Lateral cutaneous n.

Deep peroneal n.

Sural n.

LV.
ST. sp.13
sp.12 lv.12
lv. 11
lv. 10

st.33
st.34 sp.10
extra 31

extra
32
st.35 st.36

sp.9

st.42

lv.3
lv.2

Ilio-inguinal n.

Medial and intermediate
cutaneous n. of thigh

Obturator n.

Saphenous n.

Medial cutaneous n.

Infrapatellar branch of
saphenous n.

Saphenous n.

Cutaneous branch of
superficial peroneal n.

Deep peroneal n.

Table 12-1   Optimal Stimulation Sites for TENS Electrodes *(continued)*

LOWER EXTREMITY, POSTERIOR VIEW					
LOCATION	SUPERFICIAL NERVE BRANCH	ACUPUNCTURE POINT	MOTOR POINT	TRIGGER POINT	SEGMENTAL LEVEL
2" lateral to spinous process of S2	Dorsal ramus L2	B 48	Gluteus maximus (upper motor pt) (inferior gluteal L5–S2)	Gluteus maximus	L2 L5–S2
2" lateral to spinous process of S4	Dorsal rami L2-3	B 49	Gluteus maximus (lower motor pt) (piriformis directly below) (inferior gluteal L5–S2)	Gluteus maximus (piriformis directly below)	L2–3 L5–S2
At midpoint of junction between buttock and posterior thigh	Posterior cutaneous nerve of thigh, medial and lateral branches	B 50			S1–3
Popliteal fossa between biceps femoris and semitendinosus tendons	Posterior cutaneous nerve of thigh, medial and lateral branches	*B 54/40 *B 53/39 (lateral aspect of popliteal fossa medial to biceps femoris tendon)			S1–3
Midline of leg below heads of gastrocsoleus at junction of upper 2/3 and lower 1/3 of leg	Sural, communicating branch of lateral cutaneous nerve of calf (common peroneal)	B 57	Soleus (tibial nerve S1-2	Soleus	L5–S2 L4–S2
Between lateral malleolus and heelcord	Dorsal lateral cutaneous nerve-end of sural	B 60			L4–S2

*Numerical systems differ according to texts.
B 53 & 54 Acupuncture Therapy[115]
B 39 & 40 An Outline of Chinese Acupuncture[116]

Lower Extremity, Posterior View

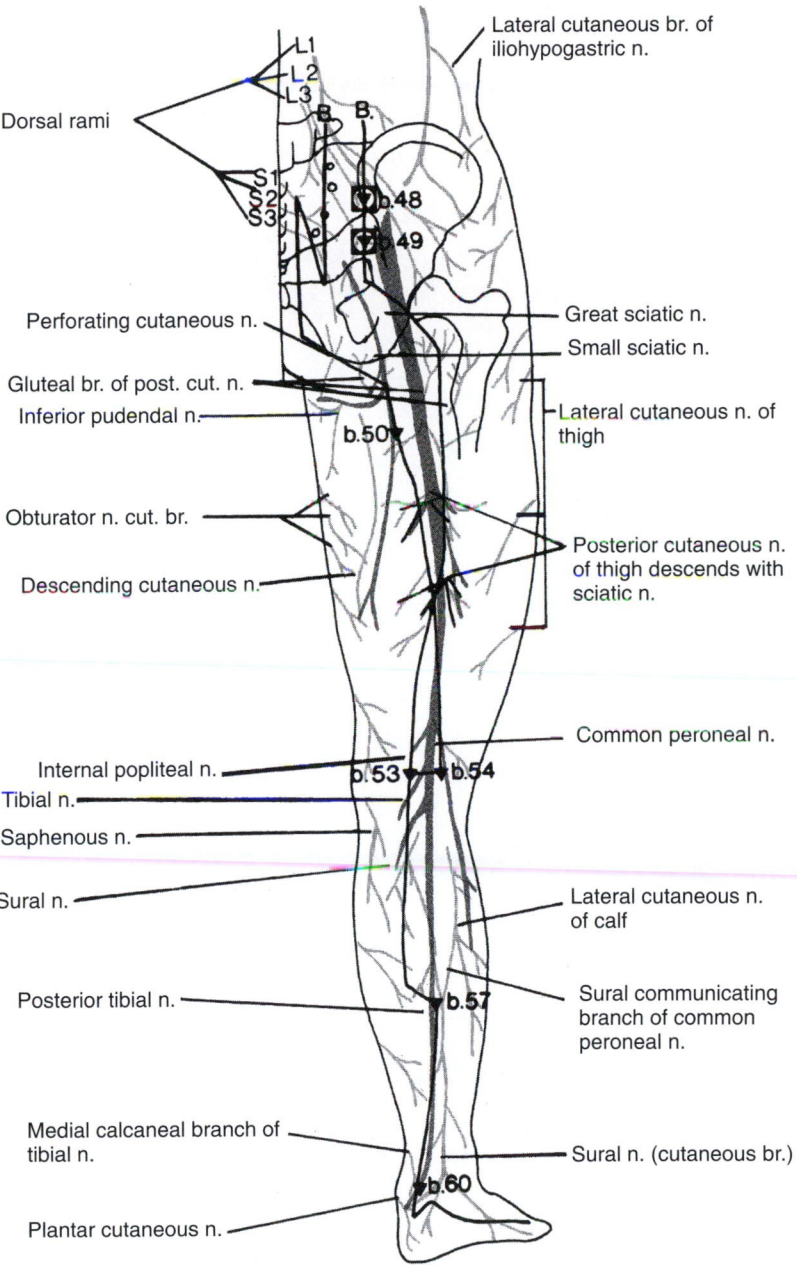

Lateral cutaneous br. of iliohypogastric n.

L1
L2
L3

Dorsal rami

B B

S1
S2
S3

b.48

b.49

Perforating cutaneous n.

Great sciatic n.

Small sciatic n.

Gluteal br. of post. cut. n.

Inferior pudendal n.

b.50

Lateral cutaneous n. of thigh

Obturator n. cut. br.

Posterior cutaneous n. of thigh descends with sciatic n.

Descending cutaneous n.

Common peroneal n.

Internal popliteal n.

b.53   b.54

Tibial n.

Saphenous n.

Sural n.

Lateral cutaneous n. of calf

Posterior tibial n.

b.57

Sural communicating branch of common peroneal n.

Medial calcaneal branch of tibial n.

Sural n. (cutaneous br.)

b.60

Plantar cutaneous n.

Objectives

- Describe the use of electrical stimulation for medication delivery.
- Describe the ionic properties of direct current.
- Outline the procedures for phoretic delivery of medications.
- Differentiate between iontophoretic drug delivery and injection.

Key Terms

Avascular
Aqueous
Biometabolism
Dermis
Elastin
Enteric

Epidermis
Integument
Iontophoresis
Isoelectric
Hepatic
Hydrophilic

Parenteral
Phonophoresis
Plasticity
Nonsteroidal anti-
    inflammatory
    drug

Steroidal anti-
    inflammatory
    drug
Turgor

Peter C. Panus, PT, PhD

Physical Agents for Transdermal Drug Delivery: Iontophoresis and Phonophoresis

Outline

"…you mean I don't have to have a shot, I can have the medication go through that pad?"

Medications or drugs may be introduced into the body by a variety of means including enteral (swallowing) or parenteral (injection) routes or through passive absorption through the skin (transcutaneously) over extended periods of time. The routes bypass the hepatic circulation, thus avoiding a major site of potential degradation.[1] Mechanisms of parenteral drug delivery include injection, passive transcutaneous delivery, and the use of electrorepulsive forces (iontophoresis) or mechanical (phonophoresis). Iontophoretic delivery is desirable for drugs that

1. Demonstrate significant hepatic metabolism or

2. Require constant plasma levels or

3. Are being used for topical or local transcutaneous tissue effects

Phonophoretic delivery may also achieve the some of the previously stated goals. This chapter reviews the biophysical and cellular composition of the skin (integument), as related to transcutaneous drug delivery, as well as the currently accepted mechanism(s) by which drugs transcutaneously per-

Patient's Perspective

Remember that your patient does not understand what you are about to do. A simple explanation using a magnet as an example, describing how like poles on a magnet repel each other might help the patient to understand how the charge of the medication will be repelled by the electrode into his or her body. This explanation will also help you to reassure yourself that you are applying the medication under the correct pole during iontophoresis.

FREQUENTLY ASKED QUESTIONS

1. What will this feel like?

2. Can I take all my medications this way?

3. If you turn it up higher, will it be better for me?

4. Shouldn't I feel something like I do with the other electrical stimulation devices?

5. Is it safe to touch that while it is on?

meate the skin under passive, iontophoretic, or phonophoretic conditions. The iontophoretic devices and electrodes currently available within the United States for human use are also discussed. Finally, the experimental and clinical evidence supporting iontophoretic and phonophoretic application in rehabilitation will be examined.

Integumentary System: Our Skin

Morphology and Function

The integument is the largest organ of the body and consists of two main layers. The epidermis is the superficial avascular layer; the dermis is a deeper vascularized layer, and the basal lamina separates the two (Fig. 13-1). The epidermis consists of five layers. The deepest layer, stratum basale, is a single layer of cells that continuously divide and differentiate as one "daughter cell" randomly migrates to the surface. The most superficial layer, stratum corneum, represents the most differentiated cells, and is composed of about 10 to 15 layers of these flattened cornified cells (corneocytes). The total thickness of skin is about 2 to 3 mm, but the thickness of stratum corneum is only about 10 to 15 μm. Most of the epidermal mass is concentrated in the stratum corneum. The stratum corneum is the major barrier to both environmental

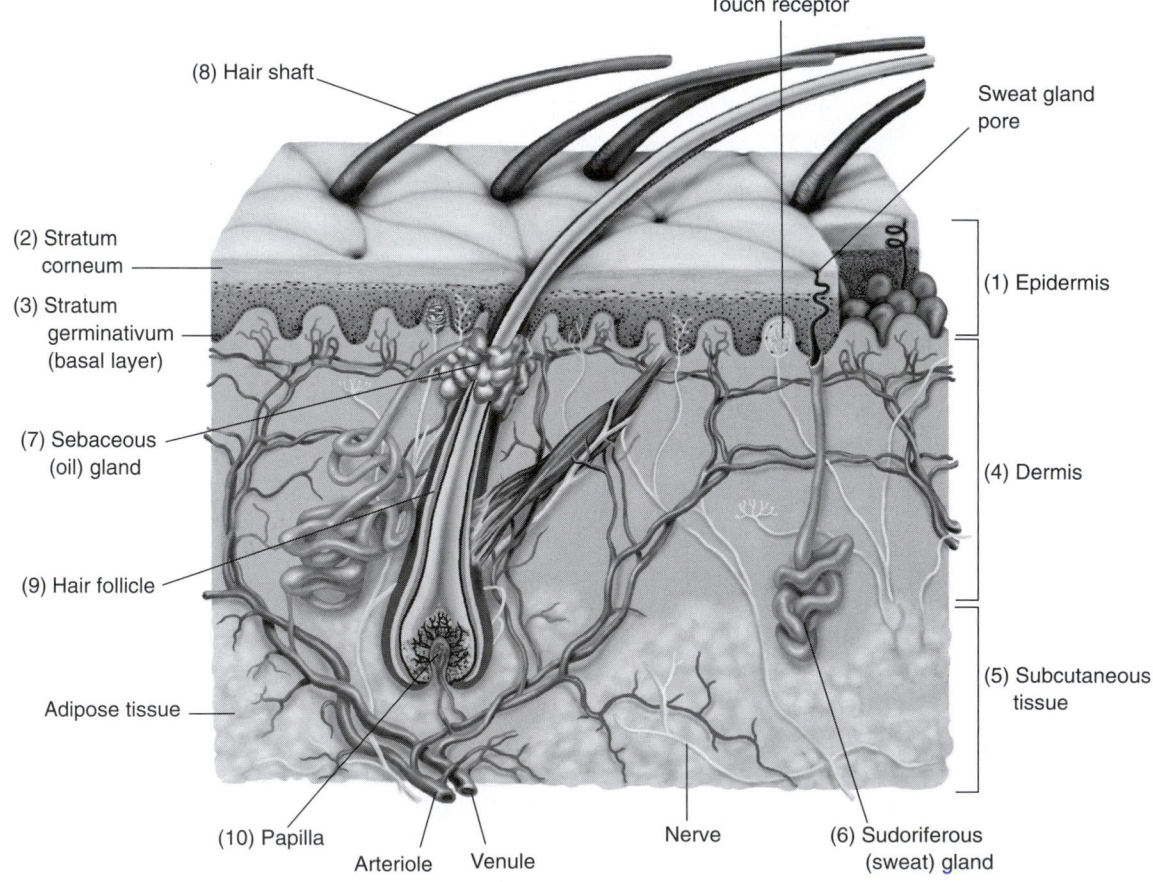

Figure 13-1   Three-dimensional view of the integument with appendages. (Reproduced with permission from Simandl G: Integumentary function. In Porth CM [ed]: Pathophysiology: Concepts of Altered Health States, ed 5. Lippincott, Philadelphia, 1998, pp 251–258.)

and infectious insults. This protection is afforded by the differentiation that occurs as the cells migrate from the stratum basale to the stratum corneum.

The cells migrating upward from the stratum basale layer differentiate and their cellular metabolism decreases, as they move away from their source of oxygen and nourishment. During this superficial migration and differentiation, the cells synthesize intracellular keratin, and extrude lipids. These lipids constitute this extracellular lamellar matrix and are composed of ceramides, cholesterol, and free fatty acids.[2] The cells maintain attachment to each other via adherens junctions (desmosomes). This intracellular keratinization and extracellular lipid secretion provide the "bricks and motor" barrier of the stratum corneum. Movement of molecules into the body requires a tortuous passage through either the aqueous or hydrophobic channels of the stratum corneum (Fig. 13-2).

The basal lamina is an irregular surface that separates the avascular epidermis from the underlying vascularized dermis. The lamina contains an interconnecting network of collagen and glycoproteins that assists in anchoring the epidermis to the underlying dermis. Additionally, the laminar surfaces increase the overall surface area for nutrient and oxygen diffusion into the epidermis.

The dermis is separated into two main regions: the more superficial papillary layer and the deeper reticular layer. The papillary layer lies directly underneath the basil lamina, the extracellular matrix providing continuity and structural support between the epidermis and deeper structures. The reticular layer is the major component of the dermis. The ground

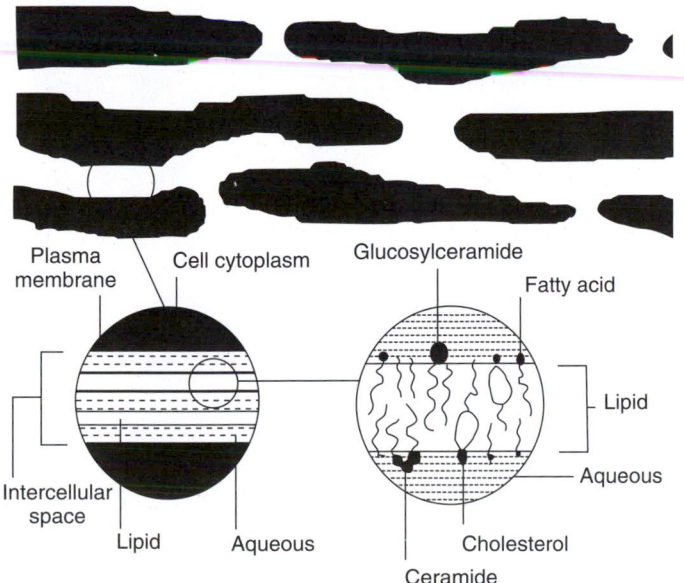

Figure 13-2 Cellular representation of the stratum corneum and the cell-lipid matrix. (Reprinted with permission of Heit, MC, and Riviere, JE: Electrically-assisted transdermal drug delivery. Pharm Res 14:687–697, 1997, Plenum Publishing Corp.)

● Why Do I Need to Know About...

HYDRATION
Hydration is a key component to the healing process. Without moisture, cells cannot migrate.

substance, collagen/elastin network, provides the turgor to the integument. This turgor is accomplished by the collagen and elastin proteins restricting the expansion when the sugar precursors attract water, much the same way thread wound around a sponge in water restrict the sponge's expansion. This ground substance also promotes the plasticity of the skin.

The integument is responsible for several non-barrier functions. The integument synthesizes vitamin D_3 from cholesterol using ultraviolet radiation and protects tissue from this same electromagnetic radiation by synthesizing melanin. Melanin was previously described in Chapter 1. Finally, the integument has an immunoregulatory role in cutaneous antigen recognition and a biometabolism role in processing cutaneously absorbed molecules.

The vasculature for the integument is divided into two major plexus. The superficial plexus is located between the papillary and reticular layers of the dermis, and the deeper vascular plexus is between the reticular layer of the dermis and subcutaneous tissue. These vascular plexi are involved in nutritional blood flow for the integument and thermoregulation of core body temperature. The epidermis is avascular.

Nerve innervations located within the dermis also provide the nervous system with information via various afferent chemical, thermal, and sensory receptors. Finally, the integument has different appendages that originate or penetrate through the dermis to the epidermis. These appendages include hair follicles and sweat glands. These glands are involved in thermoregulation, and the production and release of scent recognition in other nonhuman vertebrates.

Electrical Properties of the Skin

The role and mechanism(s) of the stratum corneum as the high resistance layer to the flow of electric current and a significant component in skin impedance have been extensively reviewed elsewhere.[3–6] (See Chapter 8, Foundations of Electrical Stimulation.)

The stratum corneum forms the high electric resistance layer and is a significant component in skin impedance.[7] The high resistance of this layer in turn is due in part to its lower water content (about 20%) compared with the normal physiological level (about 70%). The charge the skin maintains in an electric field is dependent on the pH of the solution. At a pH greater than 4, the skin maintains a negative charge when placed in an electric field, and at a pH lower than 3, the charge of the skin is positive. Thus, at the normal pH of the skin, a negative charge is present. This pH (3 to 4) about which the change in charge occurs is called the isoelectric point and is similar isoelectric point of keratin in the stratum corneum layer.[8] Biologic tissues such as skin also have a capacitance, an ability to store electrical charge, and are thus electrical capacitors. When an electric circuit contains both capacitive and resistant elements, the circuit is said to be reactive. The equivalent circuit model for the skin is that of a resistor parallel to a resistor and a capacitor.[7] A reactive circuit demonstrates impedance. The impedance represents the total electrical opposition of the circuit to the passage of a current. The human skin has an impedance to an alternating current of low frequency, but this impedance decreases as frequency of the alternating electric current is increased.[9] Due to variations in skin impedance, the current intensity of voltage-regulated stimulators cannot be easily controlled, thus most manufacturers use current regulated stimulators.[10] The loss of skin impedance with application of current may be due to a re-orientation of molecules along the ion transport pathways, such as the possible realignment of lipid molecules in hair follicles and sweat glands.[11] Also, application of current will lead to an increase in the local ion concentration, which will result in reduced impedance.[12] Thus, application of electrical current reduces skin impedance. This reduction may account for part of the enhanced transcutaneous drug delivery by application of an electrical current. The current-voltage relationship in skin is nonlinear.[13,14] The hydration status of the skin significantly influences this relationship, with higher hydration resulting in reduced impedance. Finally, temperature also affects the impedance of the skin, with reduced impedance at increasing cutaneous temperatures.[15]

 # Transcutaneous Transport

Transcutaneous Drug Penetration

As previously described, the stratum corneum acts as a barrier that minimizes transepidermal water loss. It is also the principal barrier to transcutaneous drug delivery. The transcutaneous delivery of small molecules can easily be compared to molecular diffusion through a barrier. Based on theoretical models, drugs can diffuse through the stratum corneum via a transepidermal route or transappendageal route.[3,5,16,17] Transepidermal drug delivery through the stratum corneum may occur within the lipid-rich lamellar matrix between the cells (intercellular route) or through both the transcellular route (protein-filled intracellular and intercellular domains) (Fig. 13-3). The transappendageal "shunt" pathway normally contributes little to passive transcutaneous drug delivery, due to the small fraction of the total human skin surface made up by these structures.[5,17]

The more aqueous the channels within the intercellular lamellar matrix, the more likely is the potential pathway for passive transcutaneous delivery of hydrophilic drugs. However, the hair follicles and sweat ducts can interfere and act as diffusion "shunts" for ionic molecules during iontophoretic transport.

Passive Drug Delivery

Passive drug delivery methods are used for both local and systemic indications. A broad spectrum of drugs may be de-

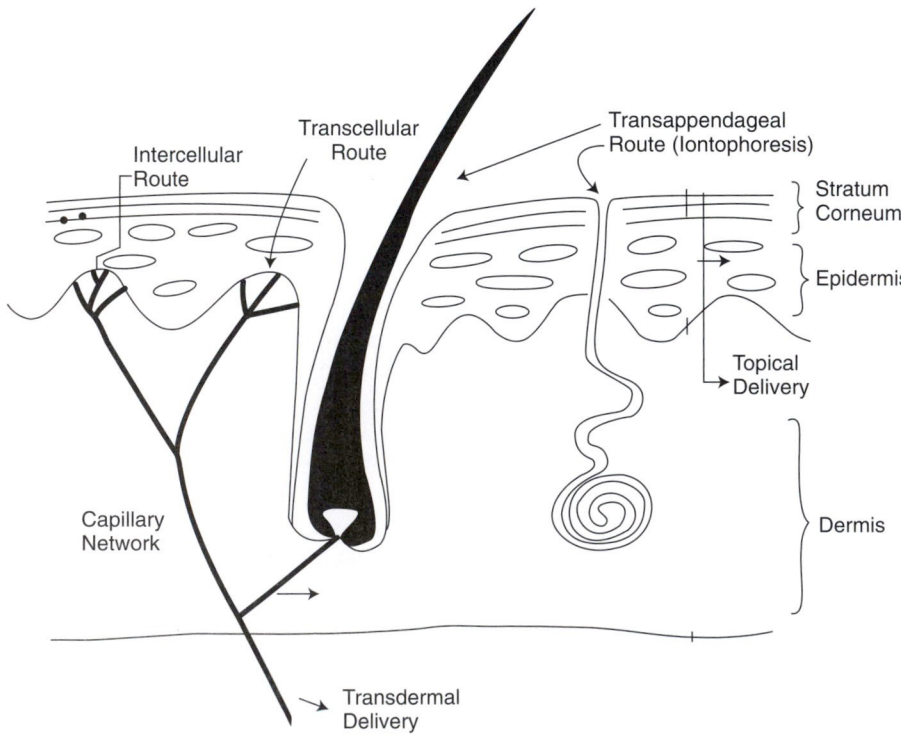

Figure 13-3 Schematic representation of the potential pathways for intracutaneous and transcutaneous drug delivery. (Reprinted with permission from Banga, AK: Electrically Assisted Transdermal and Topical Drug Delivery. Taylor and Francis, London, England, 1998.)

livered by passive delivery and range from assistance to quit smoking (nicotine) to motion sickness (scopolamine). Thus, cutaneous absorption of a variety of drugs exists. Passive intracutaneous and transcutaneous delivery of anti-inflammatory drugs have been documented in both animal and human investigations.[18–21] Passive delivery of piroxacam, a nonsteroidal anti-inflammatory drug (NSAID), into the musculature under the application site has been reported.[18] However, other investigations examining a variety of analgesics have reported that maximal depth of local tissue penetration during passive delivery, which is not attributable to systemic vasculature, occurs at the fascia to superficial muscle interface.[22–24] The consensus of these investigations is that maximal depth of delivery of these drugs is at best the superficial musculature, with deeper tissue penetration being dependent on systemic vascular absorption and redistribution.

Finally, under clinical conditions, the duration of application to achieve this tissue delivery is measured from one-half day to multiple days.[18,20,21] Thus, passive delivery for localized decrease of pain and dysfunction associated with musculoskeletal inflammation is achievable only after a prolonged period of application.

Iontophoretic Enhancement

A history of iontophoresis and the broad potential of pharmaceutics that may be transcutaneously delivered has been previously reviewed.[5,6] Topical or transcutaneous delivery of drugs, that is, drug delivery into or through the skin, can be assisted by electrical energy. The mechanism(s) involved may be iontophoresis, electro-osmosis, or electroporation.[3,5] Electro-osmosis is a phenomenon that accompanies iontophoresis and will be discussed in conjunction with iontophoresis.

Iontophoresis implies the use of small amounts of physiologically acceptable electric current to deliver drugs into the body. The technique has the potential to enhance transcutaneous permeation of both ionic (charged)[22–26] and nonionic (uncharged)[27,28] compounds several-fold over passive delivery. With iontophoresis, an electrode of the same polarity as the charge on the drug drives the drug into the skin by electrostatic repulsion (Fig. 13-4).

As examples, lidocaine, a cationic drug (positive charge), would use the anode (positive electrode) for charge-charge repulsion to deliver the drug into the body. In contrast, dexamethasone phosphate, an anionic drug (negative charge),

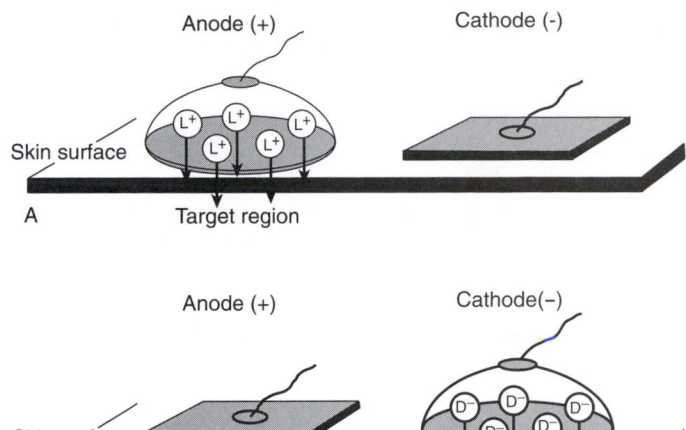

Figure 13-4 Iontophoretic concept using charge-charge repulsion to deliver drugs from both the anode "A" (positive electrode), and cathode (negative electrode) "B." Cationic drugs such as lidocaine (L^+) would be delivered from the anode. Anionic drugs such as dexamethasone phosphate (D^-) would be delivered from the cathode. (Reprinted with permission from Ciccone CD: Iontophoresis. In Robinson, AJ, and Snyder-Mackler, L [eds]: Clinical Electrophysiology, Electrotherapy, and Electrophysiologic Testing. Williams & Wilkins, Baltimore, MD, 1995, pp 333–358.)

would use the cathode (negative electrode) for delivery. Iontophoresis may be used for systemic or localized drug delivery and provides a programmed delivery as drug transport is proportional to the electric current. Patient compliance will also improve, and the dose may be adjusted to account for interpatient variability by adjusting the current.

Hair follicles and sweat glands within the skin make up only 0.1% of the surface area and represent pores within the skin with different radii, polarity, and charge concentrations.[5] As such, these pores may restrict transcutaneous permeation of compounds larger than the pore or of the opposite polarity.[26] Evidence suggests that iontophoresis transcutaneously delivers drugs through these pores, and these pores account for the previously discussed transappendageal "shunt" pathway[29,30] (see Fig. 13-3).

During iontophoresis, the greatest concentration of ionized substances is expected to move into regions of the skin where either the skin is damaged, or along the sweat glands and hair follicles. In these areas, the resistance of the skin to permeation of the drug is least. Iontophoresis may also stimulate pore formation in regions not associated with appendages.[31,32] The extracellular lipid domain and transcellular transport contribute little to hydrophilic drug transcutaneous iontophoretic transport.[31–34] The opening of the pores during iontophoresis is time dependent, as is the closing following the iontophoretic process.[17,35,36] The time required for the opening and closing of these pores depends upon the duration of current applied and the current density. Since augmented passive drug delivery continues following termination of the applied current, iontophoretic applicators should remain in place to maximize the amount of drug delivered transcutaneously. In conclusion, the iontophoretic pore pathway model is intercellular and aqueous in nature, with transcutaneous drug transport delayed after the initiation and continuing after the termination of iontophoresis.

If a voltage difference is applied across a charged porous membrane such as the skin, bulk fluid flow or volume flow, electro-osmosis, occurs in the same direction as flow of counterions. The term "iontohydrokinesis" was used in early literature to describe this water transport during iontophoresis.[37] This flow is not diffusion and involves a motion of the fluid without concentration gradients.[38] The counterions are usually cations and electro-osmotic flow occurs from anode (positive electrode) to cathode (negative electrode). The major cation transported through epidermis is Na^+. Thus, the skin and the stratum corneum in particular, is a permselective membrane with negative charge at physiologic pH.[8,39] Electro-osmosis enhances the flux of positively charged (cationic) drugs from the anode, while hindering drug flux of negatively charged (anionic) drugs or neutral drugs being delivered from the cathode. In such cases for either neutral or negatively charged drugs, transcutaneous delivery from the cathode may actually increase after the current is stopped.[28] Finally, the predicted contribution of electro-osmotic flow to total drug flux during iontophoresis depends upon additional drug formulation and skin related variables, which have been reviewed elsewhere.[5]

The biophysical parameters for electrical enhancement of transcutaneous delivery, in realistic terms, constitute a rather complex area with a large number of operating variables.

 ## Instrumentation and Application of Iontophoresis

Manufacturers market iontophoretic devices for a variety of clinical uses from hydrosis in cystic fibrosis detection to systemic delivery of opiate analgesics. The Food and Drug Administration (FDA) regards iontophoresis kits as Class III devices.[40] However, they have not undergone the clinical trials because they were marketed prior to 1976. Most were cleared under the 510(k) process that applies to grandfathered Class III devices. The iontophoretic power sources will be discussed followed by the drug delivery electrode applicators.

Iontophoretic Power Sources

Current iontophoretic systems are a combination of battery-dependent stimulators, used to provide either preprogrammed or programmable electric current for a specified time "dosage," and two electrodes. The drug applicator electrode may be selected as either the anode or the cathode. The second electrode is present only to complete the electrical circuit. The patient is also incorporated into the electrical circuit. The completed electrical circuit includes the drug delivery electrode, the patient, and the nontreatment electrode. The electrical waveform for iontophoretic devices is direct current (DC). Variations in skin impedance result in the current intensity of voltage-regulated iontophoretic devices as demonstrating intersubject variability. This results in a variable time duration required to deliver a single iontophoretic dosage with different patients, or within the same patient as two different timepoints. The iontophoretic dosage is expressed in Box 13-1.

Additionally, current through the tissue has been proposed as the most significant iontophoretic parameter.[5] Constant current devices adjust the voltage based on the skin impedance of the patient so that the current stays constant. In the event of poor electrode contact, manufacturers of constant current devices have incorporated automatic shutdowns should the voltage reach predetermined levels. This safety feature is to prevent electrical burns at the electrode sites.

To date, approximately four manufacturers market iontophoretic devices in the United States for the rehabilitation medicine profession. These manufacturers are IOMED, Empi, Life-Tech, and Birch Point Medica. The annual market for iontophoresis is about $20 million for physical therapy.[40] The first four companies market external palm-sized current-controlled devices in which the iontophoretic dosage may be programmed for each patient. These current-controlled devices are connected to separate electrodes for transcutaneous drug delivery. In contrast, Birch Point Medical Inc. uses a voltage-controlled self-contained unit with the battery and

BOX 13-1   Dosage Calculation of Milliamp* Minutes

Calculation of milliamp-minutes is based on the following formula:

$$\text{Dosage (mA*min)} = \text{Current (mA)} \times \text{time (minutes)}$$

Before You Begin

Know what the desired amount of dosage in mA*min is, and base your intensity on the patient sensation and time available, remembering that longer may be better.

electrodes designed into a single larger figure-of-eight bandage. The current amplitude for all marketed iontophoretic devices ranges from 0 to 4 mA (Table 13-1). The iontophoretic dosage (mA*min) delivered is programmable in with the Empi, Iomed, and Life-Tech devices. The iontophoretic dosage for the Birch Point Medical device is not programmable and is set at the factory at 40 or 80 mA*min. An mA-min is determined by multiplying the number of mA (intensity) by the number of minutes that the current is delivered. For example, 40 mA*min = 4 mA and a 10-minute treatment time. As the Birch Point Medical device is voltage controlled, the treatment duration for a single iontophoretic dosage may vary between patients, or for the same patient at two different times (Table 13-1). When a 20 mA*min dosage was conducted with the Birch Point Medical device, the current varied from 0.05 to 0.16 mA, and the treatment duration would vary from 2.1 to 6.7 hours. Thus, when iontophoresis is conducted in the clinic, where time commitments for treatment are constrained, current-controlled iontophoretic devices are dominant. However, the Birch Point Medical device is designed for the patient to wear after leaving the clinic. Finally, each device contains circuitry unique from those of other manufacturers. For example, the Phoresor II Auto system requires the setting of dose and current from which it calculates the treatment duration required. In contrast, the DUPEL device is a dual-channel system where the user can set the dosage and current levels for each channel independently.

Electrode Designs

Initial clinical investigations with iontophoresis used gauze or paper towels saturated with the drug.[41,42] The electric current generator was attached to these electrodes containing the drug with alligator clips. Alternatively, other investigators had their patients place the treatment site in a basin containing the drug solution. One electrode from the electric current generator was attached to the side of the basin, if metal, or placed at the bottom of the container within the solution but not in contact with the skin of the patient.[43,44] The second electrode was attached to the patient away from the basin so as to complete the electric circuit. Later commercial electrodes consisted of simple plastic bubbles that acted as fluid reservoirs.[45]

Commercially available electrode designs differ among manufacturers (Table 13-2). The general design for most electrodes is depicted in Figure 13-5. In general, the electrode design consists of an adhesive backing which allows the electrode to adhere firmly to the skin of the patient. To this backing an electrically conductive layer is added to evenly distribute the electric current over the electrode surface area. The conductor composition may be carbon or other conductor and varies by manufacturer. The drug reservoir consists of a layer to hold the drug solution during iontophoresis. The composition of this layer varies between manufacturers, but typically consists of absorptive-type materials (Table 13-2). Finally, several manufacturers use an additional outer layer that is in contact with the skin. This last layer serves to stabilize the underlying layers of the electrode and/or act as a wicking layer to absorb the applied drug solution. Empi has taken this concept further by separating the drug delivery electrode into a bilayer design that is described in greater detail later. The exception to the above electrode design is IOMED, which uses a polymerized gel (Hydrogel), either alone or

TABLE 13-1 Parameters for the Commercially Available Iontophoretic Power Sources

MANUFACTURER	AMPERAGE RANGE (MA)	MAXIMUM DOSAGE (MA*MIN)	CHANNELS	POLARITY
Dupel *EMPI* *St. Paul, MN*	0–4	160	2	+ or −
Phoresor II Auto *IOMED* *Salt Lake City, UT*	0–4	80	1	+ or −
Iontophor PM/DX	0–4	N.C.	1	+ or −
Microphor (*Check*) *Life-Tech* *Houston, TX*	0.5–4	80	1	+ or −
Iontopatch *Birch Point Medical, Inc.* *Oakdale, MN*	0.1*	40 or 80 fixed	1	+ or −

The abbreviations are as follows: polarity, cathode (−) or anode (+). Voltage-dependent device and the current (*) vary depending on patient impedance, with the range on a 20 mA-minute dosage 0.05 to 0.16 mA. N.C. no maximum dosage limits with the power source.

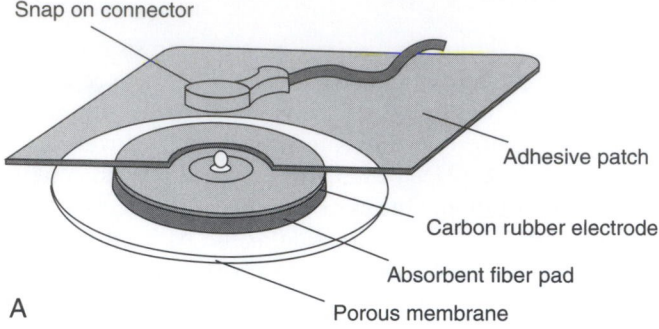

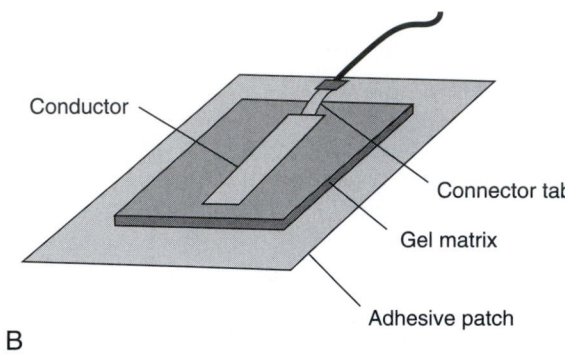

Figure 13-5 General schematics of electrode designs for fiber-based (A) and hydrogel based (B) iontophoretic electrodes. (Reprinted with permission from Ciccone CD: Iontophoresis. In Robinson, AJ, and Snyder-Mackler, L [eds]: Clinical Electrophysiology, Electrotherapy, and Electrophysiologic Testing. Williams & Wilkins, Baltimore, MD, 1995, pp 333–358.)

within a sponge matrix, as a drug reservoir. A Hydrogel formulation provides a conductive base, ease of application, and uniform current distribution at the treatment site.

Appropriate choice of electrodes is a factor that is critical to successful iontophoretic delivery of a drug.[5] The electrode material determines the electrochemistry occurring at the electrodes. Electrical current must be transferred from the electronic environment, that is, the wires, to the ionic environment, that is, the electrode aqueous solution and the body. Unless suitable mechanisms are used, iontophoresis is accompanied by electrolysis of water. This electrolysis results in a change in the pH within both the electrode and at the electrode-skin interface as follows:

$$2H_2O \rightarrow 4H^+ + O_2 + 4\,e^- \text{ (anode) } \textit{decrease pH (acid)}$$

Oxidation of water at the anode results in the production of hydrogen ion (H^+) and a decrease in pH.

$$2H_2O + 2e^- \rightarrow H_2 + 2OH^- \text{ (cathode) } \textit{increase pH (alkaline)}$$

Reduction of water at the cathode results in the formation of hydroxyl ion (OH^-) and an increase in pH. This pH change may initiate chemical irritation of the skin, or alter the skin conductivity of the electric current. Additionally, both H^+ and OH^- are mobile in the iontophoretic electric field, competing with the ionized drug to carry the current, and ultimately decreasing the transport of the drug into the underlying tissues. A pH-induced drug degradation may also occur at the electrode, decreasing the efficiency of iontophoretic drug delivery.

To avoid these pH changes in the electrode and in the skin at the application site, buffering agents may be used (see Table 13-2). Minimizing pH changes at the electrode may

TABLE 13-2 Commercially Available Electrodes

MANUFACTURER	OF SIZES	DRUG RESERVOIR COMPOSITION	BUFFER SYSTEM
BLUE[‡] Upper	4	Cotton Flannel	Ion Exchange
Lower		Polyurethane Foam	Resin
EMPI			
St. Paul, MN			
Trans-Q	2	Hydrogel	Ag/AgCl
Trans-Q E	2	Hydrogel/Sponge	Ag/AgCl
logel	3	Hydrogel/Sponge	Ag/AgCl
IOMED			
Salt Lake City, UT			
DynaPak	7	Cotton/Rayon	0.9% Saline *
Life-Tech			0.5% $NaHPO_4^-$ *
Houston, TX			
Iontopatch	1	Polypropylene	Anode: Zn/Zn++
Birch Point Medical, Inc.			Cathode: AgCl/Ag
Oakdale, MN			

The abbreviations are as follows: Ag/AgCl: silver/silver-chloride electrode, Zn:Zinc; * optional buffer addition; ‡ B.L.U.E.: Bilayer Ultra Electrode. The cathode is the negative electrode and the anode is the positive electrode.

also be accomplished by polymeric ion exchange resins,[46] such as those used by EMPI in the Bilayer Ultra Electrode (BLUE) design (see Table 13-2).

Empi has developed a bilayer drug reservoir electrode with the immobile polymeric resin impregnated into the upper fiber-type layer (BLUE). The lower layer acts as a hydrophilic matrix to absorb and retain the drug solution.

No iontophoresis electrode design is capable of delivering all drugs under every potential condition. Thus, the electrode designs and commercial availability may limit their clinical use for prolong periods or result in suboptimal iontophoretic delivery with some drugs. The use of saturated gauze or paper towels may result in a nonhomogeneous electric field due to unequal saturation of these applicators with the solution. Such unequal saturation results in higher electric current density through the parts of the towel or gauze that is wetter. This problem may also exist with current marketed iontophoretic electrodes if they are not filled with the solution volume recommended by the manufacturer. The use of a basin to iontophorese the drug removes this high current density problem. However, not all body parts are amenable to being placed in a basin containing the drug solution. Additionally, the volume required to fill the basin results in an excessive waste of the drug solution as the solution will be disposed of following the iontophoresis. The alligator clips that attached the electric current generator also may result in a high electric current density where the clip is attached to the gauze or towel. Marketed electrodes use a dispersal layer to evenly apply the electrical current over the entire surface area of the electrode applicator and through the remaining layers of the electrode. The absence of buffers in the electrode matrix may result in a pH change at both the anode and cathode.

However, a recent investigation examined pH changes in commercially available electrodes at various iontophoretic dosages, and with the cathode as the delivery electrode.[47] With an iontophoretic dosage less than 40 mA-min, no statistically significant pH changes were noted in the nonbuffered, buffered, or sacrificial electrode designs. When the iontophoretic dosage was 80 mA-min, there was an increase in the pH of the nonbuffered electrode design. These results would suggest that clinical iontophoretic dosages of 40 mA-min or less could be safely conducted in nonbuffered electrode designs.

Iontophoretic drug delivery is also proportional to the applied current.[52] In general, 0.5 mA/cm² is often stated to be the

Before You Begin

Ask the patient if he or she is allergic to the drug that is about to be administered. If there is an allergy, DO NOT administer the drug.

maximum current density that should be used on humans.[5] The charge, size, and structure of the drug will influence its potential to be an iontophoresis candidate. Ideal candidates for iontophoresis should be water-soluble, potent drugs that exist in their salt form with high charge density.[53,54] In an iontophoretic formulation, a relative increase in drug concentration compared with other ions will typically result in higher iontophoretic delivery.[55,56] In contrast, an increase in formulation viscosity may decrease the iontophoretic drug flux by hindering the mobility of the drug.[56,57] The pH of the solution will also determine whether the drug is charged or the ratio of the charged and uncharged species.[34] Thus, iontophoretic drug delivery is dependent upon electrode design, drug formulation and charge, and the barrier characteristics of the skin.

Application

Based on the previous discussions of the basic concepts of iontophoresis, specific methods should be used during application.

First, the clinician should determine the treatment area and the size of the drug delivery electrode for the application. The electrode should be large enough to cover the treatment area, but not so small that the electrical current density exceeds the 0.5 mA/cm².

Second, the clinician should saturate the delivery electrode with the drug solution. This results in the entire surface area of the delivery electrode transferring the current, and minimizes the potential that the localized current density exceeds 0.5 mA/cm². Additionally, complete contact between the electrodes and the surface of the skin will also minimize localized high current densities.

Third, the clinician should determine which drug is to be used for the specific treatment, and whether the drug is an anion or cation when ionized. The drug must be ionized at a pH used for iontophoretic application so that charge-charge repulsion will assist with the transcutaneous delivery. Additionally, the clinician should attempt to use a drug solution that has the fewest competing ions to that of the drug.

Once charge of the drug is determined, the appropriate electrode from the battery source should be attached to the delivery electrode, the cathode for anionic drugs and the anode for cationic drugs. Finally, the drug delivery site and the return electrode site should be thoroughly cleaned with an alcohol solution. This removes oils and the uppermost cells from the stratum corneum, the main barrier to iontophoretic drug delivery, and ultimately enhances iontophoretic drug

Why Do I Need to Know About...

pH CHANGES

A pH change at the cathode and the anode may result in minor skin irritation under the electrodes following the treatment intervention.

delivery. The placement of the delivery and return electrodes should be according to the manufacturer. In general, the minimal distance between the two electrodes should be 2 cm, or approximately 1 inch. Closer placement of the electrodes may result in a "short circuit current" across the stratum corneum surface without penetration of the electrical current into the deeper tissues. The removal of the drug delivery electrode following the iontophoretic treatment may be determined by the clinician on an individual patient basis. The potential for further drug delivery exists even after the battery source is removed. However, no controlled investigations have been conducted to determine if this additional application has any positive or negative effects on the treatment outcomes.

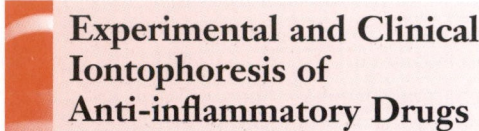

Experimental and Clinical Iontophoresis of Anti-inflammatory Drugs

Experimental Iontophoresis of Anti-inflammatory Drugs

Various pharmacologic agents have been iontophoresed to achieve both localized and systemic delivery, and have been reviewed extensively elsewhere.[5,6] Within rehabilitation medicine, the major use of iontophoresis is for the localized delivery of anti-inflammatory drugs. However, clinical investigations documenting the positive outcomes for this procedure are inconsistent. This may be due to the absence of pharmacokinetic data on experimental iontophoresis that is performed under conditions that parallel the clinic. Pharmacokinetics is the examination of the mechanism of absorption, distribution, and elimination of drugs in the body. Pharmacokinetic research examining iontophoresis to prevent local inflammation has used both steroidal anti-inflammatory drugs (SAIDs) and NSAIDs. The former are anti-inflammatory drugs derived from cholesterol and classified as glucocorticoids.[58] The latter are a chemically diverse group of drugs that inhibit the production of prostaglandin-type compounds.[59]

Dexamethasone phosphate is an anionic prodrug from the SAID class. The prodrug, dexamethasone phosphate, is converted to the active form of the drug, dexamethasone, within the tissues.[60] The initial and most commonly cited pharmacokinetic analysis of dexamethasone phosphate iontophoresis in a single Rhesus monkey calculated a 26% loss from the from the applicator electrode, supposedly into the underlying tissue. Post-iontophoretic drug penetration was documented down to submuscular tissues and intra-articular spaces. Once converted to dexamethasone, the negative charge is absent from the drug. However, the iontophoretic parameters used in this initial investigation do not parallel current clinical use of dexamethasone phosphate iontophoresis. The delivery electrode was the anode, theoretical constructs suggest the cathode as the appropriate electrode, the dosage exceeded most clinical dosages at 100 mA*min (Table 13-3), chloride

TABLE 13-3	Clinical Iontophoresis of Glucocorticoids in Musculoskeletal Dysfunction					
DYSFUNCTION	IONTO. POLARITY	PARAMETERS DOSAGE (MA* MIN)	PHARMACOLOGIC AGENT	RX	OUTCOME
Musculoskeletal inflammation	Anode	85	Dex/Lido	1–3	Subjective pain relief[127]
Musculoskeletal inflammation	?	45	Dex/Lido	4	Subjective & objective improvements[128]
Musculoskeletal dysfunction	Anode & cathode	3–7	Kenacort—A	11	56% subjects pain relief[129]
Infrapatellar tendinitis	?	40–80	Dex/Lido	6	Subjective & objective improvements[130]
Carpal tunnel syndrome	?	40–45	Dex/Lido	3	58% subjective & objective improvements[131]
Rheumatic knee	Cathode	80	Dex	3	Subjective improvement only[78]
Plantar fasciitis	Cathode	40	Dex	6	Enhanced rehabilitation[79]
TMJ dysfunction	Cathode	40	Dex/Lido	3	Conflicting results[80,81]

Abbreviations: **Dex:** Dexamethasone; **Dex/Lido:** Dexamethasone and lidocaine; **Kenacort-A:** Triamcinolone-acetonide; **Ionto:** Iontophoresis; **Rx:** Number of Treatments; **TMJ:** Temporomandibular Joint

ions were present in solution and should decrease the drug delivery efficiency, and the current density (at 0.94 mA/cm²) exceeded the previously specified safety limit (of 0.5 mA/cm².) Finally, the drug pharmacokinetics were indirectly measured by radioactivity. Subsequent in vitro research has established that optimal parameters for dexamethasone phosphate iontophoresis are from the cathode, and without competing anions such as chloride in solution.[61,62] Additionally, investigators[63] have proposed that during iontophoresis dexamethasone phosphate, and other drugs, carry the ionic current from the delivery electrode into the epidermis. Here smaller more highly mobile and numerous competing ions such as Cl^-, for dexamethasone phosphate, carry the ionic current to the other electrode in the circuit. The dexamethasone phosphate is "dropped off" in a depot in the epidermis. Deeper tissue penetration by the drug is dependent upon passive diffusion and removal by the vasculature.

Pharmacologic support exists for the concept that vasodilation at the iontophoretic site decreases localized drug delivery and increases systemic absorption, whereas vasoconstriction at the iontophoretic site has the opposite effect.[64-66] Glucocorticoids, such as dexamethasone phosphate, have a vasoconstrictive effect on the human cutaneous vasculature[20] This vasoconstriction is not observed during 40 mA-min conventional cathodic iontophoresis, at 3 mA, due to the galvanic induced erythema, but is observed following a similar cathodic iontophoresis dosage using low current (0.05 to 0.1 mA).[63] Thus, further increases in localized dexamethasone phosphate delivery may occur if iontophoretic current densities that do not cause erythema at the application site are used.

Dexamethasone phosphate was not measurable in the local venous vasculature in humans during or following 40 or 80 mA*min cathodic iontophoresis of dexamethasone phosphate at the forearm.[68]

The pharmacokinetics of anionic NSAIDs have also been examined.[6] Although the iontophoretic transport between dexamethasone phosphate and NSAIDs and their pharmacokinetics post-iontophoresis are not identical, relevant general constructs concerning the iontophoresis of anionic anti-inflammatory drugs for localized delivery may be derived. However, many newer investigations examining transcutaneous iontophoretic delivery of NSAIDs use iontophoretic parameters not clinically available. Therefore, the clinical value of these investigations is questionable and will not be discussed. Iontophoresis of several different NSAIDs under clinically relevant parameters is optimal from the cathode, and tissue penetration under the application site appears to be down to the fascia-superficial muscle interface.[22,70-72] An initial pharmacokinetic conclusion from several of the in vivo iontophoretic investigations using the NSAID, ketoprofen, was that higher current densities, 0.28 compared with 0.14 mA/cm², resulted in greater drug delivery for the same 160 mA-min dosage.[6,70,71] However, subsequent reevaluation of

the results suggest that the higher current density resulted in greater iontophoresis induced erythema and increased absorption of this NSAID from the application site into the systemic vasculature. This is based upon evidence that ketoprofen efficiently redistributes from the interstitial space under the iontophoretic site into the local vasculature and that iontophoretic currents in the range of 0.5 mA/cm² stimulate localized erythema.[73-75] Several investigations also documented a time requirement for transcutaneous transport of ketoprofen.[70,71,73,74] The time delay between initiation of iontophoresis with ketoprofen and presence in the local vasculature is due to the permeation of the drug across the epidermis. A similar time delay for transcutaneous permeation of dexamethasone phosphate may also occur. Glucocorticoids such as dexamethasone do not have extensive extravascular binding, and drug delivered to the interstitial space should redistribute quickly into the local vascular compartment.[58] However, for dexamethasone phosphate the precise time requirement for an iontophoresis treatment in order to obtain transcutaneous transport is at present undocumented. Finally, as with the dexamethasone phosphate iontophoretic investigation,[69] following an 160 mA*min cathodic iontophoresis of ketoprofen no drug was detectable in the articular space.[76]

The pharmacokinetics for iontophoresis of SAIDs and NSAIDs has been examined. What is still uncertain is the local tissue depth at which SAIDs and NSAIDs are delivered by the iontophoresis, and to what extent the systemic vasculature delivers these drugs to the deeper tissues.

Clinical Iontophoresis of Anti-inflammatory Drugs

Clinically, in the United States, the majority of iontophoresis in rehabilitation medicine is with dexamethasone phosphate. In a placebo-controlled investigation the capability of iontophoresis to prevent experimentally induced delayed-onset muscle soreness (DOMS) in 18 female subjects was examined.[77] The subjects were exposed to quadriceps eccentric exercise. Lidocaine/dexamethasone phosphate anodic iontophoresis, at a dosage of 65 mA*min, was administered 24 hours later, and final assessment was conducted 48 hours postexercise. Muscle function assessments and patient perception of soreness were conducted every day during the following 3-day trial. Although the iontophoresis-treated group demonstrated significant improvement in the subjective assessment of muscle soreness, none of the objective muscle function tests were different between the groups.

A major application of iontophoresis within rehabilitation medicine is the treatment of acute musculoskeletal inflammation. The clinical investigations examining glucocorticoid iontophoresis as a treatment for these dysfunctions, the iontophoretic parameters, pharmacologic agent used, and the clinical outcomes are reviewed in Table 13-3. As may be observed from the table, the polarity of the drug delivery electrode is absent from a number of the publications. This void would make replication of these studies difficult. Additionally, several of the investigations used drug solutions with competing ions to the dexamethasone phosphate. These competing ions would be Cl⁻ from the lidocaine, as the lidocaine is formulated as a chloride salt. The presence of Cl⁻ would result in suboptimal transcutaneous dexamethasone phosphate. The majority of investigations in Table 13-3 found improvements in both subjective and objective outcomes. However, one investigation found only an improvement in the subjective outcome, but not the objective outcome.[78] Another significant clinical observation is from an investigation treating plantar fasciitis.[79] Patients in the experimental group received dexamethasone phosphate iontophoresis in addition to the regular physical therapy regimen. The patients in the control group received placebo iontophoresis with the same physical therapy regimen. The iontophoretic group demonstrated an enhanced rate of rehabilitation. However, at the 1-month follow-up, both groups demonstrated equivalent clinical scores. These results suggest that dexamethasone phosphate iontophoresis in certain musculoskeletal dysfunction may enhance the rate of rehabilitation, but may not ultimately affect the long-term outcome. Only one musculoskeletal pathophysiology has been examined in two separate investigations. Temporomandibular joint dysfunction was examined by two investigations using similar dexamethasone phosphate iontophoretic protocols.[80,81] One investigation documented positive outcomes from the treatments,[81] whereas the other found no significant difference between the treatment and placebo groups.[80]

Finally, physical therapists are being requested to use iontophoresis for conservative nonsurgical treatment of Peyronie's disease.[82–84] However, when conducted in accordance with the literature, this is polypharmacy treatment, and should be conducted in close association with a pharmacist for formulary services. From the published controlled investigations several iontophoretic and pharmaceutical parameters are available. The anode is used for the drug delivery electrode, and is a result of the other drugs co-iontophoresed with dexamethasone phosphate. The iontophoretic dosage varies between 60 to 100 mA*min, and the number of treatments varies both between investigations and between patients with a range of 3 to 53. The other drugs co-iontophoresed with dexamethasone phosphate again vary between investigations but may include verapamil, lidocaine, and orgotein. The clinical value of this iontophoretic procedure will await further clinical examination.

In aggregate, clinical investigations suggest that dexamethasone phosphate iontophoresis may result in improved objective and/or subjective clinical outcomes in variety of musculoskeletal dysfunctions. However, interinvestigation variability makes comparisons difficult, and basic pharmacokinetic and pharmacodynamic mechanisms remain unexplained. Finally, insufficient experimental evidence exists to determine the precise depth of subcutaneous tissue delivery following iontophoresis of anionic anti-inflammatory drugs or which drugs provide the greatest potential for transcutaneous permeation by iontophoresis.

Reported Adverse Responses from Iontophoresis

Adverse reactions reported by the patients during and after iontophoresis have been related to the procedure. These adverse effects include first-degree burn, transient erythema at the drug delivery electrode, metallic taste when iontophoresis was used on the face, and one of the following during iontophoresis: tingling, burning, stinging, or a pulling sensation.[6,85,86] Additional reports of shock to patients have been documented as a result of abruptly turning the device off while the patient is still connected to the device circuit.[86] Finally, one clinical study documented contact dermatitis in a patient following iontophoresis of 5-fluorouracil, at both the site of application and a distant site.[87] This last report suggests a systemic reaction as the result of a drug iontophoresed for local application.

Phonophoresis

Phonophoresis is the use of ultrasonic mechanical energy waves to transcutaneously deliver drugs through the skin for both local and systemic tissue sites. Ultrasonic energy has been documented to transcutaneously deliver a wide variety of agents from proteins to various hydrophilic and hydrophobic drugs.[88–91] However, the mechanical energy parameters for many investigations reporting ultrasonic enhanced transcutaneous delivery are not within the 1 to 3 MHz currently available to clinicians within the United States of America. Additionally, when investigators examine these promising new ultrasonic parameters, less research is focusing on the frequencies clinically used. The current discussion will present published investigations using phonophoretic parameters currently available to clinicians.

Phonophoretic Parameters

The limitations and requirements for conducting ultrasound also exist for phonophoresis due to spatial differences in the ultrasound transducer, which must be kept in motion during treatment to prevent thermal injury to the integument. As with transfer of the mechanical energy from the ultrasound transducer to the surface of the skin, the coupling gel used during phonophoresis should allow the transfer of the mechanical energy from the ultrasound transducer to the surface of the skin. Inclusion of a drug into the coupling gel should minimize the loss of the conductance of the mechanical energy. However, not all phonophoretic couplants are equal in the conductance of the mechanical energy.[92-95] This difference in couplants transmission of the mechanical energy exists independent of the drug. Thus, clinicians should inquire about the phonophoretic gels used. Additionally, the drug being delivered should be stable in an ultrasonic field, and not provide additional resistance to the conduction of the mechanical wave in the coupling gel. Refer to Chapter 4 for a review of ultrasound and the acoustical properties of sound. Phonophoresis has one clear advantage over iontophoresis, however: the ability to deliver both ionized and nonionized drugs.[88] As with iontophoresis, the stratum corneum has been proposed as the primary impediment to transcutaneous phonophoretic drug delivery.[89,96] Several phenomena have been proposed as responsible for phonophoretic enhancement of transcutaneous drug delivery.[89,96,97] These phenomena include stable cavitation of gas bubbles within the stratum corneum; convective transport; thermal heating increasing the kinetic energy of the drug; and mechanical stresses induced by the pressure variations of the wave. Additionally, this transport may occur either within the stratum corneum itself or through hair follicles and sweat glands as with iontophoresis. Mitragotri and co-investigators[97] examined these phenomena in vitro with clinically relevant frequencies, 1 to 3 MHz, and intensities, 0 to 2 W/cm^2. The conclusion from the investigation was that phonophoretic enhancement of transcutaneous drug delivery was the result of stable cavitation occurring intracellularly at the cell membrane of the corneocytes in the stratum corneum. This cavitation appears to disorder the structures of the stratum corneum enhancing the passive movement of drugs down a concentration gradient from the exterior skin surface to deeper layers. Additionally, this cavitation enhancement of transcutaneous drug transport occurs at 1 MHz and not 3 MHz. Thus, unlike iontophoretic transcutaneous transport, transcutaneous phonophoretic transport is not transappendageal. Transcutaneous transport of all drugs may not be enhanced by phonophoresis and those that are enhanced by phonophoresis may not all be enhanced to the same extent. Mitragotri and co-investigators,[91] proposed that the phonophoretic enhancement, compared with passive delivery (e), is directly proportional to the organic

Before You Begin

Remember to check the acoustical capability of the drug by applying it to the surface of the transducer, surrounding the transducer with cellophane tape and adding water.
If the surface of the water is disturbed when the intensity of the ultrasound is increased, then the drug is acoustically conductive. If not, it is not.

solubility of the drug, and inversely proportional to the passive permeability of the drug.

The comparison supported their conclusion that variations in previously reported phonophoretic enhancement for various drugs is the result of physicochemical differences in the agents being phonophoresed. Thus, some drugs such as fluocinolone acetonide and dexamethasone demonstrate significant phonophoretic enhancement (12-fold), other drugs such as indomethacin and hydrocortisone demonstrate moderate enhancement (3- to 5-fold), and some drugs such as lidocaine and salicylate demonstrate no phonophoretic enhancement. Finally, one investigation reported enhanced back-diffusion of a drug into the phonophoretic gel when compared with passive application.[98] The drug was applied to the skin, then ultrasonic gel covered the drug and the area was sonated.

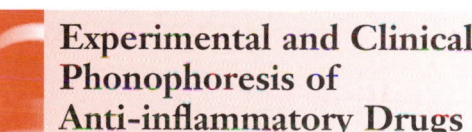

Experimental and Clinical Phonophoresis of Anti-inflammatory Drugs

Experimental Phonophoresis of Anti-inflammatory Drugs

As previously discussed, the transcutaneous permeation of all anti-inflammatory drugs is not augmented by phonophoresis. Thus, subsequent discussion will focus on those investigations using agents for which transcutaneous permeation is augmented by phonophoresis. The early phonophoretic investigations have been previously reviewed.[89] Several documented cortisol delivery at intramuscular and deeper tissue levels.[99-101] However, those experimental parameters do not parallel the clinical use of the modality, and the relevance of these results in clinical practice is debatable. Transcutaneous phonophoretic delivery of several different NSAIDs has been examined. In vivo transcutaneous indomethacin delivery was augmented by 1 MHz phonophoresis.[102-104] This augmentation was both intensity and time dependent, with higher intensity and longer times resulting in higher systemic blood drug levels. The phonophoretic enhancement also occurred with continuous and pulsed modes of ultrasound at 1 MHz. These investiga-

Why Do I Need to Know About...

ACOUSTICAL PROPERTIES
If the drug was whipped to make a paste for application onto the skin, the drug may not pass through the skin. Whipping adds air and air is not acoustically conductive.

tions do not define whether the ultrasonic transducer was moved during the application. However, due to the epidermal histologic appearance during 1 MHz at 0.75 W/cm^2 continuous ultrasound or 1.5 W/cm^2 1:2 pulsed ultrasound, the transducer may have remained stationary during the application. Finally, even after the phonophoretic application was terminated the systemic blood drug levels continued to increase. This final pharmacokinetic information demonstrates that even after clinical phonophoretic application, the augmented transcutaneous drug delivery continues. A similar time- and intensity-dependent phonophoretic enhancement of flufenamic acid using an in vitro synthetic membrane has also been documented.[105,106] However, no phonophoretic enhancement of the NSAIDs, salicylate, or benzydamine have been observed.[107,108]

In humans hydrocortisone was phonophoresed at 1 MHz continuously on the volar aspect at 1.0 W/cm^2 for 5 minutes.[111] No drug was detected in the proximal venous blood either during or up to 15 minutes postphonophoresis. Finally, the maximal tissue depth for which 1 MHz phonophoresed hydrocortisone has an anti-inflammatory effect was also examined in the pig.[112] Hydrocortisone was phonophoresed with a continuous mode at 1.5 W/cm^2 for 5 minutes. No anti-inflammatory effect was observed for the phonophoresed hydrocortisone. In these investigations, a 10% (weight/volume) hydrocortisone concentration was used for phonophoresis. In contrast to hydrocortisone phonophoretic investigations, examination of dexamethasone phonophoresis has resulted in positive outcomes. In the previous investigation by Byl in the pig,[112] dexamethasone phonophoresis, at parameters previously described for hydrocortisone, resulted in subcutaneous anti-inflammatory effects at the phonophoretic application site. However, no anti-inflammatory effects were observed in submuscular or subtendinous tissues underneath the application site. Additionally, anti-inflammatory effects were observed at tissue sites distal to the phonophoresis, suggesting a systemic delivery of the dexamethasone. In humans, 1 MHz continuous mode phonophoresis at 1.5 W/cm^2 for 8 minutes was conducted on the volar surface, and proximal venous blood samples were collected at the cubital fossa.[113] These phonophoretic parameters were similar to those previously described for hydrocortisone.[111] Forty percent of the subjects receiving the dexamethasone phonophoresis demonstrated measurable, but not quantifiable, venous drug levels. In contrast, another human investigation examined 1 MHz continuous dexamethasone phonophoresis at 1.0 W/cm^2 for 10 minutes.[114] The phonophoresis was conducted on the volar surface, and proximal venous blood samples were collected at the cubital fossa. No measurable dexamethasone was detected in the proximal venous blood. With similar phonophoretic parameters, what may account for the differing pharmacokinetic results in the human dexamethasone phonophoretic investigations. In the porcine investigation documenting

subcutaneous anti-inflammatory effect following dexamethasone phonophoresis[112] and the human investigation measuring proximal venous dexamethasone post phonophoresis,[113] the concentration of dexamethasone in the phonophoretic gel was 0.33%. In the pharmacokinetic human investigation that was unable to document measurable dexamethasone in the venous blood following phonophoresis, the concentration of drug in the phonophoretic gel was 0.017%.[114] Thus, the differences in the dexamethasone concentration in the phonophoretic gel may account for the differing results in the investigations examining dexamethasone phonophoresis.

Thus, as hypothesized,[91] phonophoresis enhancement of NSAIDs and SAIDs is selective, being in part dependent upon the chemical structure and hydrophobicity of the agent. Additionally, optimal phonophoretic delivery of the agent is dependent upon the phonophoretic frequency and intensity, treatment duration, and mechanical transmitting properties of the coupling gel.

Clinical Phonophoresis

Stronger conclusions may be based on clinical investigations using control or alternative treatment groups. Therefore, only these clinical investigations will be currently reviewed. Several different investigations have examined the clinical benefit of phonophoresis with different anti-inflammatory drugs, and the results have been mixed. Both NSAIDs and SAIDs have been used in these clinical investigations, and the phonophoretic parameters and major outcome(s) are summarized in Table 13-4. Decreases in pain perception of delayed-onset muscle soreness (DOMS) in elbow flexors by 10% trolamine salicylate phonophoresis was examined in a multicontrol investigation.[115] There was no significant reduction of DOMS when compared with sham ultrasound or passive application of 10% trolamine salicylate. However, trolamine salicylate phonophoresis reduced the DOMS when compared with an equivalent treatment with ultrasound alone, as the ultrasound treatment increased the DOMS when compared with the sham ultrasound or passive hydrocortisone application. In contrast, phonophoresis of 1% indomethacin did reduce the subjective and objective complaints of pain in patients with temporomandibular joint (TMJ) dysfunction.[116] The patients receiving comparable ultrasound therapy as treatment for their TMJ dysfunction did not demonstrate a significant reduction in their dysfunction. These results suggest that the clinical improvement in the patients receiving the indomethacin phonophoresis was the result of the addition of the drug to the ultrasound therapy. Similarly, a retrospective review compared 1% and 10% hydrocortisone phonophoresis in patients with various musculoskeletal dysfunctions.[117] The patients being treated with 10% hydrocortisone for their dysfunction required fewer treatments and demonstrated improved subjective assessment of the dysfunc-

TABLE 13-4   Clinical Phonophoresis in Musculoskeletal Dysfunction

DYSFUNCTION	MHZ	PARAMETERS W/CM²	MINUTES	PHARMACOLOGIC AGENT	RX	OUTCOME
DOMS elbow flexors	1	1.5	5	0% TS	3	Mixed results[115]
Musculoskeletal dysfunction	1	2.0 max.	9 minutes	1% Hydrocort	8–10	Effectiveness
	1	2.0 max.	maximum	10% Hydrocort	5–7	10% > 1%[117]
Musculoskeletal dysfunction	1	1.5	8	0.05% Lidex	9	Phono vs US Similar Objective Outcome[118]
Musculoskeletal Tendonitis	3	1 (20% pulsed)	5	0.015% Dex ? Lido	5	Phono vs US Similar Objective & Subjective Outcome[119]
TMJ dysfunction	1	0.8–1.5	15	1% Indo	2	Subjective & Objective Improvements[116]

Abbreviations: **Dex/Lido:** X% dexamethasone plus X% Lidocaine; **DOMS:** delay onset muscle soreness; **Hydrocort:** hydrocortisone; **Indo:** indomethacin; **Lidex:** fluocinonide; **Phono:** phonophoresis; **Rx:** number of treatments; **TMJ:** temporomandibular joint; **TS:** trolamine salicylate; **US:** ultrasound. The concentration of lidocaine in the coupling gel could not be determinded from the methods.

tion with 10% hydrocortisone phonophoresis. In contrast, the use of 0.05% fluocinonide phonophoresis was compared with a similar duration of ultrasound in the treatment of various musculoskeletal dysfunctions.[118] Both groups demonstrated similar subjective and objective improvements in the various dysfunctions. The investigators concluded that the addition of the fluocinonide to the ultrasound treatment was not significantly beneficial. Finally, phonophoresis of dexamethasone with lidocaine in the treatment of tendonitis was compared with the use of a similar treatment of ultrasound alone.[119] As with the fluocinonide phonophoretic investigation,[118] no additional improvement was observed in either the subjective or objective outcomes when dexamethasone with lidocaine was added to the ultrasound treatment. Several conclusions concerning the success of these various clinical investigations may be made based on the potential for enhancement of transcutaneous drug permeation by phonophoresis[91] and the time required for optimal phonophoretic application:[97] first, the success of the indomethacin phonophoresis in comparison to the salicylate phonophoresis.[115,116] Theoretical constructs suggest that indomethacin would be enhanced by phonophoresis, whereas salicylate would not. Additionally, the phonophoretic application duration in the indomethacin investigation was three times as long as in the salicylate investigation. Based on previously discussed phonophoretic parameters, this additional time should enhance the transcutaneous permeation of the indomethacin compared with the salicylate. In the investigations examining SAIDs,[117–119] the investigation documenting enhanced success with 10% compared with 1% hydrocortisone did not include an ultrasound only treatment group.[117] This may explain the proposed success in this investigation compared with those documenting no difference between ultrasound and

phonophoresis with an SAID.[118,119] Phonophoresis of dexamethasone would be predicted to have enhanced the delivery of the drug.[97] However, the clinical investigation demonstrated several experimental design deficiencies.[119] The phonophoretic treatment duration was just 5 minutes with pulsed (20% duty cycle) 3 MHz ultrasound. Both the short treatment duration and the 3 MHz frequency would not augment the transcutaneous transport of dexamethasone.[97] Additionally, the 0.015% dexamethasone concentration in the coupling gel may have been insufficient to provide an anti-inflammatory in the subcutaneous tissues. The final concentration of lidocaine in the coupling gel could not be determined from the methods. Finally, the authors assumed that the mechanical conduction efficiency of their coupling gel was similar to that of another steroid with efficient mechanical conduction. However, for the phonophoresis, dexamethasone tablets were crushed and mixed into the coupling gel. These crushed tablets may contain inert material, which potentially alter the mechanical conduction of the gel.

Finally, other cutaneous localized disorders may also be clinically treated with phonophoresis of anti-inflammatory drugs. A case study reported the use of phonophoresis in the treatment of cutaneous epitheloid granulomas that are associated with sarcoidosis.[120] Treatment of the nodules on the dorsal aspect of the hand with steroid anti-inflammatory drugs had previously failed. Continuous mode hydrocortisone phonophoresis at 0.5 to 0.6 W/cm² for 5 minutes was used to treat the nodules. The phonophoretic frequency was not stated. Following a month of twice per week treatments, the nodules were markedly reduced. The anti-inflammatory effect of the hydrocortisone phonophoresis was concluded to be local, as nodules in other parts of the body were not reduced. These clinical results suggest that phonophoresis of anti-inflammatory drugs may be of clinical benefit in other cutaneous conditions such as hypertrophic scarring, keloid formation, or psoriasis.

Combined Use of Iontophoresis and Phonophoresis

Experimental investigations support the enhancement of transcutaneous drug delivery by the combined use of iontophoresis and phonophoresis, although the experimental parameters are not completely reflective of those used clinically.[123,124] However, the clinical combination of these modalities may be somewhat more problematic. Two case study investigations have examined the combined use of phonophoresis and iontophoresis of SAIDs in musculoskeletal dysfunction and have reported differing results.[125,126] In the treatment of postsurgical temporomandibular dysfunction, a combination of iontophoresis and phonophoresis of hydrocortisone ointment were proposed as reducing the patient's complaints of pain and improved temporomandibular function.[125] In contrast, a combination of dexamethasone phosphate iontophoresis and triamcinolone acetonide phonophoresis were proposed as exacerbating a patient's complaints of pain and clinical symptoms in the treatment of lateral epicondylitis.[126] Whether these differing results are due to the area of treatment or drug delivery parameters is at present uncertain. Thus, the clinician should use caution with the combined use of these transcutaneous drug delivery modalities.

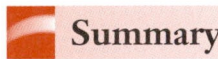

Summary

Current experimental and clinical research evidence suggests that both phonophoresis and iontophoresis possess the potential for transcutaneous delivery of anti-inflammatory pharmaceutics and potentially other medications. However, current evidence as to the pharmacokinetics of the depth of penetration and the clinical value of the pharmaceutics at these various tissue depths remains to be defined.

Discussion Questions

1. How is the dosage for iontophoresis determined and what does it consist of?
2. Why does the skin prevent the passage of electrical current into the body and what can be done to reduce that?
3. What is the difference between iontophoresis and phonophoresis?
4. What are the advantages of iontophoresis over an injection of a medication?
5. What are the disadvantages of iontophoresis over an injection of a medication?

CASE STUDY

Mary Jo is an executive secretary who was referred to the physical therapy department for recurring bilateral lateral epicondylitis. She has been treated previously with ultrasound and has had no significant reduction in her discomfort. She complains of a "gripping" sensation with active wrist extension. Mary Jo has a family history of diabetes, and both of her parents have been diagnosed with different forms of cancer within the past year.

References

1. Benet, LZ, Kroetz, DL, and Sheiner, LB: Pharmacokinetics: The dynamics of drug absorption, distribution, and elimination. In Hardman, J, Limbird, L, Editors-In-Chief: Goodman and Gilman's: The Pharmacological Basis of Therapeutics, ed 9. McGraw-Hill, New York, 1996, pp 3–28.
2. Fartasch, M: The nature of the epidermal barrier: Structural aspects. Adv Drug Del Rev 18:273–282, 1996.
3. Riviere, JE, and Heit, MC: Electrically-assisted transdermal drug delivery. Pharm Res 14:687–697, 1997.
4. Prausnitz, MR: The effect of pulsed electrical protocols on skin damage, sensation and pain. Proc Int Symp Control Rel Bioact Mater, Controlled Release Society, Inc, 1997, pp 25–26.
5. Banga, AJ: Electrically-Assisted Transdermal and Topical Drug Delivery. Taylor and Francis, London, 1998.
6. Banga, AK, and Panus, PC: Clinical applications of iontophoretic devices in rehabilitation medicine. Crit Rev Phys Rehab Med 10:147–179, 1998.
7. Yamamoto, T, and Yamamoto, Y: Electrical properties of the epidermal stratum corneum. Med Biol Eng 14:151–158, 1976.
8. Lin, RY, Ou, YC, and Chen, WY: The role of electroosmotic flow on in vitro transdermal iontophoresis. J Control Release 43:23–33, 1997.
9. Plutchik, R, and Hirsch, HR: Skin impedance and phase angle as a function of frequency and current. Science 141:927–928, 1963.
10. Boxtel, AV: Skin resistance during square-wave electrical pulses of 1 to 10 mA. Med Biol Eng Comput 15:679–687, 1977.
11. Kalia, YN, and Guy, RH: The electrical characteristics of human skin in vivo. Pharm. Res. 12:1605–1613, 1995.
12. Burnette, RR, and Bagniefski, TM: Influence of constant current iontophoresis on the impedance and passive Na+ permeability of excised nude mouse skin. J Pharm Sci 77:492–497, 1988.
13. Kasting, GB, and Bowman, LA: DC electrical properties of frozen, excised human skin. Pharm Res 7:134–143, 1990.
14. Kasting, GB, and Bowman, LA: Electrical analysis of fresh, excised human skin: A comparison with frozen skin. Pharm Res 7:1141–1146, 1990.
15. Oh, SY, Leung, L, Bommannan, D, et al: Effect of current, ionic strength and temperature on the electrical properties of skin. J Control Release 27:115–125, 1993.

16. Roberts, MS: Targeted drug delivery to the skin and deeper tissues: Role of physiology, solute structure and disease. Clin Exp Pharmacol Physiol 24:874–879, 1997.

17. Prausnitz, MR: Reversible skin permeabilization for transdermal delivery of macromolecules. Crit Rev Ther Drug Carrier Syst 14:455–483, 1997.

18. McNeill, SC, Potts, RO, and Francoeur, ML: Local enhanced topical delivery (LETD) of drugs: Does it truly exist? Pharm Res 9:1422–1427, 1992.

19. Radermacher, J, Jentsch, D, Scholl, MA, et al: Diclofenac concentrations in synovial fluid and plasma after cutaneous application in inflammatory and degenerative joint disease. Br J Clin Pharmacol 31:537–541, 1991.

20. Vickers, CFH: Existence of reservoir in the stratum corneum. Exp Proof Arch Dermatol 88:72–75, 1963.

21. Grahame, R: Transdermal non-steroidal anti-inflammatory agents. Br J Clin Pract 49:33–35, 1995.

22. Singh, P, and Roberts, MS: Iontophoretic transdermal delivery of salicylic acid and lidocaine to local subcutaneous structures. J Pharm Sci 82:127–131, 1993.

23. Singh, P, and Roberts, MS: Deep tissue penetration of bases and steroids after dermal application in rat. J Pharm Pharmacol 46:956–964, 1994.

24. Singh, P, and Roberts, MS: Skin permeability and local tissue concentrations of nonsteroidal anti-inflammatory drugs after topical application. J Pharmacol Exp Ther 268:144–151, 1994.

25. Green, P: Iontophoretic Transdermal Drug Delivery: A New Commercially Feasible Technology. Hotel International, Basel, Switzerland, October 17–18 (Organized by A. K. Banga and P. Green through Technomic Publishing), 1996.

26. Singh, P, Anliker, M, Smith, GA, et al: Transdermal iontophoresis and solute penetration across excised human skin. J Pharm Sci 84:1342–1346, 1995.

27. Li, SK, Ghanem, AH, Peck, KD, et al: Iontophoretic transport across a synthetic membrane and human epidermal membrane: A study of the effects of permeant charge. J Pharm Sci 86:680–689, 1997.

28. Kim, A, Green, PG, Rao, G, et al: Convective solvent flow across the skin during iontophoresis. Pharm Res 10:1315–1320, 1993.

29. Burnette, RR, and Ongpipattanakul, B: Characterization of the pore transport properties and tissue alteration of excised human skin during iontophoresis. J Pharm Sci 77:132–137, 1988.

30. Turner, NG, and Guy, RH: Iontophoretic transport pathways: Dependence on penetrant physicochemical properties. J Pharm Sci 86:1385–1389, 1997.

31. Menon, GK, and Elias, PM: Morphologic basis for a pore-pathway in mammalian stratum corneum. Skin Pharmacol 10:235–246, 1997.

32. Craane Van Hinsberg, IW, Verhoef, JC, Spies, F, et al: Electroperturbation of the human skin barrier in vitro: II. Effects on stratum corneum lipid ordering and ultrastructure. Microsc Res Tech 37:200–213, 1997.

33. Hinsberg, WHMC, Verhoef, JC, Bax, LJ, et al: Role of appendages in skin resistance and iontophoretic peptide flux: Human versus snake skin. Pharm Res 12:1506–1512, 1995.

34. Cullander, C: What are the pathways of iontophoretic current flow through mammalian skin? Adv Drug Del Rev 9:119–135, 1992.

35. Turner, NG, Kalia, YN, and Guy, RH: The effect of current on skin barrier function in vivo: Recovery kinetics post-iontophoresis. Pharm Res 14:1252–1257, 1997.

36. Li, SK, Ghanem, AH, Peck, KD, et al: Characterization of the transport pathways induced during low to moderate voltage iontophoresis in human epidermal membrane. J Pharm Sci 87:40–48, 1998.

37. Gangarosa, LP, Park, N, Wiggins, CA, et al: Increased penetration of nonelectrolytes into mouse skin during iontophoretic water transport (iontohydrokinesis). J Pharmacol Exp Ther 212:377–381, 1980.

38. Pikal, MJ: The role of electroosmotic flow in transdermal iontophoresis. Adv Drug Del Rev 9:201–237, 1992.

39. Burnette, RR, and Ongpipattanakul, B: Characterization of the permaselective properties of excised human skin during iontophoresis. J Pharm Sci 76:765–773, 1987.

40. Gwynne, P: Companies developing more uses for iontophoresis. Scientist 11:1, 1997.

41. Kahn, J: Acetic acid iontophoresis for calcium deposits. Phys Ther 57:658–659, 1977.

42. Kahn, J: A case report: lithium iontophoresis for gouty arthritis. J Orthop Sports Phys Ther 4:113–114, 1982.

43. LaForest, NT, and Cofrancesco, C: Antibiotic iontophoresis in the treatment of ear chondritis. Phys Ther 58:32–34, 1978.

44. Saggini, R, Zoppi, M, Vecchiet, F, et al: Comparison of electromotive drug administration with ketorolac or with placebo in patients with pain from rheumatic disease: A double-masked study. Clin Ther 18:1169–1174, 1996.

45. Wieder, DL: Treatment of traumatic myositis ossificans with acetic acid iontophoresis. Phys Ther 72:133–137, 1992.

46. Johnson, MTV, and Lee, NH, inventors; Empi, assignee. PH Buffered Electrodes for Medical Iontophoresis. MN, USA 4,973,303. 1990.

47. Guffey, JS, Rutherford, MJ, Payne, W, et al: Skin pH changes associated with iontophoresis. J Orthop Sports Phys Ther 29:656–660, 1999.

48. Sage, BH: Iontophoresis. In Swarbrick, J, and Boylan, JC: Encyclopedia of Pharmaceutical Technology. Marcel Dekker, New York, 1993, pp 217–247.

49. Lelawongs, P, Liu, J, Siddiqui, O, et al: Transdermal iontophoretic delivery of arginine-vasopressin (I): Physicochemical considerations. Int J Pharm 56:13–22, 1989.

50. Brand, RM, Duensing, G, and Hamel, FG: Iontophoretic delivery of an insulin mimetic peroxovanadium compound. Int J Pharm 146:115–122, 1997.

51. Hollinger, MA: Toxicological aspects of topical silver pharmaceuticals. Crit Rev Toxicol 26:255–260, 1996.

52. Phipps, JB, Padmanabhan, RV, and Lattin, GA: Iontophoretic delivery of model inorganic and drug ions. J Pharm Sci 78:365–369, 1989.

53. Gangarosa, LP, Park, NH, Fong, BC, et al: Conductivity of drugs used for iontophoresis. J Pharm Sci 67:1439–1443, 1978.

54. Lattin, GA, Padmanabhan, RV, and Phipps, JB: Electronic control of iontophoretic drug delivery. Ann N Y Acad Sci 618: 450–464, 1991.

55. Miller, LL, and Smith, GA: Iontophoretic transport of acetate and carboxylate ions through hairless mouse skin: Cation exchange membrane model. Int J Pharm 49:15–22, 1989.

56. Thysman, S, Preat, V, and Roland, M: Factors affecting iontophoretic mobility of metoprolol. J Pharm Sci 81:670–675, 1992.

57. Chu, DL, Chiou, HJ, and Wang, DP: Characterization of transdermal delivery of nefopam hydrochloride under iontophoresis. Drug Dev Ind Pharm 20:2775–2785, 1994.

58. Schimmer, B, and Parker, K: Adrenocorticotropic hormone; adrenocortical steroids and their synthetic analogs; inhibitors of the synthesis and actions of adrenocortical hormones. In Hardman, J, Limbird, L, Editors-In-Chief: Goodman and Gilman's The Pharmacological Basis of Therapeutics, ed 9. McGraw-Hill, New York, 1996, pp 1459–1485.

59. Insel, P: Analgesic-antipyretic and antiinflammatory agents and drugs employed in the treatment of gout. In Hardman, J, Limbird, L, Editors-In-Chief: Goodman and Gilman's The Pharmacological Basis of Therapeutics, ed 9. McGraw-Hill, New York, 1996, pp 617–658.

60. Glass, JM, Stephen, RL, and Jacobson, SC: The quantity and distribution of radiolabeled dexamethasone delivered to tissue by iontophoresis. Int J Derm 19:519–525, 1980.

61. Petelenz, TJ, Buttke, JA, Bonds, C, et al: Iontophoresis of dexamethasone: Laboratory studies. J Control Release 20:55–66, 1992.

62. Anderson, CR, Morris, RL, Boeh, SD, et al: Quantification of total dexamethasone phosphate delivery by iontophoresis. Int J Pharm Compound 7:115–159, 2003.

63. Anderson, CR, Morris, RL, Boeh, SD, et al: Effects of iontophoresis current magnitude and duration on dexamethasone deposition and localized drug retention. Phys Ther 83:161–170, 2003.

64. Riviere,, JE, Monteiro Riviere, NA, and Inman, AO: Determination of lidocaine concentrations in skin after transdermal iontophoresis: Effects of vasoactive drugs. Pharm Res 9:211–214, 1992.

65. Riviere, JE, Sage, B, and Williams, PL: Effects of vasoactive drugs on transdermal lidocaine iontophoresis. J Pharm Sci 80:615–620, 1991.

66. Singh, P, and Roberts, MS: Effects of vasoconstriction on dermal pharmacokinetics and local tissue distribution of compounds. J Pharm Sci 83:783–791, 1994.

67. Nowicki, KD, Hummer, CD 3rd, Heidt, RS Jr, et al: Effects of iontophoretic versus injection administration of dexamethasone. Med Sci Sports Exerc 34:1294–1301, 2002.

68. Smutok, MA, Mayo, MF, Gabaree, CL, et al: Failure to detect dexamethasone phosphate in the local venous blood postcathodic Iontophoresis in humans. J Orthop Sports Phys Ther 32: 461–468, 2002.

69. Blackford, J, Doherty, TJ, Ferslew, KE, et al: Iontophoresis of dexamethasone phosphate into the equine tibiotarsal joint. J Vet Pharmacol Ther 23:229-236, 2000.

70. Panus, PC, Campbell, J, Kulkarni, SB, et al: Transdermal iontophoretic delivery of ketoprofen through human cadaver skin and in humans. J Control Release 44:113–121, 1997.

71. Panus, PC, Campbell, J, Kulkarni, B, et al: Effect of iontophoretic current and application time on transdermal delivery of ketoprofen in man. Pharm Sci 2:467–469, 1996.

72. Panus, PC, Ferslew, KE, Tober-Meyer, B, et al: Ketoprofen tissue permeation in swine following cathodic iontophoresis. Phys Ther 79:40–49, 1999.

73. Tashiro, Y, Kato, Y, Hayakawa, E, et al: Iontophoretic transdermal delivery of ketoprofen: novel method for the evaluation of plasma drug concentration in cutaneous vein. Biol Pharm Bull 23:632–636, 2000.

74. Tashiro, Y, Kato, Y, Hayakawa, E, et al: Iontophoretic transdermal delivery of ketoprofen: effect of iontophoresis on drug transfer from skin to cutaneous blood. Biol Pharm Bull 23:1486–1490, 2000.

75. Grossmann, M, Jamieson, MJ, Kellogg, DL Jr, et al: The effect of iontophoresis on the cutaneous vasculature: Evidence for current-induced hyperemia. Microvasc Res 50:444–452, 1995.

76. Eastman, T, Panus, PC, Honnas, CM, et al: Cathodic iontophoresis of ketoprofen over the equine middle carpal joint. Equine Vet J 33:614–616, 2001.

77. Hasson, SM, Wible, CL, Reich, M, et al: Dexamethasone iontophoresis: Effect on delayed muscle soreness and muscle function. Can J Sport Sci 17:8–13, 1992.

78. Li, LC, Scudds, RA, Heck, CS, et al: The efficacy of dexamethasone iontophoresis for the treatment of rheumatoid arthritic knees: A pilot study. Arthritis Care Res 9:126–132, 1996.

79. Gudeman, SD, Eisele, SA, Heidt, RS Jr, et al: Treatment of plantar fasciitis by iontophoresis of 0.4% dexamethasone. A randomized, double-blind, placebo-controlled study. Am J Sports Med 25:312–316, 1997.

80. Reid, KI, Dionne, RA, Sicard Rosenbaum, L, et al: Evaluation of iontophoretically applied dexamethasone for painful pathologic temporomandibular joints. Oral Surg Oral Med Oral Pathol 77:605–609, 1994.

81. Schiffman, EL, Braun, BL, and Lindgren, BR: Temporomandibular joint iontophoresis: A double-blind randomized clinical trial. J Orofac Pain 10:157–165, 1996.

82. Riedl, CR, Plas, E, Engelhardt, P, et al: Iontophoresis for treatment of Peyronie's disease. J Urol 163:95–99, 2000.

83. Schroeder-Printzen, I, Hauck, EW, et al: New aspects in Peyronie's disease—a mini-review. Andrologia. 31 Suppl 1:31–35, 1999.

84. Montorsi, F, Salonia, A, Guazzoni, G, et al: Transdermal electromotive multi-drug administration for Peyronie's disease: Preliminary results. J Androl 21:85–90, 2000.

85. Lener, EV, Bucalo, BD, Kist, DA, et al: Topical anesthetic agents in dermatologic surgery. A review. Dermatol Surg 23:673–683, 1997.

86. Lesions and shocks during iontophoresis. Health Devices 26:123–125, 1997.

87. Anderson, LL, Welch, ML, and Grabski, WJ: Allergic contact dermatitis and reactivation phenomenon from iontophoresis of 5-fluorouracil. J Am Acad Dermatol 36:478–479, 1997.

88. Levy, D, Kost, J, Meshulam, Y, et al: Effect of ultrasound on transdermal drug delivery to rats and guinea pigs. J Clin Invest 83:2074–2078, 1989.

89. Byl, NN: The use of ultrasound as an enhancer for transcutaneous drug delivery: phonophoresis. Phys Ther 75:539–553, 1995.

90. Mitragotri, S, Blankschtein, D, and Langer, R: Ultrasound-mediated transdermal protein delivery. Science 269:850–853, 1995.

91. Mitragotri, S, Blankschtein, D, and Langer, R: An explanation for the variation of the sonophoretic transdermal transport enhancement from drug to drug. J Pharm Sci 86:1190–1192, 1997.

92. Cameron, MH, and Monroe, LG: Relative transmission of ultrasound by media customarily used for phonophoresis. Phys Ther 72:142–148, 1992.

93. Benson, HAE, and McElnay, JC: Topical non-steroidal anti-inflammatory products as ultrasound couplants: Their potential in phonophoresis. Physiotherapy 80:74–76, 1994.

94. Benson, HAE, and McElnay, JC: Transmission of ultrasound energy through topical pharmaceutical products. Physiotherapy 74:587–589, 1988.

95. Docker, MF, Foulkes, DJ, and Patrick, MF: Ultrasound couplants for physiotherapy. Physiotherapy 68:124–215, 1982.

96. Simonin, JP: On the mechanisms of in vitro and in vivo phonophoresis. J Control Release 33:125–141, 1995.

97. Mitragotri, S, Edwards, DA, Blankschtein, D, et al: A mechanistic study of ultrasonically-enhanced transdermal drug delivery. J Pharm Sci 84:697–706, 1995.

98. Meidan, VM, Walmsley, AD, Docker, MF, et al: Ultrasound-enhanced diffusion into coupling gel during phonophoresis of 5-fluorouracil. Int J Pharm 185:205–213, 1999.

99. Griffin, JE, and Touchstone, JC: Effects of ultrasonic frequency on phonophoresis of cortisol into swine tissues. Am J Phys Med 51:62–78, 1972.

100. Griffin, JE, and Touchstone, JC: Ultrasonic movement of cortisol into pig tissues. Am J Phys Med 42:77–85, 1963.

101. Griffin, JE, and Touchstone, JC: Low-intensity phonophoresis of cortisol in swine. Phys Ther 48:1336–1344, 1968.

102. Miyazaki, S, Mizuoka, H, Kohata, Y, et al: External control of drug release and penetration. VI. Enhancing effect of ultrasound on the transdermal absorption of indomethacin from an ointment in rats. Chem Pharm Bull Tokyo 40:2826–2830, 1992.

103. Miyazaki, S, Mizuoka, H, Oda, M, et al: External control of drug release and penetration: enhancement of the transdermal absorption of indomethacin by ultrasound irradiation. J Pharm Pharmacol 43:115–116, 1991.

104. Asano, J, Suisha, F, Takada, M, et al: Effect of pulsed output ultrasound on the transdermal absorption of indomethacin from an ointment in rats. Biol Pharm Bull 20:288–291, 1997.

105. Hippius, M, Smolenski, U, Uhlemann, C, et al: In vitro investigations of drug release and penetration-enhancing effect of ultrasound on transmembrane transport of flufenamic acid. Exp Toxicol Pathol 50:450–452, 1998.

106. Hippius, M, Uhlemann, C, Smolenski, U, et al: In vitro investigations of drug release and penetration-enhancing effect of ultrasound on transmembrane transport of flufenamic acid. Int J Clin Pharmacol Ther 36:107–111, 1998.

107. Benson, HAE, McElnay, JC, and Harland, R: Use of ultrasound to enhance percutaneous absorption of benzydamine. Phys Ther 69:113–118, 1989.

108. Oziomek, RS, Perrin, DH, Herold, DA, et al: Effect of phonophoresis on serum salicylate levels. Med Sci Sports Exerc 23:397–401, 1991.

109. Muir, WS, Magee, FP, Longo, JA, et al: Comparison of ultrasonically applied vs. intra-articular injected hydrocortisone levels in canine knees. Orthop Rev 19:351–356, 1990.

110. Davick, JP, Martin, RK, and Albright, JP: Distribution and deposition of tritiated cortisol using phonophoresis. Phys Ther 68:1672–1675, 1988.

111. Bare, AC, McAnaw, MB, Pritchard, AE, et al: Phonophoretic delivery of 10% hydrocortisone through the epidermis of humans as determined by serum cortisol concentrations. Phys Ther 76:738–745, 1996.

112. Byl, NN, McKenzie, A, Halliday, B, et al: The effects of phonophoresis with corticosteroids: A controlled pilot study. J Orthop Sports Phys Ther 18:590–600, 1993.

113. Conner Kerr, TA, Franklin, ME, Kerr, JE, et al: Phonophoretic delivery of dexamethasone to human transdermal tissues: A controlled pilot study. Eur J Phys Med Rehabil 8:19–23, 1998.

114. Darrow, H, Schulthies, S, Draper, D, et al: Serum dexamethasone levels after Decadron phonophoresis. J Athl Train 34:338–341, 1999.

115. Ciccone, CD, Leggin, BG, and Callamaro, JJ: Effects of ultrasound and trolamine salicylate phonophoresis on delayed-onset muscle soreness. Phys Ther 71:666–675, 1991; discussion 675–678.

116. Shin, SM, and Choi, JK: Effect of indomethacin phonophoresis on the relief of temporomandibular joint pain. Cranio 15:345–348, 1997.

117. Kleinkort, JA, and Wood, F: Phonophoresis with 1 percent versus 10 percent hydrocortisone. Phys Ther 55:1320–1324, 1975.

118. Klaiman, MD, Shrader, JA, Danoff, JV, et al: Phonophoresis versus ultrasound in the treatment of common musculoskeletal conditions. Med Sci Sports Exerc 30:1349–1355, 1998.

119. Penderghest, CE, Kimura, IF, and Gulick, DT: Double-blind clinical efficacy study of pulsed phonophoresis on perceived pain associated with symptomatic tendinitis. J Sport Rehabil. 7:9–19, 1998.

120. Gogstetter, DS, and Goldsmith, LA: Treatment of cutaneous sarcoidosis using phonophoresis. J Am Acad Dermatol 40:767–769, 1999.

121. Fang, J, Fang, C, Sung, KC, et al: Effect of low frequency ultrasound on the in vitro percutaneous absorption of clobetasol 17-propionate. Int J Pharm 191:33–42, 1999.

122. Harris, DW, and Hunter, JA: The use and abuse of 0.05 per cent clobetasol propionate in dermatology. Dermatol Clin 6:643–647, 1988.

123. Ueda, H, Ogihara, M, Sugibayashi, K, et al: Change in the electrochemical properties of skin and the lipid packing in stratum corneum by ultrasonic irradiation. Int J Pharm 137:217–224, 1996.

124. Kost, J, Pliquett, U, Mitragotri, S, et al: Synergistic effect of electric field and ultrasound on transdermal transport. Pharm Res 13:633–638, 1996.

125. Kahn, J: Iontophoresis and ultrasound for postsurgical temporomandibular trismus and paresthesia. Phys Ther 60:307–308, 1980.

126. Panus, PC, Hooper, T, Padrones, A, et al: A case study of exacerbation of lateral epicondylitis by combined use of iontophoresis and phonophoresis. Physiother Can 48:27–31, 1996.

127. Harris, PR: Iontophoresis: Clinical research in musculoskeletal inflammatory conditions. J Orthop Sports Phys Ther 4:109–112, 1982.

128. Bertolucci, LE: Introduction of antiinflammatory drugs by iontophoresis: double blind study. J Orthop Sports Phys Ther 4:103–108, 1982.

129. Chantraine, A, Ludy, JP, and Berger, D: Is cortisone iontophoresis possible? Arch Phys Med Rehabil 67:38–40, 1986.

130. Pellecchia, GL, Hamel, H, and Behnke, P: Treatment of infrapatellar tendinitis: A combination of modalities and transverse friction massage versus iontophoresis. J Sport Rehabil 3: 135–145, 1994.

131. Banta, CA: A prospective, nonrandomized study of iontophoresis, wrist splinting, and antiinflammatory medication in the treatment of early-mild carpal tunnel syndrome. J Occup Med 36:166–168, 1994.

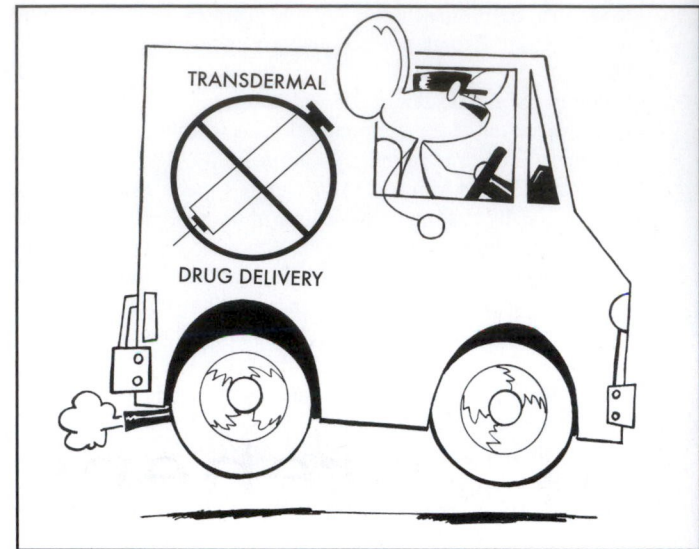

Comprehensive Approach to Treatment

Objectives

- Discuss the impact of the Food and Drug Administration on medical device development.
- Describe how clinicians can find evidence to support their choice in a treatment intervention.
- Select the best interventions for a given patient based on the patient's goals, treatment goals, safety, time constraints, cost efficiency, and availability of equipment.
- Sequence modality interventions to complement and enhance other treatment interventions.
- Describe the essential information to be included when documenting the objective portion of a SOAP note.

Key Terms

Assessment	Indication	Preparatory treatment
Compliance	Objective	Reliability
Contraindication	Plan	Subjective
Documentation	Precaution	Tolerate

Barbara J. Behrens, PTA, MS   *Stacie Larkin, PT, MEd*

Integration of Physical Agents: Clinical Decision Making

Outline

> *Why should I care? What does it mean to me in my practice?*

The practice of physical therapy is forever changing. According to the APTA *Guide to Physical Therapist Practice* (2001), a document developed and reviewed by a contingent of more than 600 physical therapists, treatment interventions using electrotherapeutic modalities, physical agents, and mechanical modalities are used for the purpose of (1) reduction of a symptom or (2) promotion of a response. This includes the promotion of tissue healing,[1-4] increasing blood flow to an injured area,[5,6] muscle strengthening,[7-9] increasing tissue extensibility,[10-12] and the promotion of pain relief.[13-16] These treatment goals have therapeutic benefits that can be visually observed and manually or mechanically measured.

These goals can often be interdependent. For example, a modality used for the reduction of pain may reduce the level of discomfort enough to decrease the protective muscle guarding in the area. If the guarding subsides, then the potential exists that the blood flow into or from the area will no longer be impeded by the muscle guarding, and metabolite retention in the area will have a chance to diminish, resulting in less chemical irritation (from the metabolite retention), and ultimately less pain. Pain can also be considered a protective

Patient Perspective

Remember that if your patient has previously received physical therapy for an injury, your patient is probably one of your best resources for information regarding what works for them and what does not. Your patient must be included in the treatment intervention process. You must be considerate of their time as well as your own. Instructions must be stated in terms that your patient or significant other will be able to understand. If you are asking your patient for feedback, make sure that your patient knows how to provide appropriate feedback. Some patients may have the misconception that "no pain, means no gain." It is your responsibility to explain what you are doing and why this philosophy does not apply to physical therapy treatment interventions with physical agents.

FREQUENTLY ASKED QUESTIONS

1. Why can't you just do everything at the same time?

2. Why do I need to have ice after exercise, I really want to leave sooner?

3. Why don't you do the same thing with every patient? That patient seemed to "get more" than I did and our bills were the same.

4. Yesterday when I had the traction without the heat, my neck hurt.

response, warning the individual not to further stress the injured area. The area is no longer as strong as it once was. Pain perception may intensify because of the muscle guarding and the resulting metabolite retention in the injured tissue.

Many of the individual techniques presented throughout this text address the three sides of the *Pain Triangle*—pain, dysfunction, and muscle guarding—but to different degrees (see Chapter 1).

Some techniques primarily target the pain, or the muscle guarding, and indirectly address the dysfunction. Others specifically target the dysfunction by promoting tissue healing and experience a resultant decrease in pain perception and muscle guarding as the area heals. One important consideration in the selection of physical agents is the concept of causal factors. The mark of excellence in clinical practice is the attention paid to the cause-and-effect relationship and acknowledgment of the importance of understanding the relationship. Clinicians treat the patient considering "the patient," and the normal courses of response to therapeutic interventions. By identifying the cause of the patient's problems, effective treatment interventions can be used, decreasing the potential of reoccurrence. Technicians treat the individual symptom, without regard for causal factors. Patients treated in the manner are more likely to get frustrated as their symptom relief is often temporary.

Skilled clinicians must select the appropriate treatment intervention to fit: (1) the diagnosis of the patient, (2) the medical stability of the patient, (3) the anticipated goals of the intervention, (4) the experience of the clinician, and (5) the choices available to the clinician. The influence of each of these factors will vary from individual to individual. Patient safety must remain foremost in this aspect of the decision-making process.

This chapter will focus on each of the anticipated outcomes from direct treatment interventions identified within the APTA *Guide to Physical Therapist Practice* resulting from electrotherapeutic modalities, mechanical modalities, and physical agents (Box 14-1). In order to determine whether a goal has been accomplished, the clinician must be able to collect the appropriate information from the patient through tests and measures. The clinician must also recognize that his or her overall approach to the treatment intervention and to the patient will affect his or her results. The clinician's approach in treating a patient experiencing pain involves the recognition of the pain and assessment of its impact on functional activities and the patient's life in general.[17,18] Determining what factors contributed to the patient's symptoms and how to help the patient limit the potential for the return of symptoms is essential. The technician who merely applies a modality indicated for the treatment of pain may not have lasting success if the cause of the pain is not addressed. This is where patient education becomes an important component of the treatment plan.

There are several different approaches to treatment interventions that will result in favorable responses from and for the patient. The clinician must be a good observer and know what tests and measures to apply before and after performing any therapeutic treatment intervention to determine if the chosen intervention had a positive outcome.

Food and Drug Administration (FDA)

The past has taught us that we can no longer take "for granted" that something works, without really asking the basic science questions regarding the "why and how?" Before May 1976, medical devices were regulated as a new drug, and due to their use and lack of specific scrutiny within that division, those in existence were "grandfathered" in as safe and effective. Now they are regulated by the FDA's Center for Devices and Radiological Health, which manages and facilitates a highly structured process for medical devices including regulations, classifications, premarket approvals, investigational device exemptions, and labeling and tracking guidelines. Essentially, these regulations require manufacturers to first prove that a device is not only safe for use on human subjects but also effective before it is marketed to the clinical community. This process requires that testing take place to determine exactly what results can be expected from the application of the device to a patient.[19]

Very few "new" devices have gone through this scrutiny, which can take years. An excellent example is the recent introduction and premarket approval of low-level or "cold"

BOX 14-1 Direct Interventions and the Anticipated Goals

Electrotherapeutic Modalities
- Biofeedback
- Electrical muscle stimulation
- Functional electrical stimulation (FES)
- Iontophoresis
- Neuromuscular electrical stimulation (NMES)
- Transcutaneous electrical nerve stimulation (TENS)

Anticipated Goals from Electrotherapeutic Modalities
- Ability to perform physical tasks is increased.
- Ventilation, respiration (gas exchange), and circulation are improved.
- Complications are reduced.
- Edema, lymphedema, or effusion is reduced.
- Motor function (motor control and motor learning) is improved.
- Muscle performance is increased.
- Pain is decreased.
- Joint integrity and mobility are improved.
- Risk of secondary impairments is reduced.
- Soft tissue swelling, inflammation, and restriction are reduced.
- Wound and soft tissue healing is enhanced.

Direct Interventions: Physical Agents and Mechanical Modalities
Physical Agents
- Cryotherapy (cold pack, ice massage)
- Deep thermal modalities (ultrasound, phonophoresis)

- Superficial thermal modalities (heat, paraffin baths, hot packs, Fluidotherapy)
- Hydrotherapy (aquatic therapy, whirlpool tanks, contrast baths, pulsatile lavage)
- Phototherapy (ultraviolet)

Mechanical Modalities
- Traction (sustained, intermittent, or positional)
- Compression therapies (vasopneumatic compression devices, compression bandaging, compression garments, taping, total contact casting)
- Tilt table or standing table
- Continuous passive motion (CPM)

Anticipated Goals from Physical Agents and Mechanical Modalities
- Ability to perform movement tasks is increased.
- Complications from soft tissue and circulatory disorders are decreased.
- Edema, effusion, or lymphedema is reduced.
- Motor function (motor control and motor learning) is improved.
- Pain is decreased.
- Joint integrity and mobility are improved.
- Risk of secondary impairments is reduced.
- Soft tissue swelling, inflammation, or restriction is reduced.
- Tolerance to positions and activities is increased.
- Independence in airway clearance is increased.

From the APTA *Guide to Physical Therapist Practice*, ed 2.

LASER devices for adjunctive use in the temporary relief of hand and wrist pain associated with carpal tunnel syndrome. Although LASER (acronym for Light Amplification of Stimulated Emission of Radiation) has been commonly used outside the United States for many years, in 2002 only one manufacturer was granted 510(k) approval for this application. Using a medical device for interventions that are not preapproved by the FDA is not reimbursable by insurance carriers and are termed "off label" applications. This policy and procedure was put into place to protect the public from unsafe or unfounded claims being made and equipment from being used in an untested manner and billed to a patient's insurance carrier.

Additionally, the FDA has implemented a Medical Device User Fee and Modernization Act of 2002 (MDUFMA), which charges a fee to those companies who apply for pre-market approval for a new device. The goal of the MDUFMA is to fund the FDA's medical device directives to "ensure that safe and effective new products get to consumers as quickly as possible."[20]

Evidence-Based Practice

The impact of the FDA on the practice of physical therapy may seem remote to some clinicians, but in reality, it helped spark a movement leading toward evidence in practice. Evidence-based practice has been defined as "the conscientious and judicious use of current best evidence in making decisions about the care of individual patients."[21]

When a profession places more value on past practice or previous experience rather than evidence-based practice, the potential exists for negative outcomes to be interpreted as a failure of physical therapy, when in reality, the intervention was at fault. Reliance on evidence-based practice to set the standard for care should eliminate potential negative outcomes.[22] Evidence is more than just the experience of a clinician; it is based upon the documented outcomes of multiple clinicians with standardized sets of patient groups, symptoms, and treatment parameters. Additionally, the measurement tools for evidence based practice tend to be more objective than personal experience.

"Hooked on Evidence"

The need for evidence has grown considerably stronger through the efforts of the American Physical Therapy Association (APTA), which developed an online searchable database entitled "Hooked on Evidence." This database is a compilation of article extractions related to physical therapy interventions submitted by members of the APTA. Those who submit an extraction use a prescribed detailed template to extract the following information from a published research article: general information, study design, study details, methods, treatment, and outcomes. At time of writing of this text, there were approximately 1500 article extractions included in the database.[23] Part of the process involves an attempt to take a body of preexisting work and attempt to quantify the results using the same markers, some taken from the APTA *Guide to Physical Therapist Practice*. For example, the following headings are highlighted for each reviewed article[23]:

- Target Condition
- Element of Patient/Client Management Model
- Practice Pattern
- Design Type
- Study Population
- Population Location
- Inclusion Criteria
- Exclusion Criteria
- How were subjects selected?
- How many subjects were contacted initially?
- How many subjects were eligible to participate?
- How many subjects agreed to participate?
- Nonclinical characteristics of study participants
- Clinical characteristics of study participants
- Blinded clinicians
- Blinded subjects
- Same person providing treatment and testing measures
- Intention-to-treat analysis
- Treatment groups
- Authors' stated purpose interventions
- Study outcomes
- Authors conclusions
- Reviewer's comments

Other Online Databases

Databases or online resources vary significantly in the types of information that they search. There are online data-bases that cover business-related journals to help researchers track business conditions (ABI Inform) through PsycINFO, which contains articles from more than 1700 journals that deal with psychology-related topics. Although it would seem logical to find all things "medical" in the MEDLINE database (the National Library of Medicine's electronic database), this is not the case. Each of the databases has its own inclusion and exclusion criteria, which is one of the reasons that it is better to consult more than one online database. It is important to remember that these services are subscription services, unlike Google, which is a nonspecific meta-search engine that is available to everyone and provides all "hits" with the key terms. Items retrieved through a nonsubscription service must be carefully evaluated for their value. Not all articles published on the Web are reviewed, so it is important when looking at these articles that you consider the source and currency of the information presented. Just because something can be accessed via the Web does not make it reliable or valuable. Articles published in professional journals that are peer reviewed are still the most reliable sources of information regarding patient and treatment intervention information. Table 14-1 depicts online databases and the types of information that can be accessed through them.

Therapeutic Treatment Goals: Is a Physical Agent Appropriate?

The physical agents that this text addresses are used in the management of numerous soft tissue injuries and some selected neurologic conditions. These conditions are associated with symptoms that may include pain, altered sensation, edema, muscle guarding, muscle weakness, decreased soft tissue extensibility, or lack of muscle function. Each of these symptoms may be managed in part through the application of one or several physical agents as components of a physical therapy treatment intervention. Many of the aforementioned signs and symptoms can also be addressed through the use of therapeutic exercise, manual techniques, pharmacologic agents (medications), and rest as a part of the total care of the patient. However, physical agent approaches can be used in combination with any or all of the other approaches to help facilitate recovery for the patient. The ultimate question for all clinicians will remain the same: "Am I doing all that I can do to improve the condition of the patient safely, efficiently, and cost-effectively?"

The overzealous or inexperienced clinician may use a "shotgun" approach. This involves the use of multiple techniques both manual and mechanical to accomplish a goal. Unfortunately, the patient may report a negative treatment outcome that then could not be traced back to any individual source, because all of the pieces were administered together. For example, suppose a patient is receiving a therapeutic treatment intervention for a primary complaint of pain,

TABLE 14-1   Online Databases and the Types of Information That Can Be Accessed Through Them

ONLINE DATABASE	TYPE OF INFORMATION
PubMed	The National Library of Medicine's premier bibliographic database covering the fields of medicine, nursing, dentistry, veterinary medicine, the health care system, and the preclinical sciences. The database contains over 12 million citations dating back to the mid-1960s. (www.ncbi.nlm.nih.gov/pubmed)
The American Physical Therapy Association's (APTA's) "Hooked on Evidence"	APTA's "Hooked on Evidence" website represents a "grassroots" effort to develop a database containing current research evidence on the effectiveness of physical therapy interventions. This database is available to all APTA members. (www.hookedonevidence/com)
CINAHL (owned by Ebsco Host)	Index with abstracts from 1200 of the leading journals in nursing and allied health
Ebsco Host—Academic Search	Provides full text for nearly 3200 scholarly publications covering academic areas of study, including social sciences, humanities, education, computer sciences, engineering, language and linguistics, arts and literature, medical sciences, and ethnic studies
Ebsco Host—Health Source, Consumer Edition	Indexing and many full text for over 270 health periodicals, over 1100 health pamphlets, and 20 health reference books
Ebsco Host—Nursing Academic	Provides over 520 scholarly full-text journals focusing on many medical disciplines. Also featured are abstracts and indexing for over 560 journals
Educational Resource Information Center ERIC	Contains citations and abstracts from over 980 educational and education-related journals, as well as full text of more than 2200 digests
Lexis Nexis—Academic Universe: Medical	Full text and abstracted medical and health information
PsychINFO	Indexing and abstracts for over 1 million articles in 1700 journals dating back to 1887 with some full-text articles available through PscArticles

Some of these databases require subscription fees or are limited access and may be available through college or university libraries.

which upon examination is thought to be attributed to protective muscle guarding throughout the cervical musculature, limiting the motion and thus protectively guarding the injured area from further trauma. The therapeutic treatment interventions that were used included hot packs, traction, electrical stimulation, ultrasound, massage, joint mobilization, and therapeutic exercises. Several of the chosen treatment techniques would address the primary complaint of pain, and several of the techniques might be capable of relieving the cause underlying pain or protective muscle guarding. The combination of treatment techniques may or may not relieve the symptoms. The patient's symptoms may increase if any one of the techniques used is not appropriate for this patient, and with this approach, it will not be possible to determine which technique is at fault.

Clinicians can also get lost in the multitude of symptoms that a patient may offer. Prudent practitioners will identify the primary functional goals and address the impairments that are limiting the patient's ability to perform a given functional activity. When a selected intervention is used, the therapist must assess the patient's response following the individual treatment intervention to determine if a positive change has occurred. If there are remaining impairments, another physical agent or treatment intervention might be indicated. Reduction of the patient's "chief complaint" may result in reductions of his or her other symptoms, but this will be evident only to the observant clinician. If, for example, pain is worsened by the underlying muscle guarding, reduction of the guarding should reduce the pain. It may or may not be

true that relieving the pain will reduce the muscle guarding. This is why it is important to focus treatments on what is causing the pain rather that just trying to treat pain in isolation. Pain is a symptom that may affect a patient's ability to perform functional tasks. It is the ability to perform these tasks that must also be reassessed to determine if physical therapy was successful.

Available Treatment Time

Patients receive physical therapy in a variety of settings, including hospitals, outpatient clinics, skilled nursing facilities, schools, and their own homes when they are well enough to be home but cannot easily commute to an outpatient clinic. The time constraints and support mechanisms will vary significantly between these settings. It is important to consider the patient's needs and goals when designing a treatment program. Patients will realistically not devote every waking hour to their recovery. Time management in the accomplishment of therapeutic treatment goals must be a consideration. Treatment sessions that involve physical agents may require approximately 10 to 20 minutes with the remaining treatment time dedicated to manual techniques, patient education, therapeutic exercise, and reassessment. Although there are exceptions, based upon the diagnosis and other related factors, most treatment sessions usually last approximately 1 hour.

During this time, the goals that have been established and negotiated with the patient need to be addressed. This is where true integration must take place. Many of the techniques will treat the primary patient complaints, and indirectly address the other patient problems. It is not necessary or realistic to use every modality that could possibly be used to treat a patient because of this overlapping of responses. Time management and intervention assessment revolve around carefully limited choices to accomplish a goal, assessing the outcome of a given physical agent, and then making modifications when indicated.

Use of every "unattended" physical agent conceivable for an impairment could involve several hours of time with no more significant results than the careful selection of one of the physical agents used for 15 to 20 minutes. The general guideline that therapists should follow is to choose the minimum treatment interventions that will achieve the maximal response. Whenever possible, treatments should be combined in order to be more efficient. For example, a patient with an edematous knee could receive ice, compression, and elevation at the same time. Another example is combining active range of motion exercises while receiving a whirlpool treatment. It is important to be judicious in the selection of interventions, and conscious of time requirements to use them as this will directly impact your schedule and ability to treat other scheduled patients. Also, reimbursement can be an issue depending on how a third-party payer reimburses physical therapy treatment sessions. Some carriers may pay for their patients to receive up to three different treatment interventions. Others carriers may pay a flat rate for treatment, regardless of the number of individual treatment interventions used or the amount of time spent with a patient. Remember that patients, too, desire and deserve efficient use of their time. If the treatments become excessively long, the patient may become frustrated and not return for future appointments. Box 14-2 provides the clinician with questions to consider when treating patients with physical agents.

Some treatment interventions that might be indicated for a given patient, based upon their condition, may produce comparable results through completely different mechanisms. The approach taken may be more reflective of the individuality of the patient and his or her responses to previous treatment intervention techniques than a specific technique itself. If, for example, a patient had read an article in a magazine that outlined the successes of the use of electrical stimulation for the relief of "muscle tension" via pain relief, he or she may respond better to electrical stimulation than to traction. Their beliefs may influence the potential benefits of the selected physical agent (see Box 14-2).

Before You Begin

Choose the minimum treatment interventions that will achieve the maximal response.

BOX 14-2 Clinical Considerations When Treating with Physical Agents

- What is the available treatment time? How much time will it take? (more or less than 1 hour?)
- How long has it been since the actual injury?
- What is the medical stability of the patient?
- What expectations does the patient have about the treatment?
- What modalities are available to accomplish the treatment goals in the time available for treatment?

Acuity of the Injury

When treating an acute injury, the emphasis of treatment is focused on maintaining mobility and preventing further injury while the impairments of pain, edema formation, and muscle guarding are addressed.[24] Severely involved patients with multiple trauma and those with neurologic impairment will most often be seen for treatment initially in an acute care hospital setting and then be transferred to a rehabilitation facility for a more intensive approach to their recovery. Generally, when there is more tissue destruction, the recovery time will be longer. In these instances, the patient may be seen by a clinician twice daily in an inpatient setting. Even there, the focus on careful selection of treatment intervention techniques should not change. Because these patients have experienced a significant change in their functional ability, they will be involved in a more broad-based therapeutic program. There will be a greater emphasis on therapeutic exercise and adaptive skills for functional independence. Physical agents as treatment interventions will be chosen as an adjunct to their treatment plan to reduce symptoms and to enhance their return to function. Overall, time management and goal optimization in the utilization of therapeutic agents should remain the same regardless of the treatment setting.

Medical Stability of the Patient

Therapeutic treatment interventions are performed to promote optimal recovery of the patient, not the symptom. Patients with comorbidities might limit your potential choices of physical agents as treatment interventions. Suppose, for example, that a patient sought out physical therapy for the treatment of a cervical strain and sprain, and her primary complaints included pain with limited motion in the cervical spine due to muscle guarding. The patient's medical history reveals that she has osteoporosis. Although cervical traction may be beneficial for the relaxation of the cervical musculature, it would be contraindicated for this patient. The intervention choice may change to one of managing the pain with a portable electrical stimulation device and focusing predominantly on the patient's pain to decrease the muscle guarding rather than the opposite.

Another example of an alteration in treatment intervention selection arising from medical stability issues would be the patient who is referred to therapy for lower extremity edema. Upon assessment of the lower extremity, there are no palpable pedal pulses. Although one of the treatment interventions that might have been used for the management of the edema could have been intermittent compression, it would be contraindicated for this patient. The lack of pedal pulses would indicate a decrease in the blood supply to the lower extremity and may be indicative of further medical complications that would need to be evaluated by a physician. It is important to be sure that the cause of the edema is known and that it is appropriate to receive physical therapy interventions. When edema is the result of medical conditions such as congestive heart failure or kidney dysfunction, treating the edema can cause undesirable responses. Box 14-3 will teach you indications, contraindications, and precautions and "why."

The Impact of Patient Compliance on Recovery

Patient compliance plays a crucial role in the recovery process. The patient must be able to understand the purpose of the therapeutic interventions so that there is follow-through during the times he or she is not in therapy. Most treatment plans incorporate patient education and/or a home exercise plan so that gains made in therapy can be maintained or further developed at home. Those who are too young or have impaired ability to follow instructions may need to rely on a family member to help with a home program. When progress is slowed or when gains that were made in therapy are not present in the next treatment session, it becomes evident that compliance is not happening. Patients and their families must understand that the therapy that they receive is only for about 1 hour three times each week. The other 23 hours of those days and the 24 hours of the days without therapy are the responsibility of the patient.

Suppose, for example, that a pediatric patient is with her parents seeking physical therapy to assist in the reduction of the lateral curvature of her scoliosis. The therapist may suggest a trial use of electrical stimulation on the concave side of the curvature to fatigue the musculature and on the convex side for strengthening. The optimal time for the application is at night while the child sleeps. Success with this intervention may obviate the need for surgical correction of the curvature. Unfortunately, the parents feel sorry for their child and use the device every other night rather than the recommended nightly protocol. This course of therapy was unsupported by the parents and deemed a failure, resulting in the child requiring corrective surgery. The intervention may have been appropriate and effective if it had been applied as instructed, but without parental support, it is failure (Box 14-4).

Patient Expectations

Another problem that exists is the perpetuation of the phrase among fitness fanatics and athletes of "no pain, no gain." It is important to realize that when administering a

---

BOX 14-3 Know Your Indications, Contraindications, and Precautions! Why?

- *Indications:* If you do not have a sound physiologic rationale for why you are doing something, then you should not be doing it.

- *Contraindications:* Check the patient's medical record for possible contraindications. For example: if treating over the lower back region of a female patient, ask her if she is pregnant or if there is any chance that she is pregnant. Pregnancy is a common contraindication for many physical agents. It is better to be safe than sorry. Do not assume someone else asked the patient these questions yet!

- *Precautions:* Be familiar with your patient's medical history and review the medications he or she is taking. Precautions are conditions that need to be closely monitored when providing a specific intervention. If the patient is taking analgesics, he or she may not be able to accurately report painful sensations, so you would need to be more cautious when working with them. Another example: if your patient has a pacemaker, the heart rate will not change in the same way that a patient without a pacemaker would respond.

BOX 14-4 Enhancing Patient Compliance

Patient Education

- If you don't know what to expect, how will you know if you are getting it?

- If you don't know what you should be feeling, how will you know if you are feeling it?

- If you don't understand what you shouldn't be feeling, how will you protect yourself?

Significant Others/Family Members

- Do they understand the intent of the intervention and that it is not painful?

- Do they understand that the intervention is not a form of punishment?

- Do they understand the importance of managing the symptoms when the patient is not in the clinic? And that a "break" from the activities may cause a patient setback?

treatment intervention or physical agent, the appropriate responses to the treatment must be explained to the patient, as well as the inappropriate responses to treatment. Let us use the example of an athlete who seeks physical therapy for the treatment of a contusion to the quadriceps. Ultrasound has been recommended for the alteration of the scar tissue that is now limiting the athlete's torque production. During the application of the ultrasound, the patient thinks of the "no pain, no gain" philosophy. The patient begins to feel a prickling sensation leading to a burning sensation, and thinks: "OK, now it's really working, it's really beginning to burn now," without ever making a comment to the clinician delivering the intervention. The patient probably experienced a periosteal burn, which is detrimental to the tissue. The outer lining of bone, the periosteum is highly innervated and rich in collagen. The patient should have been informed about ultrasound and what it should and should not feel like and told to report any perceived sensation to the clinician during the delivery of ultrasound. Instruction needs to be clear prior to applying the physical agent, and the patient's ability to respond appropriately needs to be assessed to determine whether the selected physical agent will be safe for the patient (Box 14-5).

The Physical Agents Available

Because there is a wide degree of overlap of many clinical physical agent treatment interventions for the accomplishment of therapeutic goals and because several of the agents address primary complaints as well as secondary complaints, it is important to recognize what "tools" are available. Patients may plateau with their progress after repeated attempts with a given treatment intervention. It is also feasible that when a patient arrives in the department for treatment, the specific physical agent that was used during the last treatment session may not be available. Clinicians need to understand how to accomplish the same treatment goals using alternate methods if their first choice is unavailable (Box 14-6).

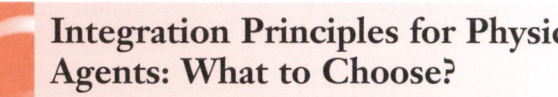

BOX 14-6   **The Physical Agents Available**

- What are the goals that I need to accomplish?
- Which modalities are capable of accomplishing the goals?
- What is presently not in use by someone else?
- Can more than one goal be accomplished with what is available?
- Is there another way to address the goal with the modalities that are available?

Integration Principles for Physical Agents: What to Choose?

Indications: Primary and Secondary

The first step in determining what physical agent or agents lies in the indications. What are the direct effects, and what are the secondary benefits of selecting a given physical agent? Is it primarily used to reduce edema: will it reduce pain indirectly because of the decreased edema? By establishing a list of the primary and secondary indications of a physical agent and comparing that list with the treatment goals for a patient, you can determine which physical agents might be of benefit for that patient.

Safety Considerations: Precautions and Contraindications

After this initial list is compiled, review each of the physical agents selected, and compare them with the medical condition of the patient. Determine whether there are any safety concerns, such as impaired cognition, compromised sensation, or peripheral vascular disease that could eliminate any of the physical agents as potential treatment options. It is the responsibility of the clinician to know the contraindications and precautions for each specific treatment intervention with or without physical agents and to screen for them.

Equipment Availability

Next, look at the availability of the potential physical agents that you have selected. There are multiple pieces of equipment in any therapy department that can accomplish a multitude of goals—some better than others. Determine exactly what is available by looking at the necessary parameters for the protocol that you have selected. Do any of the pieces of equipment available meet the parameter requirements?

Equipment Reliability

Of the pieces of equipment available to you that are not contraindicated for your patient and meet the appropriate

BOX 14-5   **Previous Patient Experience with Selected Physical Agents**

- Has your patient ever been treated with this physical agent before?
- What was his or her experience with it?
- Was it ever explained to the patient, and did the patient understand what to expect?
- Is your patient willing to try your use of the physical agent again?
- You will explain what they should expect.
- Make sure your patient understands normal and adverse responses that he or she needs to report to you.

parameters for you to accomplish your treatment goals, how many are reliable? When was the last inspection date from the biomedical engineering department? Most electrical equipment should be professionally inspected at minimum once a year and the date of the inspection should be identified with a sticker on the device. The clinician must inspect the equipment and its accessories to determine whether it is complete and operating properly BEFORE applying it to a patient. Any device that appears faulty should be labeled so and removed from the treatment area. Also, make sure that you are familiar with all of the unit's controls and parameters BEFORE applying it to a patient.

Previous Patient Experience with the Selected Physical Agent

One valuable resource that can easily be overlooked is the patient! Many patients who are receiving therapy have received physical therapy previously. The patient may have had a memorable experience with a physical agent. Ask your patient about his or her previous experiences with therapy and with physical agents. Knowing what has worked well for the patient in the past may help you decide what to use. Likewise, if a patient has a particular aversion to a certain physical agent, as often seen with cryotherapy, then you might want to suggest other appropriate alternatives.

What Does the Rest of the Plan of Care Include?

It is important to look at your choices in terms of efficient use of time and expected outcomes. If you selected a physical agent that will address only the primary complaints requiring 20 minutes to apply and you identify that you will also need to use something else to address additional symptoms, can you combine two physical agents and apply them simultaneously? If you do, would this compromise the therapeutic benefit of either one? This is often done with cold packs and electrical stimulation, when the treatment goal is to decrease pain and inflammation.

Preparatory Treatment

Is your goal for the physical agent one that involves preparation for another activity within the plan of care? For example, heat is often used prior to interventions that focus on increasing the extensibility of connective tissue, such as joint mobilization, soft tissue mobilization, and traction. The heat serves to relax the patient and heat the superficial structures, which can enhance the patient's response to the mobilizing techniques that follow.

Follow-Up to an Activity or Treatment Approach

Treatment sessions may involve a wide variety of treatment techniques, some of which may result in some minor levels of discomfort to the patient. Therapeutic exercise may increase the amount of friction in the joint structures, which may result in some localized edema following the activity. Ice may be applied postexercise to reduce the localized inflammation that was just caused by the increased activity level of the injured area. If the plan involves the application of a physical agent to reduce inflammation after an activity, it is important for the clinician to explain the process to the patient so that the discomfort can be understood and not offset fear of the activity in the future.

Putting It All Together: The Decisions and The Evidence

There is a great deal of decision making involved when choosing and incorporating a physical agent into a patient's treatment program. As discussed above, clinicians must consider many issues when deciding which intervention is best for a particular patient. Part of the decision-making process includes knowing what evidence is credible and available to support a particular intervention with a physical agent. Finding evidence is getting easier and easier as electronic databases are making the search quicker for clinicians to find up-to-date information, but the strength of that information must be carefully evaluated as to the source, reproducibility, and adherence to published guidelines established by licensing agencies where applicable, such as the FDA.

Observation of the initial condition and then reassessment of the patient following any therapeutic intervention will justify either their continuation, modification, or the termination of a treatment. Without a carefully constructed process for these assessments, it is difficult to ascertain whether progress is being made (refer to Chapter 2 for assessment techniques). If a patient is beginning to regain strength, experiences a decrease in pain, has less edema, or has less muscle guarding, then he or she will likely resume functional activities. Return to function is the cornerstone of therapeutic interventions (Box 14-7).

Documentation

Documentation is an essential form of communication that serves the needs of the patient, the physical therapist, the physical therapist assistant, third-party payers, and other health care providers involved with the care of the patient

---

BOX 14-7   Keys to Success with Physical Agents

- Review the published literature.
- Explain treatment techniques to your patients.
- Keep treatment plans simple.
- Observe your patient and record those observations.
- Portray confidence to your patients.
- Reassess after every individual treatment technique and intervention.
- Observe again! And continue to record your observations.

---

including nursing, other therapists, and the physician.[25] It is the legal document that serves to substantiate the treatments provided, and they are often used by third-party payers to determine reimbursement for the interventions. It also provides the details necessary for someone else to reproduce the treatment. For these reasons, it is essential that documentation is clear, concise, and accurate. All pertinent information must be recorded for it to be useful as a record.

SOAP Notes

One common documentation format is the SOAP note format. SOAP is an acronym for Subjective, Objective, Assessment, and Plan. A SOAP note is a form of progress note used to document both the treatment and the patient's responses to the treatment. This form of documentation is recorded in the patient's chart and becomes a permanent record of therapy for that patient. It is these progress notes that will answer the basic questions of how a patient responded to a given treatment technique when the chart is reviewed. The chart should present a clear and concise record of exactly what was done and how the patient responded so that anyone reading the chart would understand exactly why the particular course of actions took place upon subsequent patient visits. When documenting a treatment intervention with a physical agent, the details of the treatment must be readily apparent to whoever reads it. This would include the type of physical agent, the parameters chosen (for example, duration, intensity/temperature, frequency), patient positioning (if unusual), and the body part or structure treated. These details are typically found in the objective portion of the treatment note. The patient's response to treatment and suggestions for progressing or modifying the treatment should also be documented, usually in the assessment and plan sections of the progress note. Box 14-8 outlines the components of a SOAP note. Please remember the key to documentation, "If it wasn't documented, it didn't happen."

BOX 14-8   SOAP Notes

- *S = Subjective:* Subjective information refers to the information offered by the patients pertaining to how they "feel." Personal biases and emotional background influence subjective information. It may encompass physical complaints and emotional or psychological difficulties. The comments by the patient are entered into the patient record in quotation marks and identified by the phrase "the patient stated that... ."Asking patients how they feel lets them report their perception of their current state, and can also orient the clinician as to what questions should be asked next.

- *O = Objective:* Objective information, unlike subjective information, is unbiased, impersonal, unprejudiced, and truly factual information. This is the portion of the documentation that includes all relative parameters of the treatment approach so that anyone reading the chart could duplicate the treatment. Examples of objective entries for each modality are listed with the modality to which they pertain:

Thermal Modalities

Ultrasound

Hydrotherapy

CPM

Intermittent compression

Electrical Stimulation

- *A = Assessment:* The assessment portion of the documentation deals with the patient's response to treatment. The tendency for the use of the phrase "pt. tolerated treatment well" MUST be avoided, because the word "tolerated" provides little information regarding the response to the treatment. To tolerate something literally means to bear up under or to endure without injury. It offers no positive or negative comments regarding the treatment effectiveness. The assessment is your professional judgment of how the patient is progressing with the plan of care.

- *P = Plan:* The plan should involve a description of anticipated treatment sessions, based upon the assessment of the present treatment intervention. It also includes information regarding potential discharge or new techniques or exercises for the next session.

Summary

Tools are wonderful to have, but without the knowledge to know what to do with them they are useless. In physical therapy as in other areas, this is also true. If we do not stop and take the time to think about what we need to accomplish or the most efficient way to accomplish it, we will fail. This is especially true if we neglect to reassess what we have done and document it. Throughout this chapter, we have presented a way to integrate the information from this text and to find credible sources of new information for new tools. We have also provided a systematic approach to documenting what you have done with your patients.

CASE STUDY

Case Study 1

Richard is a 55-year-old retired truck driver who has been referred to physical therapy for treatment to relieve pain and stiffness in his right knee. X-rays revealed arthritic changes in both knees. He had a medial meniscectomy in the right knee 2 years ago. His recent complaints of pain and stiffness are related to his present leisure and work activities. Richard is an avid golfer, country and western dancer, and chauffeur.

Case Study 2

Charlotte is a 50-year-old secretary who has been referred to physical therapy for treatment to relieve symptoms associated with the automobile accident that she was involved in 3 weeks ago. She is having difficulty maintaining an upright posture due to severe headaches, back pain, and intermittent paresthesias in her dominant right hand. She is a frail woman, who taught aerobics classes five nights a week. She is unable to teach at all now. There were no fractures, and she is otherwise healthy.

Discussion Questions

1. Using an electronic database find evidence to support the use of electrical stimulation to facilitate wound healing.
2. A patient you are treating presents with edema due to a recent ankle sprain. List all the interventions that you could consider for treating the edema. What must you consider when deciding the best intervention to decrease her swelling?
3. As a therapist, how would you monitor patient compliance for a home exercise program?
4. Search the World Wide Web for websites that would be helpful to you as physical therapy student. Your search results should include the address that you visited, how you found the address, the date you visited it, and what you found useful about it. You will also need to consider the validity of the content by identifying the source of information—for example, did the information come from the National Institutes of Health's website or from a commercial vendor? And when was the website last updated? The course director will keep all search results in a resource notebook. You may have future access to the sites that each of your classmates found.
5. Your mother is scheduled to see a physical therapist after her recent car accident. She has heard you speak about electrical stimulation and is terrified. How could this impact the results that she is able to attain? What could be done to help alleviate her fears of this modality? (written assignment or class discussion)
6. A colleague has stated that there is no time in the clinic for patient explanations to take place regarding treatment. The colleague stated that they just want patients to come in, receive treatment, and leave and that this has been successful so far. How would you respond to this and what if anything would you suggest to the colleague. (written assignment or class discussion)

References

1. Houghton, PE, Kincaid, CB, Lovel, M, et al: Effect of electrical stimulation on chronic leg ulcer size and appearance. Phys Ther 83:17–28, 2003.
2. Debreceni, L, Gyulai, M, Debreceni, A, et al: Results of transcutaneous electrical stimulation (TES) in cure of lower extremity arterial disease. Angiology 46:613–618, 1995.
3. Karba, R, Semrov, D, Vodovnik, L, et al: DC electrical stimulation for chronic wound healing enhancement. Part 1. Clinical study and determination of electrical field distribution in the numerical wound model. Bioelectrochem Bioenerg 43:265–270, 1997.
4. Gentzkow, G, Pollack, S, Kloth, L, et al: Improved healing of pressure ulcers using Dermapulse, a new electrical stimulation device. Wounds 3:158–170, 1991.
5. Field-Fote, EC, and Tevavac, D: Improving intralimb coordination in people with incomplete spinal cord injury following training with body weight support and electrical stimulation. Phys Ther 82:707–715, 2002.
6. Griffin, JW, et al: Reduction of chronic post-traumatic hand edema: A comparison of high voltage pulsed current, intermittent pneumatic compression, and placebo treatments. Phys Ther 70:279, 1990.
7. Fitzgerald, GK, Piva, SR, and Irrgang, JJ: A modified neuromuscular electrical stimulation protocol for quadriceps strength training following anterior cruciate ligament reconstruction. J Orthop Sports Phys Ther 33:492–501, 2003.
8. Snyder-Mackler, L, Delitto, A, et al: Strength of the quadriceps femoris muscle and functional recovery after reconstruction of the anterior cruciate ligament. A prospective, randomized clinical trial of electrical stimulation. J Bone Joint Surg Am 77:1166–1173, 1995.
9. Lewek, M, Steven, J, Snyder-Mackler, L: The use of electrical stimulation to increase quadriceps femoris muscle force in an elderly patient following a total knee arthroplasty. Phys Ther 81:1565–1571, 2001.
10. Peres, SE, Draper, DO, Knight, KL, et al: Pulsed shortwave diathermy and prolonged long duration stretching increase dorsiflexion range of motion more than identical stretching without diathermy. J Athl Train 37:43–50, 2002.
11. Knight, CA, Rutledge, CR, Cox, ME, et al: Effect of superficial heat, deep heat, and active exercise warm-up on the extensibility of the plantar flexors. Phys Ther 81:1206–1214. 2001.
12. Funk, D, Swank, AM, Adams, KJ, et al: Efficacy of moist heat pack application over static stretching on hamstring flexibility. J Strength Cond Res 15:123–126, 2001.

13. Jarit, GJ, Mohr, KJ, Waller, R, et al: The effects of home interferential therapy on post-operative pain, edema, and range of motion of the knee. Clin J Sport Med 13:16–20, 2003.

14. Hurley, DA, Minder, PM, McDonough, SM, et al: Interferential therapy electrode placement technique in acute low back pain: A preliminary investigation. Arch Phys Med Rehabil 82:485–493, 2001.

15. Albright, J, Allman, R, Bonfiglio, RB, et al: Philadelphia panel evidence-based clinical practice guidelines on selected rehabilitation interventions for knee pain. Phys Ther 81:1675–1700, 2001.

16. Moore, SR, and Shurman, J: Combined neuromuscular electrical stimulation and transcutaneous electrical nerve stimulation for treatment of chronic pain: A double-blind, repeated measures comparison. Arch Phys Med Rehabil 78:55–60, 1997.

17. Waddell, G, and Richardson, J: Observation of overt pain behavior by physicians during routine clinical examination of patients with low back pain. Psychosom Res 36:77, 1992.

18. Vlayen, JWS, et al: Assessment of the components of observed chronic pain behavior: The Checklist for Interpersonal Pain Behavior (CHIP). Pain 43:337, 1990.

19. Device Advice: Device Advice is CDRH's self service site for medical device and radiation emitting product information. Device advice is an interactive system obtaining information concerning medical devices. Available at www.fda.gov/cdrh/deadvice/ 2004.

20. FDA Talk Paper: FDA Meets with Stakeholders to Address Issues Related to the Implementation of the Medical Device User Fee and Modernization Act of 2002 (MDUFMA). Available at www.fda.gov/bbs/topics/ANSWERS/2003/ANSO 2004.

21. Sackett, DL, Rosenberg, WM, Gray, JA, et al. Evidence based medicine: What it is and what it isn't. BMJ 312:71–72, 1996.

22. Fritz, JM, and Wainner, RS: Perspective examining diagnostic tests: An evidence-based perspective. Phys Ther 81:1546–1564, 2001.

23. "Hooked on Evidence." Available at http://www.hookedonevidence.com.

24. Soderberg, GL: Skeletal muscle function. In Currier, DP, and Nelson, RM (eds): Dynamics of Human Biologic Tissues. FA Davis, Philadelphia, 1992, pp 92–93.

24. Miller, CR, and Webers, RL: The effects of ice massage on an individual's tolerance level to electrical stimulation. J Orthop Sports Phys Ther 12:105, 1990.

25. Kettenbach, G: Writing SOAP Notes—With Patient/Client Formats, ed 3 FA Davis, Philadelphia, 2004, p 2.

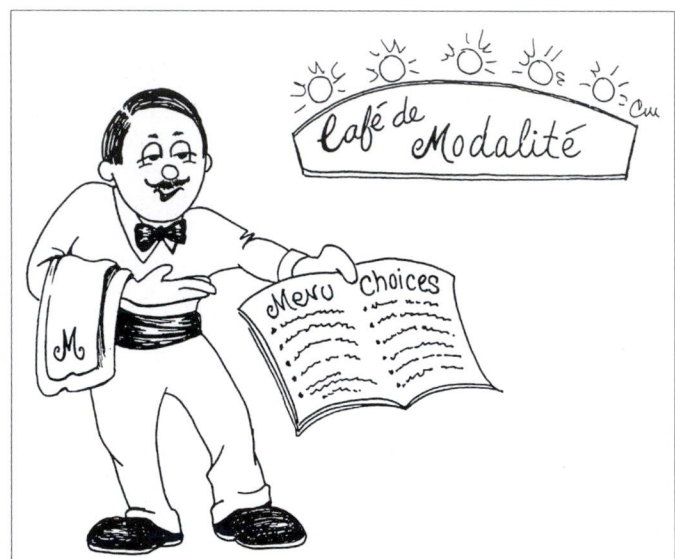

Index

Page numbers followed by "f" denote figures, "t" denote tables, and "b" denote boxes